# Pathomechanics of Lower limb dysfunctions: Prevention and Manual Therapy, 2nd edition.

- ➢ **Ethically Approved Case Study:** This book features a meticulously detailed case study titled "Knee Dysfunction Leading to Medial/Varus Knee Arthritis: Pathomechanics, Early Diagnosis, and Manual Therapy Treatment." The case study has received ethical approval from the BMMRC Ethics Committee, Hyderabad, Telangana, under reference number 939/BMMRC/IEC approval/2020.

- ➢ **Comprehensive Pathomechanics:** The book explores pathomechanics, linking knee dysfunctions to various forms of arthritis, including Medial/Varus knee arthritis and Lateral/Valgus knee arthritis. The intricate interplay of the above and below-knee kinetic chain is elucidated for a holistic understanding.

- ➢ **Dynamic Knee Movement Analysis:** The text delves into the relationship between full arc movements of the knee and the resultant pressure variations within the joint. By elucidating the mechanics of synovial fluid influx and efflux, the analysis provides insights into how manual therapy can potentially reverse knee arthritis, offering an alternative to major knee replacement surgeries.

- ➢ **Innovative Assessment and Treatment Approaches:** A novel approach to assessment using spring tests is introduced, accompanied by manual therapy treatments tailored for Hip, Knee, Ankle, and Foot dysfunctions. This inclusion enhances the reader's toolkit with effective techniques for diagnosing and addressing these specific issues.

**By**
**Dr. Naveen Kumar P**
**B.P.T (SVNIRTAR), M.P.T (Orthopedics), MISCP(Ireland)**

Naveen Institute of Orthopaedic Manual Therapy (Physio 4 knee and pain)
Main branch: shop no-G13&14, Agarwal Chambers, King Koti Road, Abids.
Branch 2: Flat no- 402, Block no- 5, Malaysian Township, Hyderabad, India.
Cell: 9392403507; www. physio4kneenpain.com
E-mail: nimt@physio4kneenpain.com

**Pathomechanics of Lower limb dysfunctions: Prevention and Manual Therapy, 2nd edition**

© 2020, Dr. Naveen Kumar P

All rights reserved. No part of this publication should be reproduced, stored in a retrieval system, or transmitted in any form or by any means: electronic, mechanical, photocopying, recording, or otherwise, without the prior written permission of the author and publisher.

This book has been published in good faith that the material provided by contributors is original. Every effort is made to ensure the accuracy of the material, but the publisher, printer, and Author will not be held responsible for any inadvertent error(s). In case of any dispute, all legal matters are settled under Hyderabad (India) jurisdiction only.

Second Edition: 2020

ISBN: 9798632513609

**Editors of the book:** Dr. Naveen Kumar
Dr. Monalisa
Dr. Athya Saba

# ABOUT THE AUTHOR
## Dr. Naveen Kumar (PT), M.P.T (Ortho), MISCP (Ireland)

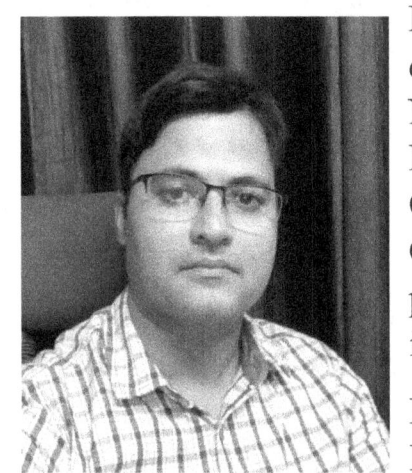

Dr. Naveen Kumar (PT), MISCP (Ireland), MIAP, is a distinguished graduate of the Swami Vivekananda National Institute of Rehabilitation Training and Research (SVNIRTAR), completing his M.P.T in Orthopaedics in 2009. His groundbreaking work in Orthopaedic Manual Therapy focuses on the unique pathomechanics of lower limb dysfunctions, particularly in the context of knee arthritis.

Dr. Naveen's approach to Medial/Varus and Lateral/Valgus knee arthritis has revolutionized the understanding of the exact causes of these conditions. Through his extensive clinical experience, he has successfully treated thousands of patients, providing a comprehensive understanding of the pathomechanics involved. This knowledge enables early diagnosis and precise treatment of knee dysfunctions, potentially avoiding the need for knee replacement surgeries.

The book explores the Hesch method of spring test, applied to knee, hip, and foot dysfunctions, facilitating accurate diagnosis and treatment. Recent research articles support the mechanics of synovial fluid dynamics, Condylar cartilage nutrition, joint stability, and vascular flow concerning joint movement and pressure variations inside the joint.

By restoring normal mechanics and range of motion in joints, Dr Naveen demonstrates how Orthopaedic Manual Therapy can potentially reverse knee arthritis, offering an alternative to invasive surgeries. The lower limb pathomechanics discussed in the book provides valuable insights into how Varus and Valgus knees impact hip and foot mechanics, offering a holistic approach to treating lower limb dysfunctions.

Dr. Naveen Kumar's expertise extends beyond clinical practice, teaching, and management. He has conducted Orthopaedic Manual Therapy courses and organized workshops, contributing significantly to the field.

# PREFACE

The physiotherapy field is becoming a more advanced skilled profession and continuously changing due to new advances. The book aims to help final year B.P.T(Bachelor Physiotherapy) students, D.P.T(Doctor of Physiotherapy), clinicians, and those doing PhDs in lower limb dysfunctions, mainly on knee arthritis. With new innovative concepts, It also gives an insight into the aims and means of physiotherapy advances in manual therapy.

With one decade of clinical experience and research, I have written this book to make the subject of manual therapy easy and comprehensive for physiotherapists.

The author has proposed pathomechanics of knee dysfunctions to Medial/Varus knee arthritis and Lateral/Valgus knee arthritis or severe extension and/ flexion loss of the Knee, which are different forms of OA knee. The book's uniqueness is that it contains specific spring tests to diagnose Knee, hip, and foot joint dysfunctions more accurately and treat them with manual therapy. Moreover, it also includes associated soft tissue assessment and treatment using Cyriax deep friction.

In the preventive aspect, analyzing physical stress acted upon specific tissue from a person's lifestyle and advising progressive strengthening proportionate to physical stress using theory-"physical stress VS tissue strength, adaptation and progressive strengthening" is included.

Recent research on the human model of the Knee proved that normal human knee motion causes intra-articular joint space and pressure change that subserve the regulation of synovial fluid inside the joint: mechanics of synovial fluid influx and outflux, Condylar cartilage nutrition, Joint stability, and vascular flow. That gives insight into how arthritis can be improved or reversed to normal depending on early and chronic conditions.

Although I have taken great care in writing this book, the author might have committed some errors. Hence, comments and criticism from teachers and students will be highly appreciated and rectified in subsequent editions. I wish you a happy reading and learning.

**Dr. Naveen Kumar P, M. P. T (Orthopaedics)**

# ACKNOWLEDGEMENTS

Behind every endeavour stand able and enthusiastic minds and sources of inspiration. I want to take this opportunity to thank all those whose instructions, support, and encouragement contributed to this book. Dr. P.P. Mahonty is a HOD-Physiotherapy of SVNIRTAR (Swami Vivekananda National Institute of Rehabilitation Training and Research) who inspired and taught us manual therapy concepts. All of my colleagues at Naveen Institute of Orthopaedic Manual therapy, Hyderabad, India, participated in implementing single group pre and post-test experimental design research to help refine the techniques in this book. Most of all, my clients were always ready to try anything new which might help. I want to thank Dr Athiya Saba (PT) for assisting in editing this book and Dr Sonali (PT) for her contributions to artwork and for being a model in this book. My sincere appreciation is extended to my best friends and colleagues, Dr Melchi Sedec and Dr Praveen, who have shared and assisted in my research and development of new material for many years. My best efforts could not have produced this text without their intervention.

I want to thank Mahaveer Hospital and the Research ethics committee for allowing me to present my research proposal on **"Knee dysfunction leading to Medial/Varus Knee Arthritis: it's Pathomechnics, Early diagnosis, and Treatment with Manual Therapy."**
Ethics committee approval no- **N0: 939/BMMRC/IEC approval/2020**

Much is owed to my colleagues, Dr. Shravan and Dr. Madhuri, for their dedication and enthusiasm despite their hectic work and family responsibilities. Their clinical and technical support has indeed made this book a possibility.


Jai Sat chit Anand

# ABOUT CLINICAL RESEARCH AND THIS TEXT

I would love to describe in depth the clinical research that guided me to publish the contents of this book. Hundreds of patients have received all of the therapeutic interventions presented in this book.

Thousands of patients have received some of the therapies outlined in this book by myself, my associates and other practitioners of manual therapy. The material in this text is almost all unique, the outcome and synthesis of my knowledge, skills, and passion for manual therapy. My experience with all patient populations- orthopaedic, neurologic, chronic pain, pediatric, and geriatric- has granted me an exceptional learning opportunity.

Single-group pre- and post-test experimental design studies have been performed on severely impaired joints with impartial "pre-and post-testing," using deep friction and the 3-planar spring test and treated with various manual therapy approaches. In the learning and research process, I have proposed the important concept of pathomechanics for Medial/Varus knee arthritis and Lateral/ Valgus knee arthritis.

In the concept of prevention and prevention of recurrence of dysfunction after treatment, applying the theory- of "physical stress VS tissue strength, adaptation, and progressive strengthening" is an essential aspect of the book.

My preference was to publish this book now; within it is important information for the health care consumer. I sincerely hope that practitioners will use this information to meet their individual needs with their clients.


Good luck and health.
**Dr. Naveen Kumar P, M.P.T (Orthopaedics)**

## Table of Contents

**Case study: Knee Dysfunction to Medial/Varus Knee Arthritis: Its Pathomechanics and Manual Therapy treatment**..........................1

Chapter 1: **Prevention of Injury and Dysfunction: Theory- Physical Stress acted upon the tissue Verses Strength, adaptation, and strengthening of the tissue.** ........................................... 23

Chapter 2: **Progressive strengthening and fitness of the desired tissue: Knee joint specific.** ...............................................40

Chapter 3: **Variable factors affecting the level of the physical stress on the tissue or the adaptive response of the tissue to physical Stress: Knee joint specific.** ...............................................68

Chapter 4: **Synovial Mechanics: Concepts of etiologies and effects of normal human knee pressure variations with movement.** ................89

Chapter 5: **Soft tissue: Injury, healing, soft tissue adhesions, assessment, and treatment.** ...............................................109

Chapter 6: **Anatomy and Biomechanics of the tibio-femoral joint.** ........129

Chapter 7: **Tibio-Femoral joint: Its Dysfunctions and Pathomechanics...140**

Chapter 8: **Assessment and Treatment methods: Knee joint Complex Specific.** ...............................................158

Chapter 9: **Assessment and Treatment of Tibio-Femoral joint dysfunctions of knee**...............................................172

Chapter 10: **Anatomy, Biomechanics, and Pathomechanics of Patella-Femoral joint**...............................................195

Chapter 11: **Assessment and Treatment of Patellar dysfunctions.** ..........204

Chapter 12: **Proximal Tibio-Fibular joint: Biomechanics, Pathomechanics, and Treatment.** ...................................................................212

Chapter 13: **The Soft tissue of Knee: Palpation and Treatment.** ...............226

Chapter 14: **Ankle and Foot: Biomechanics, Pathomechanics, and Treatment.** ..........................................................................................246

Chapter 15: **Hip joint: Biomechanics, Pathomechanics, and Treatment**....295

Index: 311

# CASE STUDY

## Knee dysfunction leading to Medial/Varus Knee Arthritis: It's Pathomechanics, Early diagnosis, and Treatment

**Principal Investigator:** Dr. P. Naveen Kumar, M.P.T. (Orthopedics) - Naveen Institute of Orthopaedic Manual Therapy.
**Ethics committee approval:** Mahaveer hospital and research, Hyderabad, Telangana. India. N0: 939/BMMRC/IEC approval/2020

## ABSTRACT

**Objective:**
To evaluate if the assessment with Spring test and interventions with Manual Therapy, strengthening, and orthosis, which are designed according to the proposed pathomechanics, can improve Varus Knee knee dysfunction, a precursor of medial knee arthritis.

**Design:**
It is a single case pre-and post-test experimental study with a duration of 10 weeks with five treatment sessions per week.

**Method:**
Diagnosis of this dysfunction is made by three planar Spring test. The intervention includes manual therapy consisting of Three planar mobilizations and manipulation, sustained glide, taping, and deep friction. Strengthening exercises are prescribed to prevent a recurrence, and stands are given to do self-sustained medial and anterior glides of the proximal tibia twice a day at home.

**Results:**
Upon intervention, the spring test became negative in the pre-assessment range and showed an increase in R.O.M. (Internal rotation: right Knee and left Knee by $3^0$ and $2^0$, respectively. Extension: right and left Knee by $4^0$ and $3^0$, respectively). On x-ray, the right and left medial joint space increased by 1.5mm and 2mm, respectively. The right and left lateral joint spaces decreased by 1mm and .5mm, respectively. The right and left proximal tibia medially shifted by 2mm and 1mm with respect to the distal femur. The medial tilt of the right and left Knee decreased from $4.8^0$ to $1.6^0$ and from $3.7^0$ to $1.4^0$, respectively. There is a significant decrease in pain in the right and left Knee by six and four points (NPRS), respectively, and an increase in the overall functional abilities of the subject by 35 points.

**Conclusion:**
Diagnosis with spring test and interventions based on pathomechanics have improved the medial joint space and ROM, which improved the alignment and synovial fluid in varus knee dysfunction.

## Background

Knee osteoarthritis is the most common joint disease, and the cause is idiopathic[1]. Most believe that **causes** of osteoarthritis of the Knee are: (but with counter questions)

**Ageing**- (Are all other joints not ageing at the same time ?)[28]
**Obesity**- (Do thin people not have OA knee?)
**Hereditary** - (Is it always applicable?)
**Wear and tear** - (On X-ray, it is seen that joint space is reduced in one compartment, but in another compartment, there is gapping; will it not tilt rather than wear and tear?)

What would be the Primary Cause, then?
Analysis of the Primary Cause of the problem is best answered by "**Physical stress theory**"[16]

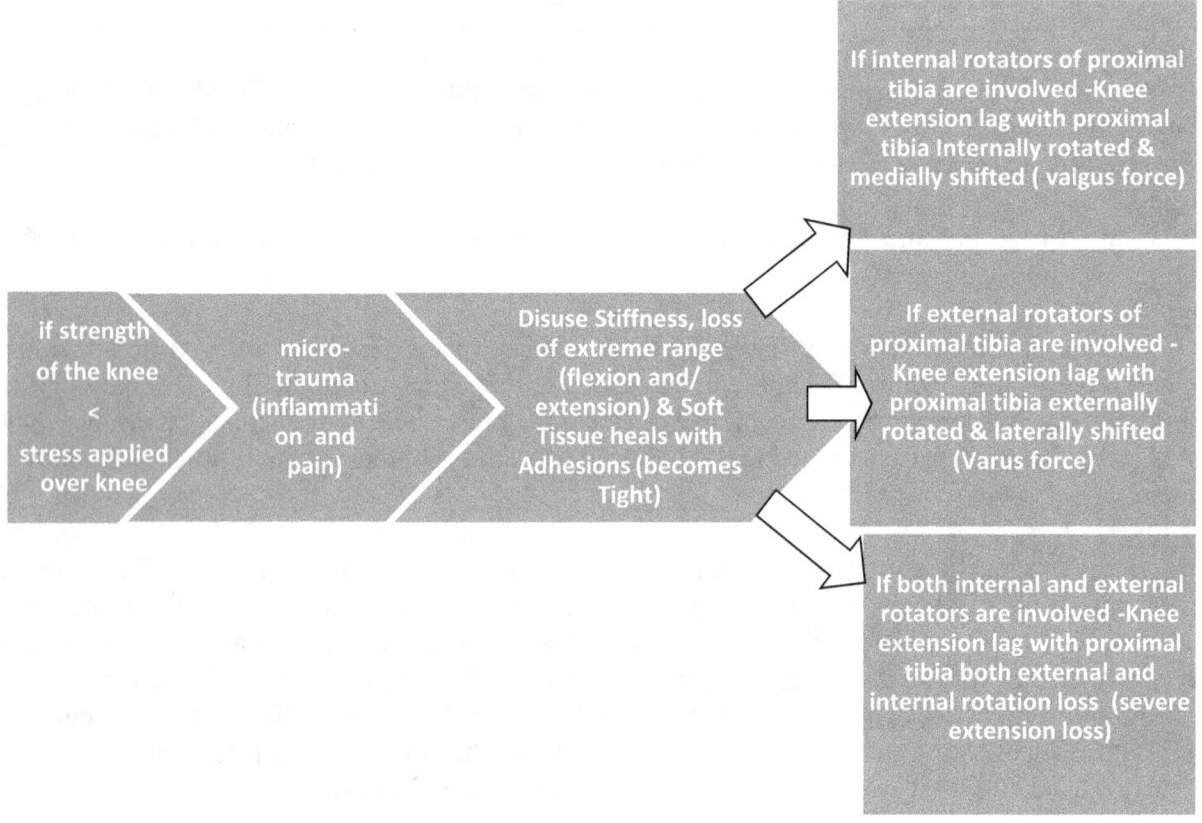

As knee dysfunctions that lead to different forms of O.A. Knee are a vast subject, this study proposes to take up one of the common and largely affected possibilities of OA Knee[5,6], varus knee arthritis. It is a Knee dysfunction wherein knee extension lag with the proximal tibia externally rotated and laterally shifted, leading to Medial/Varus knee arthritis. Pathomechanics of the same is depicted in the flowchart.

Flowchart:

### Pathomechanics of Knee dysfunction leading to Varus Knee:

**Physical Stress Theory:**
**Physical Stress on a Knee tissue > Strength of the Knee tissue**

↓

**Injury/Dysfunction:**
The relative threshold value of the knee tissue is negative, therefore results in injury → pain and inflammation → disuse glides loss of terminal extension and /flexion (stiffness) → soft tissue heal with adhesions(becomes tight) - if external rotators; Tensor Fascia Latae, bicep femoris, lateral gastrocnemius, vastus lateralis (lateral patellar retinaculum, lateral part of ligamentum patellae) of the tibia are involved later they heal with adhesions/become tight, then that will rotate the proximal tibia externally and shifts laterally (due to anatomical position) leading to Varus knee.

↓

**Extension lag**

-Range of motion will decrease, which in turn will reduce synovial fluid influx and outflux.

**Flexion lag**

-Range of motion will decrease, which in turn will reduce synovial fluid influx and outflux.

**Both flexion and extension lag:**

-If both extension and flexion lag is involved, as an extension lag component will come into play during the weight-bearing cycle of the gait, the knee will be under varus pressure.
-As there is pain and loss of range, synovial influx and outflux will be reduced.

↓

**Knee extension lag with proximal tibia** externally rotated and laterally shifted.
- As an extension lag component will come into play during the weight-bearing cycle of the gait, the knee will be under varus pressure.
-If not diagnosed early and treated leads to Varus/Medial knee arthritis.
-As there is pain and loss of range, synovial influx and outflux will be reduced.

**Knee flexion lag with proximal tibia** externally rotated and laterally shifted.

-This dysfunction does not contribute to Varus/Medial knee arthritis as terminal flexion of the knee is not involved during the weight-bearing cycle of the gait.
- As there is pain and loss of range, synovial influx and outflux will be reduced.

## Objective:

Upon post-intervention to see whether any change in
- Increase in Range of Motion, especially extension and internal rotation.
- On x-ray: Increase medial joint space, decrease lateral joint space, and shift of proximal tibia medially with respect to the distal femur will decrease medial tilt.
- Decrease pain and restoration of functional abilities.
- Spring test becoming negative at the pre-test range.

## Methodology

1. Single case study.
2. The type of research study is pre and post-test experimental design.
3. Inclusion criteria:
   - Male/Female age groups of 20 to 75 years.
   - Bilateral knee pain.
   - Positive clinical spring test for Varus knee dysfunction and x-ray correlation.
   - Acute, sub-acute, and chronic stages
4. Exclusion Criteria:
   - Infective Arthritis.
   - Bone Tumors.
   - Non-united and mal-united fractures around the knee.
   - Post Total Knee Replacement cases.
   - Acute bruises, Acute ligamentous injury/laxity
5. Sampling and setting: non-randomized, primary level, outpatient physiotherapy department.
6. Treatment duration: five treatment sessions per week (Wednesday and Sunday were break days) up to 10 weeks.

## Methods / Measures:

- Spring test.[8,9,10]
- X-ray imaging (joint space, tilt, shift).[14,13,16]
- NPRS (Numeric Pain Rating Scale for pain intensity).[17]
- Range Of Motion - Active and Passive [18,28]
- Functional disability testing by modified Cincinnati Rating System Questionnaire.[19]

## I. INTRODUCTION

Osteoarthritis is the most common joint disease in adults around the world; it is a progressive disease resulting in chronic joint pain and significant disability. The knee is one of the most frequently affected joints of OA[28]. So far, it is known that the cause of OA is idiopathic. Varus knee alignment has been identified as a risk factor for the progression of medial knee OA[3]. Valgus knee alignment is knock knee and is less common than varus knee[1].

This study proposes that based on "physical stress theory"[15] if physical Stress is dominant over the strength of knee tissue in a given activity, it leads to injury[28,29]. Soft tissue micro (non-visible) or macro (visible) trauma occurs according to the extent of the injury. Later, it heals with adhesions/tightness, which leads to dysfunction. If not diagnosed and treated early, it may fall into pathomechanics and end up as a deformity of either varus/valgus or severe extension and/or flexion loss of the knee, which are different forms of OA knee.

This study focuses on pathomechanics of Medial/Varus knee arthritis. If the soft tissues like external rotators of the proximal tibia (TFL-tensor fascial lata, vastus lateralis, Bicep Femoris, Lateral Gastrocnemius, lateral patellar retinaculum, lateral part of liagmentum patellae) are involved in the injury, later they heal[4,5] with adhesions/tightness. That, in turn, will pull the proximal tibia into external rotation and laterally shift because of the anatomical position. That, in turn, again leads the Knee into varus stress with medial compartment compression and lateral gapping, causing varus knee if left untreated. With this knowledge, one can diagnose and treat the dysfunction early, preventing Medial/Varus Knee Arthritis and possibly most knee replacement surgeries.

## II. KNEE JOINT

The native knee is a synovial joint that functions as a complex hinge, permitting rotational, antero-posterior, and medial/lateral translational movement with 6 degrees of freedom.[6,7,12]

- **Multiple Degrees of Freedom of Joint Motion**

The movement of the knee joint is governed by its ligaments, other supporting soft tissue structures and the geometric constraints of the articular surfaces. The knee is capable of movement in six degrees of freedom: three rotations and three translations. Knee motion can be described by relating movement to three principal axes: the tibial shaft axis, the epicondylar axis, and the antero-posterior axis, which is perpendicular to the other axes (Figure 1 & figure 2). Translations along these axes are referred to as proximal-distal, medial-lateral, and anterior-posterior translations. Rotations about these axes are referred to as internal-external rotation, flexion-extension, and varus-valgus rotation, respectively.[4,12]

**Figure 1:** Schematic diagram illustrating the six degrees of motion of the human knee joint. (Reproduced from Woo SL-Y, Livesay GA, and Smith: Kinematics, Knee Surgery. Baltimore, Williams & Wilkins, 1994, pp 155–173.

**Figure 2:** Six degree motion of knee [7]

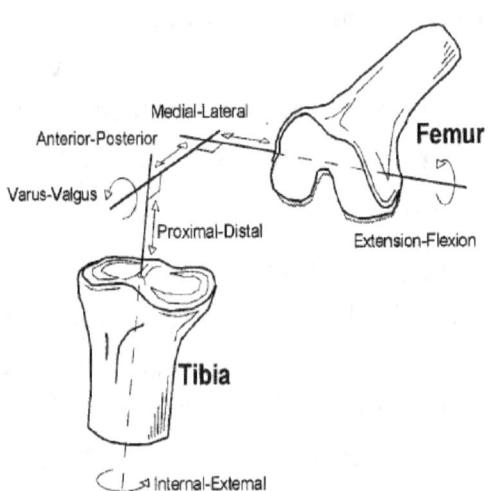
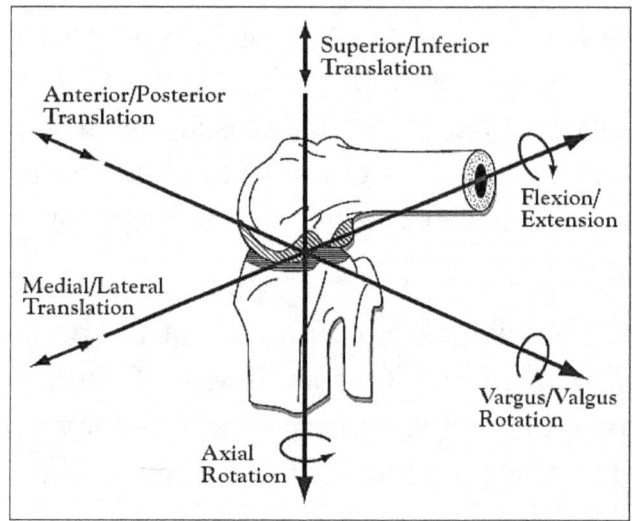

- **Mechanics of knee function**

Knee function may be viewed analytically as the balanced interaction of mechanical and biological factors. The mechanical factors can be static or dynamic, although there can be no clear distinction in functional terms. Static factors include alignment of the limb segments, the surface geometry of the articulating bones, and joint laxity. Dynamic factors include the distribution of load during different aspects of gait, affected by proprioceptor feedback, and other neuromuscular control mechanisms that help regulate force levels in the joint. If the various mechanical factors fail to operate in concert, the joints may become dysfunctional; Biological factors may compound the effect of mechanical ones. These include the state of the bone and connective tissues, in which disease or congenital deficiency may accelerate wear and deterioration even under normal loading patterns.[1]

Axes of knee motion: The femur, tibia, and patellofemoral mechanisms work together as a composite, tri-compartment linkage. The knee's flexion/extension (F/E) range may be 160° or more. The motion axes correspond closely, if not exactly, to the bones' mechanical axes: the femur's passing from the femoral head centre to the knee centre and the tibia's passing from mid-plateau to mid-ankle. In F/E, these axes have biaxial movement, which is not parallel throughout the range. Put another way, there is an element of valgus/varus rotation in F/E so that the movement is not confined within the sagittal plane[1].

## III. OSTEOARTHRITIS:

Osteoarthritis (OA) is the most common joint disease in adults around the world; it is a progressive disease resulting in chronic joint pain and significant disability. The knee is one of the most frequently affected joints by OA. According to Metcalfe et al. 2013, more than 40% of people over 60 years have symptomatic knee OA, and more than 50% have bilateral knee OA. In Knee OA, the Medial Compartment (MC) is the most commonly distressed as during the stance phase of gait, more than 70% of the load applied to the knee joint passes through the MC, as seen in Figure 3, as the centre of mass passes through the medial to the centre of the Knee joint[1].

## IV. VARUS KNEE:

Varus knee alignment has been identified as a risk factor for the progression of medial knee osteoarthritis.[3] Genu varus deformity can lead to medial compartment overload and a progression of ipsilateral compartment osteoarthritis.[2] Varus alignment is the most common alignment in OA; 75% of all patients have it. Regarding cartilage degradation of the tibio-femoral compartments, the medial side is usually the worst affected. Subjects with varus knee alignment are bowlegged and have negative HKA angles (angle b/w femoral and tibial mechanical axes)[1].

Geometry and alignment: The **Weight-Bearing Axis** describes the knee's normal 'frontal alignment' in the coronal plane. It extends from the centre of the hip down to the centre of the ankle. Understanding this principle helps define varus and valgus malalignment (refer to Figure 3).[6]

Limb alignment abnormalities and functional disorders are common and do not impose functional restraints unless the varus is severe. However, varus alignment can lead to knee instability and anterior cruciate ligament (ACL) deficiency. Forces in gait cause a typical lateral thrust of the knee, reflecting the failure of the ACL to effectively control the medial displacement of the tibia during extension and failure to stabilize the knee against anterior displacement of the tibia coupled with internal rotation, ACL reconstruction may be a partial answer for such cases, which require realignment as well. Varus limb alignment is accompanied by both joint surfaces having an exaggerated **lateral-to-medial downward inclination**--the oblique varus knee. The sloping joint surfaces facilitate subluxation under load. The tibia is prominent (proximally and laterally), and typically, there is a lateral thrust of the knee during gait. Many cases show osteoarthritis (OA), with deterioration concentrated in the medial compartment. The patella is often displaced laterally because of coexistent malrotation at the distal femur and/or the proximal tibia.[1]

**Figure 3:** Alignment of genu varum and genu valgum[6]

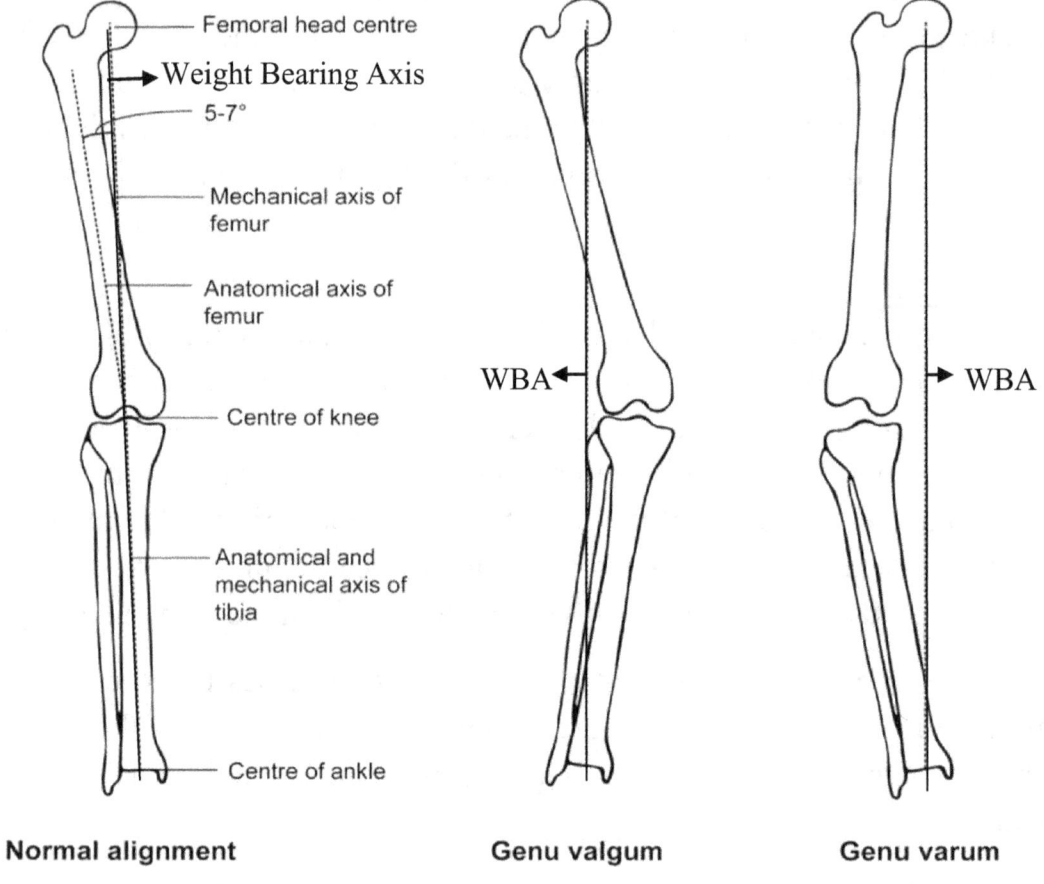

## V. BIOMECHANICS:
- **Biomechanics of tibio-femoral joint**[12]

Proximal component - Femur (convex femoral condyle)
Distal component - Tibia (proximal concave surface of the tibial plateau)
**Motion:** 3-Planar Movements: figure 1&figure 2
> Flexion and Extension are Sagittal Plane movements.
> External and Internal Rotations are Transverse Plane movements.

> Abduction and Adduction are Coronal Plane movements.
> Compression-retraction or proximal-distal movement of the joint

**Biomechanics of the Knee during gait cycle[11]:**

The three linear motions describing the tibia's translational behaviour with respect to the femur were medial/lateral shift, anterior/posterior drawer, and compression/distraction. Shift and anterior-posterior drawer and internal and external rotation are affected by passive knee structures and/or muscle action. Compression and distraction are affected by a weight-bearing stance, non-weight-bearing swing, and shift of the load-bearing axis of the limb.

- **Tibial shift**

The pattern of tibial shift during the stance phase indicates an initial medial shift followed by a lateral shift of similar duration but a higher amplitude. During the swing phase, the tibia continued the medial shift initiated before toe-off some 35 ms after maximum knee flexion was reached. The shifts occurring during the stance and swing phases produce tibial excursions of 5.6 mm. The tibia's shift closely matched the flexion/extension of the tibiofemoral joint, i.e., when the joint flexed, the tibia slid medially, and when it extended, the tibia moved laterally with respect to the femur.

- **Distraction/compression**

The distraction/compression of the tibiofemoral joint shows a pattern similar to both shift and drawer, with a magnitude greater than shift but lesser than a drawer. The joint distracts during flexion and is compressed during extension. From the stance phase to the swing phase, a total distance of 0-7mm varies according to the weight and position of the weight-bearing axis of the limb.

- **Flexion/ Extension:**

The average pattern of flexion/extension of the tibio-femoral joint during walking is biphasic: a slight flexion followed by an extension during the stance phase and a large flexion followed by an extension during the swing phase. In more detail, as the heel struck the ground, the knee flexed and reached an initial peak value $20^0$ in approximately 190ms. In the following 300 ms, the tibiofemoral joint extended to a mean position just $1.3^0$ short of full extension (defined as $0^0$). After that, the flexion of the joint began. It reached $35^0$ by toe-off and peaked at $60^0$ early into the swing phase. In the last 30 ms of the gait cycle, the tibio-femoral joint reached almost full extension ($-0.5^0$) in preparation for the next heel strike.

- **Abduction/adduction:**

The average pattern of abduction/adduction of the tibio-femoral joint (rotation around the floating axis) was uniphasic and was limited to $5^0$ (1.7). From heel

Strike until shortly before toe-off, no abduction/adduction movement took place, and the tibiofemoral joint remained abducted at approximately $1.2^0$

- **External/internal rotationt[6]**

Recent studies indicate that in the transverse plane, the screw-home movement occurred as expected during the pre-swing and late-swing phases at an angle of about 17°. However, the tibia rotated externally with respect to the femur rather than internally. At the same time, the knee joint started to flex during the loading response (paradoxical screw-home movement[12]), and the angle was 6°.

## VI. CASE DESCRIPTION:

- A 65-year-old female came to our clinic with chief complaints of severe bilateral knee pain for four years with gradual onset.
- **Aggravating factors:** Difficulty while walking, stair climbing, cross-leg sitting, and getting up from the floor.
- **Relieving factors:** Rest and flexed knee position.
- No medical, family, or surgical history.
- **Treatment history:** Consulted physician; she was advised to exercise.

## VII. KEY ASSESSMENT:

**SPRING TEST:**

"Spring Tests," a fundamental concept of Manual Therapy, have been improved by Dr. Jerry Hesch, MHS, PT, DPT. Within the Hesch Method, the spring testing method is an enhancement referred to as "Springing with Awareness." Specifically, this approach allows the clinician to experience and interpret the visco-elastic joint structure's recoil instead of simply letting go of the spring. This refined testing is fundamental to experiencing hypo-mobility and hypermobility with confidence empirically. In this way, the therapist will find that the application of the Hesch Method techniques will enhance clinical palpatory literacy. "Springing with Awareness" has applications throughout the body in joints and dense connective tissue[11].

By enhancing traditional spring tests, the Hesch Method allows the therapist to evaluate true motion loss in each plane instead of perceived loss. There is precision in assessment and ultimately greater success in restoring normative joint function through precisely targeted treatment.

Treatment is based on the viscoelastic creep model of connective tissue and thoroughly addresses movement dysfunction in all planes of the body. Treatment is, therefore, much more effective when addressing the dysfunction in all three planes[9].

## VIII. EXAMINATION:

### a) Spring test for varus knee dysfunction

**Position of the patient:** As shown in Figure 4, the position of the patient is supine, and the right knee is to be assessed.

**Position of the therapist and procedure:** The therapist approaches from the right side of the patient. The therapist's left-hand Pisiform is placed on the proximal-lateral surface close to the tibial tuberosity. Then, with internal rotation (transverse plane) glide, medial glide (coronal plane), and anterior glide (sagittal plane) of the proximal tibia, three planar movement barriers are reached. Simultaneously, the therapist's right wrist is slightly extended with fingers flexed, grasping the distal posterior surface of the tibia; internal rotation, abduction[28,] and upward force are applied to reinforce the three planar movement barriers at the proximal tibia. After reaching the three planar movement barriers, extension slack is taken with (4-6)kg force. Furthermore, (4-6)kg force is applied in extension to feel the spring. If it does not, spring indicates dysfunction.

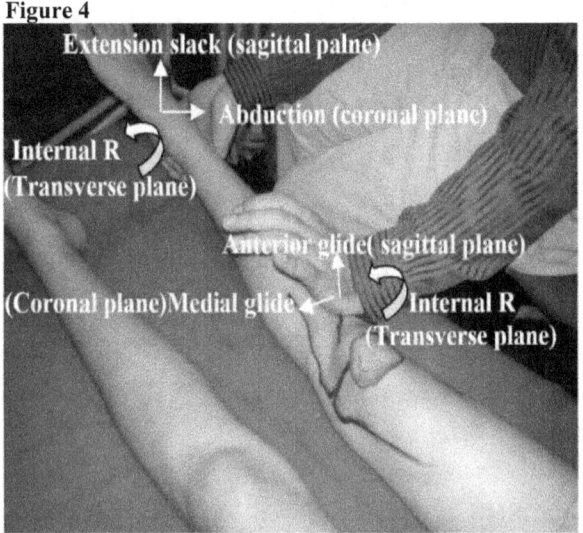

Figure 4

### b) Palpation of soft tissue:
external rotators of the proximal tibia for adhesions/trigger points are done by Cyriax deep transverse friction massage.

## IX. TREATMENT:

### 1. Three planar Mobilizations and Manipulations[20]

- As shown in Figure 4, the therapist and patient positions are the same as mentioned above in assessing varus knee dysfunction using a spring test.
- After reaching three planar movement barriers, extension glides are given according to the grades of mobilization.

### 2. Deep Friction / Soft Tissue release[21-22] 
given to the affected external rotators of the proximal tibia- TFL, Vastus lateralis (including lateral retinaculum and ligamentum patella), biceps femoris, and lateral part of the gastrocnemius.

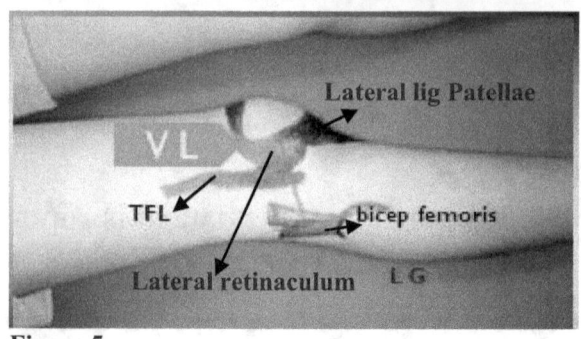
Figure 5

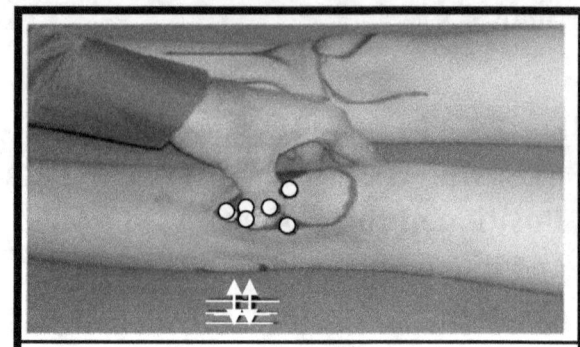
Figure 6

**Figure 5:** Depicts the palpatory landmarks of the external rotators of the proximal tibia.

**Figure 6:** Palpation with the thumb[31]: Patellar tendon divided into three rows, and each row is again divided into points with a distance of 1cm so that the entire affected portion of the tendon will be covered for the deep friction. Horizontal lines represent the alignment of patellar tendon fibre. Bilateral vertical arrow lines represent the application of deep friction perpendicular to the alignment of the fibres[32].

**3. Sustained Glide[23]:** these are unidirectional glides given for a certain duration of time[30].

i). Sustained lateral to medial glide of the proximal tibia at the extension barrier, as shown in Figure 7.

- The stand consists of a rectangular base (length 15 inches, breadth 5.5 inches, thickness of half an inch), and at the centre, there is a projection (height 2", length 10" and thickness of half an inch)
- the patient is side-lying; the proximal lateral surface of the tibia is placed on the projected part of the stand.
- With the help of body weight, the proximal tibia glides medially on the femur.
- Duration: 2-5 minutes can be kept; weight can be added to the tibia's distal medial surface according to the patient's tolerance and condition.

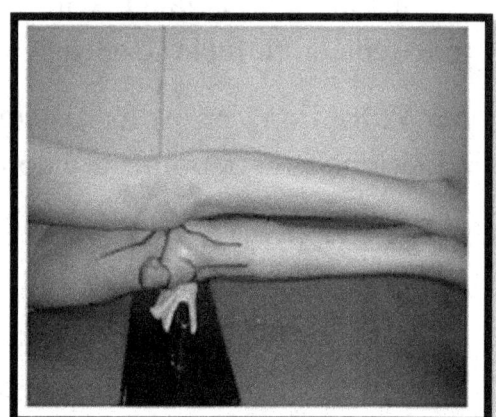
Figure 7

ii). Sustained anterior glide of the proximal tibia (knee extension). The patient is in prone-lying

- The distal anterior surface of the femur is placed on the projected part of the stand, as shown in Figure 8.
- With the help of body weight, the proximal tibia glides anteriorly on the femur.
- Duration: 2-5 minutes can be kept; weights can be added to the tibia's distal posterior surface according to the patient's tolerance and condition.

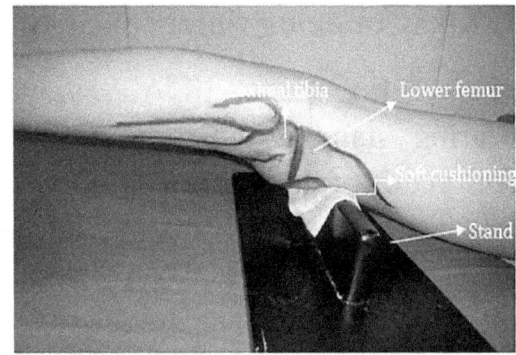

Figure 8

**Note:** Self-sustained glides on knee stands are advised to be done twice daily for 2- 5 minutes, depending on the condition and tolerance of the patient.

4. **Progressive strengthening exercises:** Passive to active assisted, then active and progressed to resisted exercises are suggested according to the patient's condition and tolerance.

5. **Orthotics[24]:** to correct the varus knee dysfunction/deformity, lateral raise for the footwear can be advised. $1^0$-$4^0$ of the wedge is added on the lateral plantar side of the footwear, as shown in Figure 9. In this dysfunction, the patient walks with the supinated foot; that is, the weight falls on the lateral border of the foot. Footwear with lateral wedge puts valgus force on the knee, the reverse of varus[33] force.

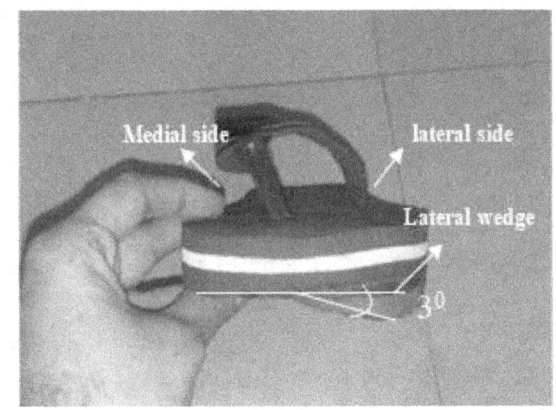

Therefore, it will enable self-correction with one's body weight.

Figure 9

**Note:** It was advised to use gradually, starting with 1 hour in the morning and 1 hour in the evening and progressing for the entire day according to the patient's tolerance.

## X. RESULTS: PRE AND POST-TREATMENT COMPARISON

**1. Spring test:** became negative; that is, joint end feel at pre-treatment range is springing after treatment, indicating improvement after post-treatment.

**2. X-ray imaging (joint space, tilt, shift)** [13,14,16]

**a)     Joint space:** In A.P. view, pre-and-post-x-rays were taken in a weight-bearing standing position, between the anterior surface of the knee and the collimator of the x-ray, a 50-inch distance was kept[15]. Joint space is measured from the mid-point of the medial and lateral tibial joint surfaces to the projection point on the femur's medial and lateral joint surfaces. The pre-treatment x-ray of the right knee shows that the lateral joint space was 3mm and the medial joint space was 0 mm, whereas the left knee's lateral joint space was 2.5mm and the medial joint space was .5mm. Compared with the post-treatment x-ray, right knee lateral joint space decreased from 3mm to 2mm, and medial joint space increased from 0mm to 1.5mm. In the same way, left knee lateral joint space decreased from 2.5mm to 2mm, and media joint space increased from .5mm to 2.5mm.

**Pre-treatment X-ray**

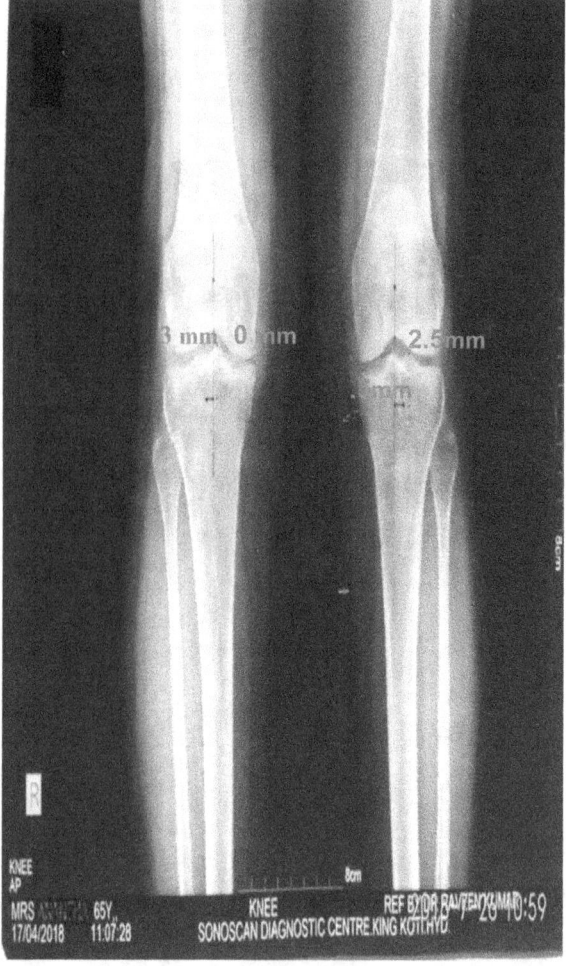

**Post-treatment X-ray**

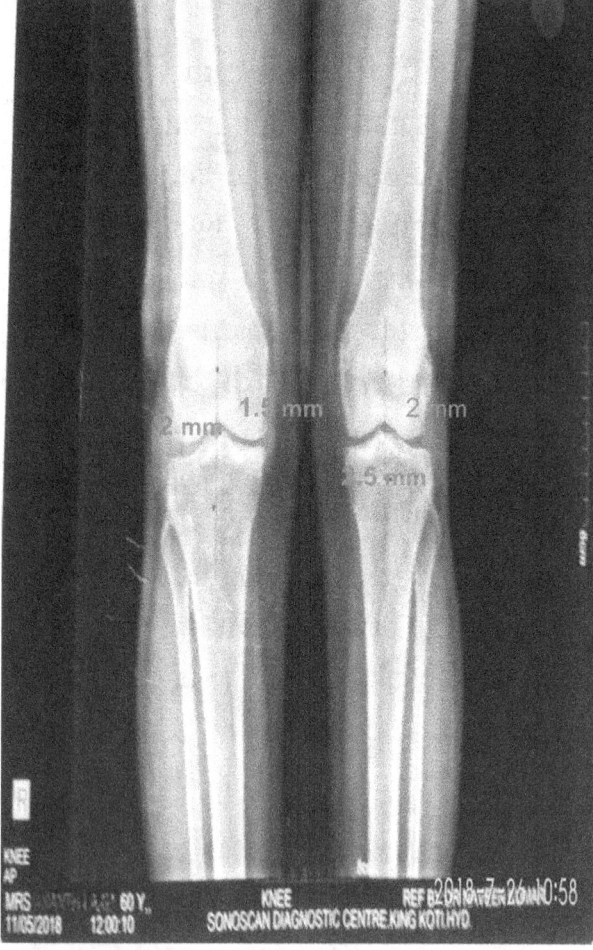

**NOTE:** On comparing the pre and post-treatment x-ray findings of medial joint space increment and lateral joint space decrement, it is evident that total joint retraction also occurs after treatment. All x-ray findings were evaluated by blinding the radiologist experienced in the diagnostic field over 15 years.

**b) Tilt**[1,27]:

Right knee      (Pre-treatment)      Left knee

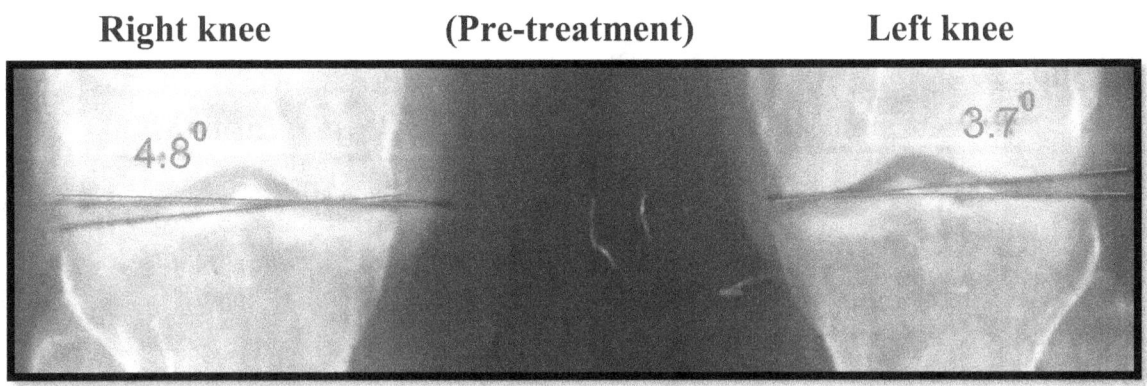

Right knee      (Post-treatment)      Left knee

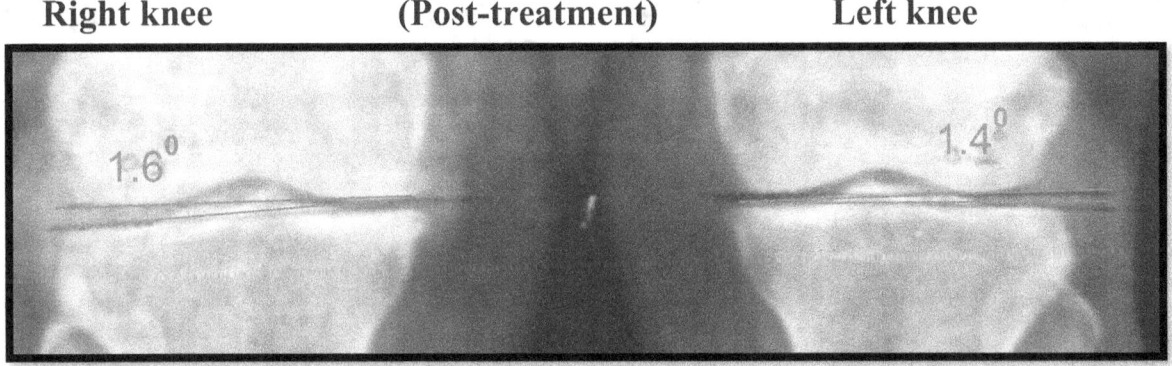

External rotation and lateral shift (adduction) of the tibia create medial tilt (lateral to medial downward inclination). It is measured by a line joining the highest points of both femoral and tibia joint surfaces. Pre-treatment of the right knee's medial tilt was about $4.8^0$, and the left knee was about $3.7^0$ (indicating the load-bearing axis of the limb shifting towards the medial compartment). If it is compared with post-treatment tilt, it has decreased to $1.6^0$ and $1.4^0$, respectively (Indicating the Load Bearing Axis[27] of limb shifting towards the Centre of the Knee joint after post-treatment.)

**c) Shift:** Proximal tibia position with respect to distal femur[16,28]

The standard reference to calculate proximal tibia position with respect to the femur: From the Centre of the femoral inter-condylar notch 1 cm above, the centre point of the femur is taken, and from the lateral tibial spike of joint 1cm below the centre point of the tibia is taken. The horizontal distance between these two points is measured. Upon comparing pre and post-treatment x-rays of the Right Knee, the proximal tibia moved medially by 2mm, and in the left knee, the proximal tibia moved medially by 1mm with respect to the femur.

**Pret-reatment**

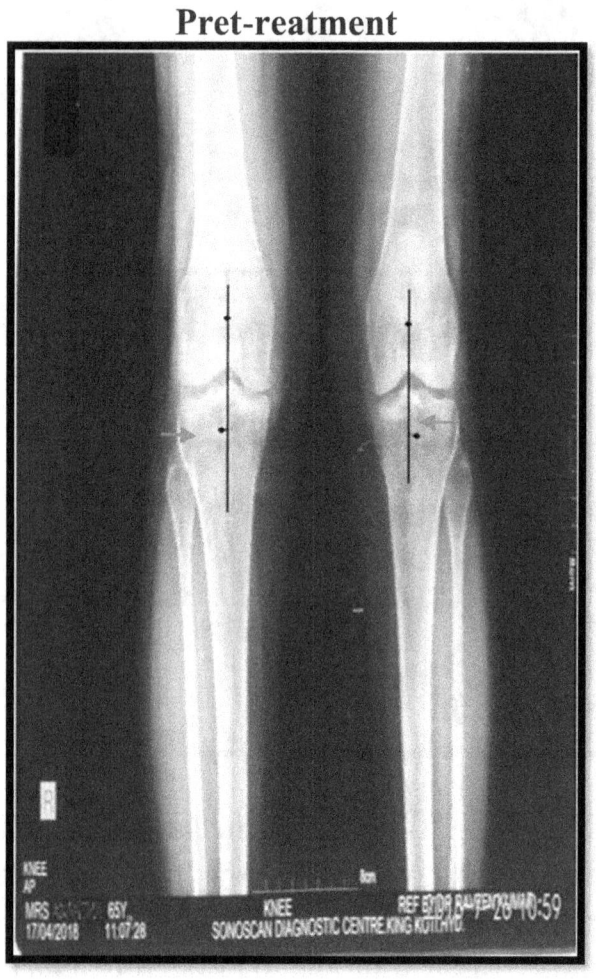

**Post-treatment**

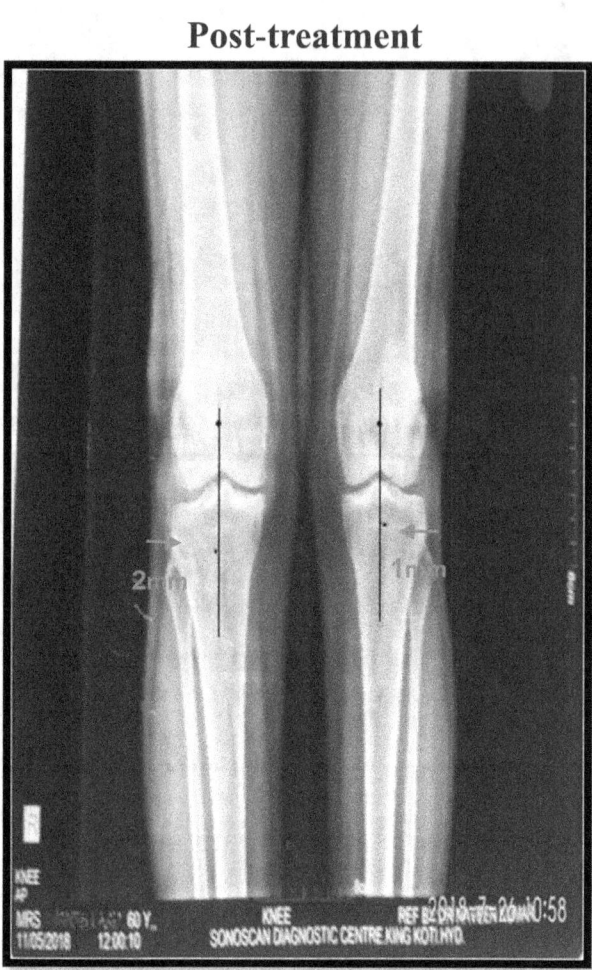

**3. NPRS** (Numeric Pain Rating Scale for pain intensity)[18]. Refer to Table 1

Pre-treatment NPRS of the right knee was 8/10, the left knee was 6/10 on day 1, and it decreased to 2/10 and 0/10, respectively, after post-treatment on day 70, indicating a significant reduction of pain.

Table 1

| Numeric Pain Rating Scale DAY-1 | | DAY-70 |
|---|---|---|
| Right Knee | 8/10 | 2/10 |
| Left Knee | 6/10 | 0/10 |

**4. Range Of Motion**: Active and Passive range in degrees.[19](Refer to table 2)
Normal range of motion of knee: Flexion ($140°$) - extension ($0°$) - hyperextension ($-5°$)[27].

As it is known, the loss of this range is the major contributor to the dysfunction of the Varus/Medial knee arthritis. There is a significant increase in the pre-and post-treatment of the left and right Knee's active and passive range of motion, especially in internal rotation and extension range.

Table 2. Range of motion in degrees

|  | Right knee Before intervention (degrees) | Right knee After intervention (degrees) | Right knee Difference (degrees) | Left knee Before intervention (degrees) | Left knee After intervention | Left knee Difference (degrees) |
|---|---|---|---|---|---|---|
| **Active** | | | | | | |
| Extension lag | 6 | 2 | 4 | 3 | 0 | 3 |
| **Passive** | | | | | | |
| Extension lag | 6 | 2 | 4 | 2 | -3 | 5 |
| Internal rotation | 2 | 5 | 3 | 3 | 5 | 2 |

**5. Functional disability testing by modified Cincinnati Rating System Questionnaire** [20]:

Pre: 48(fair)                    Post: 83(excellent)

Upon comparing the pre- (48-fair) and post-treatment (83-excellent) questionnaire scores of functional disability testing by the modified Cincinnati Rating System. There is a significant increase in the patient's functional ability after treatment.

## XI. **OUTCOME OF THE CASE STUDY:**

In Medial / Varus knee arthritis, the loss of joint range of motion and pain are the major clinical findings affecting the patient's functional ability in daily living. Treatment with three planar mobilizations and manipulation has reduced the stiffness by increasing the joint range of motion, specifically in internal rotation and knee extension, eventually improving synovial fluid influx and outflux[25]. After the interventions, which were designed based on pathomechanics, had potentially restored the normal alignment, that in turn may have caused the WBA (Weight weight-bearing axis) of the limb to shift from the medial compartment towards the centre of the joint and soft tissue release also contributed in increasing internal rotation medial shift by reducing the lateral pull caused by tight external rotators of proximal tibia restoring normal alignment.

On comparing the pre and post-x-ray, it is evident that medial joint compartment gapping increased and lateral joint compartment gapping maintained instead of decreasing as there is joint retraction. The proximal tibia shifted from lateral to medial, thereby reducing the varus (adduction of the tibia) and medial slope (medial tilt), improving normal joint space and alignment of the Knee. Lateral wedge orthosis helped to maintain the effect achieved by manual therapy and deep friction by creating valgus force at the joint. Knee strengthening improved the dis-use loss of strength and assisted in the prevention of recurrence. Thus, all the multi-model interventions synergistically assisted one another in achieving an improved range of motion, thereby improving synovial fluid, increasing the medial joint space and decreasing cartilage compression. The above explanation potentially proves the proposed pathomechanics, diagnosis, and treatment of Varus knee dysfunction.

**Note:** Research is going on in the large study group, and it will be published soon.

**References:**

1. T. derek v. cooke, Allan scudamore, William greer. Axial alignment of the lower limb and its association with disorders of the knee. Operative Techniques in Sports Medicine, Vol 8, No 2 (April), 2000: pp 98-107

2. Jorge Chahla, M.D., Chase S. Dean, M.D., Justin J. Mitchell, M.D., Gilbert Moatshe, M.D., Raphael Serra Cruz, M.D., and Robert F. LaPrade, M.D., Ph.D. Medial Opening Wedge Proximal Tibial Osteotomy. Arthroscopy Techniques, Vol 5, No 4 (August), 2016: pp e919-e928

3. Amir Ali Jafarnezhadgero1, Morteza Madadi Shad, Mahdi Majlesi, Urs Granacher. A comparison of running kinetics in children with and without genu varus: A cross sectional study. https://doi.org/10.1371/journal.pone.0185057 September 19, 2017

4. Savio L-Y. Woo, Richard E. Debski, John D. Withrow, Marsie A. Janaushek. Biomechanics of Knee Ligaments. The American journal of sports medicine, Vol. 27, No. 4 © 1999 American Orthopaedic Society for Sports Medicine.

5. Savio L.-Y. Woo, Steven D. Abramowitch, Robert Kilger, and Rui Liang. Biomechanics of knee ligaments: injury, healing, and repair. S.L.-Y. Woo et al. / Journal of Biomechanics 39 (2006) 1–20.orthopaedics and trauma 33:4

6. R Shenoy, PS Pastides, D Nathwani. Biomechanics of the Knee and TKR. Osama Aweid, Humza Osmani, Joel Melton. Biomechanics of the Knee. Orthopaedics and trauma.

7. Ahmed Aljawadi*, Mohammed Elmajee, Noman Niazi, Noman Jahangir, Omar Alsawaf, and Anand Pillai. Current Evidence for Biome-chanical Principles in the Management of Knee Osteoarthritis, Review of Literature. Aljawadi A, et al., J Orthop Res Physiother 2019, 5: 045

8. Jerry Hesch PT. Evaluating sacroiliac joint play with spring test. J OB/GYN PT, 20:3, SEP,1996

9. Jerry Hesch, B.S.PT., Jeannie A. Aisenbrey, M.S,PT., John Guarino, B.S., PT. Manual therapy evaluation of the pelvic joints using palpatory and articular

spring tests. National conference of the American physical therapy association in Anaheim, California, in June 1990.

10. Olson, L., Kraemer, TJ. Establishing the reliability of the Hesch method's spring and positional tests in patients with low back pain. rr-pl-2274 Sunday 13:10, Palau de Congressos, Hall 5, Room 7

11. M. A. lafortune, t p. r. cavanagh,h . j. sommer 111a4n d a. kalenak~i. three-dimensional kinematics of the human knee during walking. j. &mechanics vol. 25, no. 4, pp. 347-357. 1992.

12. Ha yong kim, kap Jung Kim, Dae Suk Yang, Sang Wook Jeung, Han Gyeol Choi, Won Sik Choy. Screw-Home Movement of the Tibiofemoral Joint during Normal Gait: Three-Dimensional Analysis. Clinics in Orthopedic Surgery 2015; 7:303-309.

13. J. Sanfridsson, L. Ryd, G. Svahn, T. Fridén & K. Jonsson. Radiographic measurement of femorotibial rotation in weight-bearing: The influence of flexion and extension in the knee on the extensor mechanism and angles of the lower extremity in a healthy population. Acta Radiologica 42 (2001) 207–217

14. Ismail Anas, Tabari Abdulkdir Musa, Isyaku Kabiru, Abdulkadir Adekunle Yisau, Idris Sulaiman Kazaure, Suwaid Muhammad Abba, Saleh Muhammad Kabir. Digital radiographic measurement of normal knee joint space in adults at Kano, Nigeria. The Egyptian Journal of Radiology and Nuclear Medicine (2013) 44, 253–258.

15. Michael J Mueller, Katrina S Maluf. Tissue Adaptation to Physical Stress: A Proposed "Physical Stress Theory" to Guide Physical Therapist Practice, Education, and Research. Physical Therapy. Volume 82. Number 4. April 2002.

16. Kenneth A. Krackow. The measurement and analysis of axial deformity at the knee. Copyright © 2008 Stryker

17. Sara R. Piva, Alexandra B. Gil, Charity G. Moore, G. Kelley Fitzgerald. Responsiveness of the activities of the daily living scale of the knee outcome survey and numeric pain rating scale in patients with patellofemoral pain. J Rehabil Med 2009; 41: 129–135.

18. Prem p. gogia, James h. braatz, Steven j. rose, and Barbara j. Norton. Reliability and Validity of Goniometric Measurements at the Knee. Volume 67 / Number 2, February 1987.

19. Sue D. Barber-Westin, Frank R. Noyes, John W. McCloskey. Rigorous Statistical Reliability, Validity, and Responsiveness Testing of the Cincinnati Knee Rating System in 350 Subjects with Uninjured, Injured, or Anterior Cruciate Ligament-Reconstructed Knees. The American journal of sports medicine, vol. 27, no. 4© 1999 American Orthopaedic Society for Sports Medicine.

20. Brent C. Mangus, Laura A. Hoffman, Mark A. Hoffman, and Peter Altenburger. Basic Principles of Extremity Joint Mobilization Using a Kaltenborn Approach. Florida Intl University on 09/22/16, Volume 11, Article Number 4.

21. Janet McMurray, Scott Landis, Kris Lininger, Russell T. Baker, Alan Nasypany, Jeff Seegmiller. A Comparison and Review of Indirect. Myofascial Release Therapy, Instrument-Assisted Soft Tissue Mobilization, and Active Release Techniques to Inform Clinical Decision Making. 30, September 2015 international journal of Athletic Therapy & training

22. Salvi Shah, Akta Bhalara. Myofascial Release. International Journal of Health Sciences & Research (www.ijhsr.org) 69 Vol.2; Issue: 2; May 2012.

23. Ahmed Mohamed El-Sodany, Mohamed Salaheldien Mohamed Alayat, Ayman Mohammed Ismail Zafer. Sustained natural apophyseal glides mobilization versus manipulation in the treatment of cervical spine disorders: a randomized controlled trial. International Journal of Advanced Research (2014), Volume 2, Issue 6, 274-280.

24. Isabel A. C. Baert, Jo Nijs, Mira Meeus, Enrique Lluch, Filip Struyf. The effect of lateral wedge insoles in patients with medial compartment knee osteoarthritis: balancing biomechanics with pain neuroscience. Clin Rheumatol (2014) 33:1529–1538.

25. William O Irvine. Concepts of Etiologies and Effects of Normal Human Knee Pressure Variations. Irvine, Anat Physiol 2015, 5:2.

26. Christian Egloff, Thomas Hügle, Victor Valderrabano, Biomechanics and Pathomechanisms of osteoarthritis. Swiss Med Wkly. 2012; 142: w13583.

27. A Kapandji.The physiology of joints, Vol 2, 5th edition.

28. Ackerman IN, Kemp JL, Crossley KM, Culvenor AG, Hinman RS. Hip and Knee Osteoarthritis Affects Younger People, Too. J Orthop Sports Phys 2017; 47(2): 67±79.

29. Caine D, DiFiori J, Maffulli N. Physeal injuries in children's and youth sports: reasons for concern? Brit J Sport Med 2006; 40(9): 749±60.

30. Ahmed Mohamed El-Sodany, Mohamed Salaheldien Mohamed Alayat, Ayman Mohammed Ismail Zafer. Sustained natural apophyseal glides mobilization versus manipulation in the treatment of cervical spine disorders: a randomized controlled trial. International Journal of Advanced Research (2014), Volume 2, Issue 6, 274-280.

31. Alessandro Pedrelli, Carla Stecco, Juli Ann Day. Treating patellar tendinopathy with fascial manipulation, J Bodyw Mov Ther. 2009 jan;13(1):73-80.

32. Cesar Fernandez, Cristina Aloso-Blanco, et al. The immediate effect of ischemic compression technique and transverse friction massage on the tenderness of active and latent myofascial trigger points: A pilot study. 2005, ScienceDirect. Vol 10, pages 3-9.

33. D. Casey Kerrigan, Jennifer L Lelas, et al. Effectiveness of a lateral-wedge insole on knee varus torque in patients with knee osteoarthritis. Arch Phy Med Rehabil: 2012 July;83(7):889-93.

# CHAPTER 1
## Prevention of injury and dysfunction

**Theory – "Physical Stress Acted Upon the Tissue Vs Strength, Adaptation and Strengthening of Tissue**

Physical Stress is defined as the force applied to a given area of biological tissue[1]. The theory explains that when Physical Stress acts upon the tissue, it may get injured or maintain its homeostasis, get strengthened (hypertrophy), or get atrophied (weakened) depending on the relative amount of physical Stress acted upon the tissue versus the relative amount of tissue strength. The theory will guide the understanding of mechanisms of injury and prevention of a broad range of patients' musculoskeletal problems. The main principle of the theory is based on the relationship between physical Stress acting upon a particular tissue, tissue strength, and its adaptive behaviour. Based on the adaptive behaviour of tissue, it can be strengthened without injury.

Exercise interventions that modify physical Stress have been shown to decrease impairments, functional limitations, disability, and pain in various patient populations.[2-4]. The same interventions can help people with or without disease by increasing muscle performance[5], bone mineral density[6], and fitness levels[4]. Increased evidence indicates exercise can positively affect disease processes such as diabetes[7], arthritis[2-4] and coronary artery disease[8].

The application of force over a given area of the tissue during movement results in Stress on the tissue.
[Stress = force per unit area – where force may be applied in any direction, tension, shear, compression.][1]

Although the movement is a major source of physical stress on the tissue, other forces, such as isometric muscle contraction, generated inside the body, and gravity, generated outside the body, may contribute to tissue stress.

This concept is well supported by PST (**Physical Stress Theory**), proposed by Michael j Muller and Katrina S. Maul[9].

**The effect of physical stress on tissue adaptation: "physical stress theory"[9] The present concept is the modification of physical stress theory and further steps ahead by applying the principle specifically to the knee joint.** This modification gives rise to a new theory called **"Physical Stress on a tissue vs. strength of the tissue".**

## MAJOR COMPARATIVE STUDIES

The theory is based on three major comparative studies on the strength of tissue and how physical stress acts on it.

I. The relationship between physical Stress acted upon the tissue vs tissue strength.

II. The relationship between physical Stress acted upon the tissue vs tissue adaptation.

III. The relationship between physical Stress acted upon the tissue vs tissue strengthening.

### I. RELATIONSHIP BETWEEN PHYSICAL STRESS ACTED UPON THE TISSUE VS TISSUE STRENGTH

Every tissue has the relative strength to withstand physical Stress. Likewise, every joint in our body has strength contributed by bone, ligaments, tendons, and peri-articular muscles surrounding it. Suppose physical Stress acts upon the tissue through a particular activity that exceeds the tissue's strength. In that case, it decreases the tissue's tolerance to the physical stress acted upon it, leading to micro/micro-traumas of one or more ligaments, tendons, or muscles of the particular joint[2]. If the Stress acting upon the tissue is more than the strength, it can cause major injury. For example, the surrounding soft tissue of the knee joint, i.e., muscles, tendons, ligaments, and bone, should be strong enough to take the physical stress acted upon by joint activities like standing, walking, etc. If the surrounding soft tissues are strong, there will be no injury. In short, the strength of the tissue surrounding the joint should be more than or at least equal to mechanical stress acting upon it to avoid any injury/dysfunction. A thorough scientific analysis of the relationship between relative physical Stress and the relative strength of the tissue plays a vital role in predicting the tissue response to injury, adaptation, and strengthening. The term "relative" is used for physical Stress as it can be increased or decreased or become equal to tissue strength and vice versa. This analysis is further utilized in physical therapy intervention to prevent and treat musculoskeletal dysfunctions.

Figure 1: Flow chart of the theory: "Physical Stress on a tissue VS Strength of the tissue"

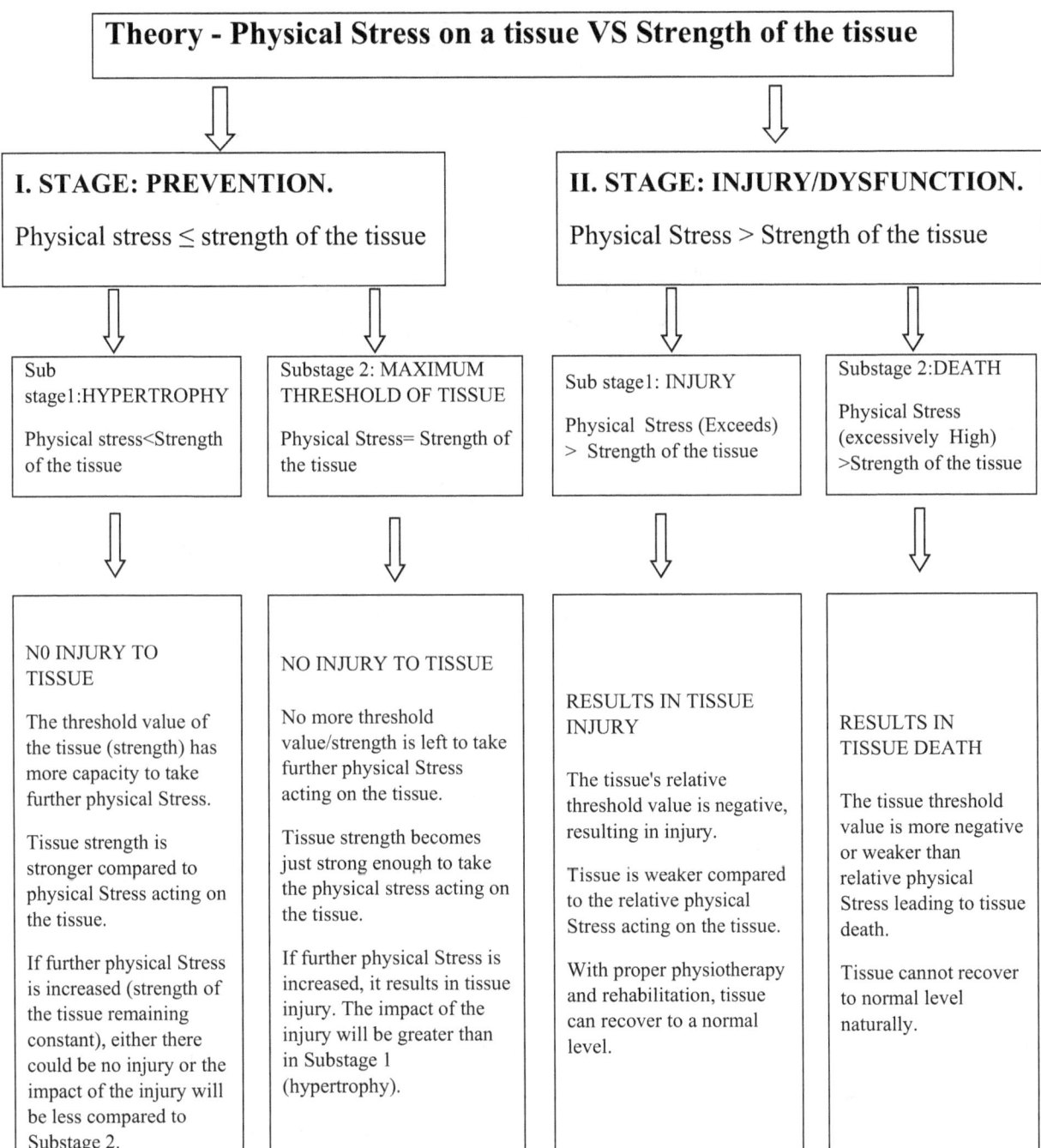

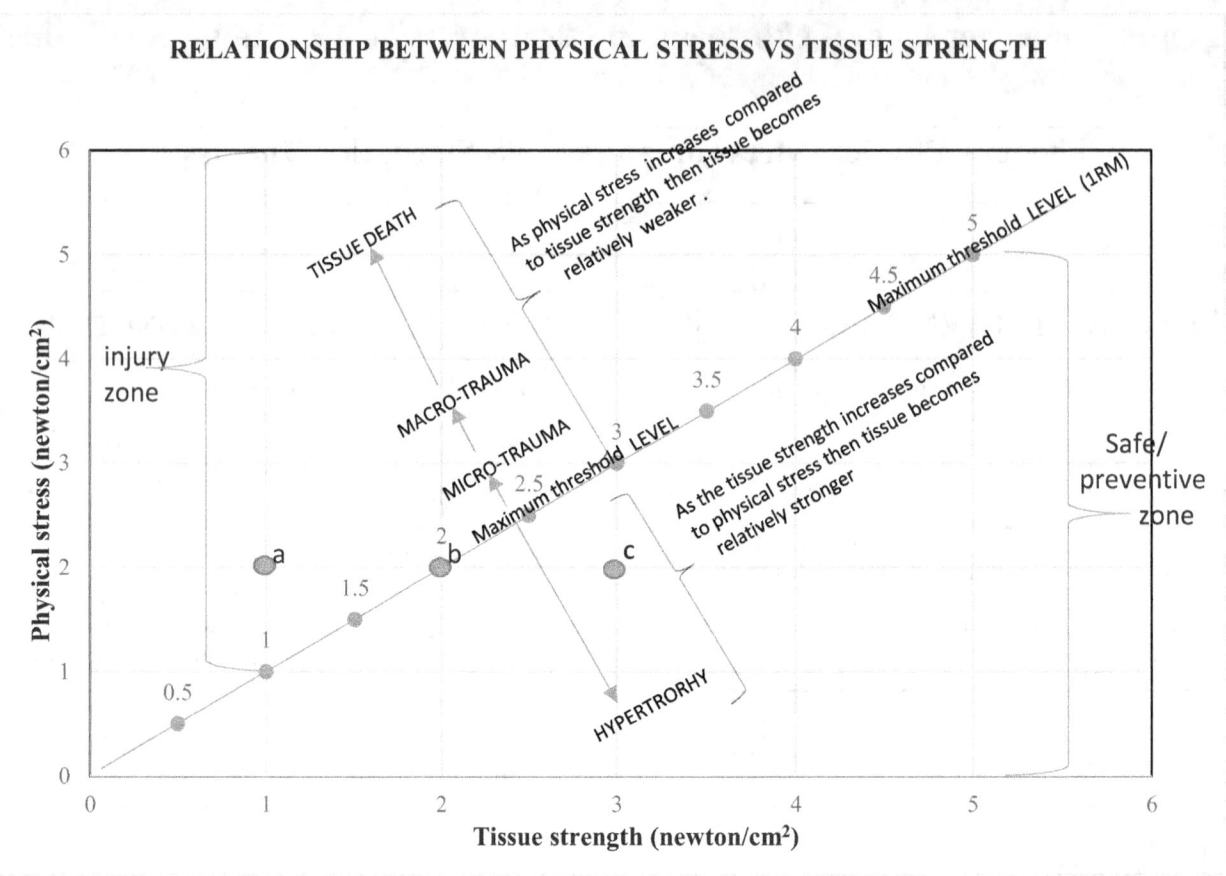

**Graph 1**: It depicts a direct relationship between physical stress acted upon the tissue versus tissue strength in the prospective of tissue injury (injury zone) and prevention of injury (preventive/safe zone and threshold level). The X-axis represents tissue strength; the y-axis represents physical Stress acting on the tissue.

**I. Prevention stage**: When physical Stress applied over the tissue is proportional to tissue strength that results in no injury/dysfunction; it is called the **Maximum threshold level** (represented as an oblique line).

If the physical Stress < strength of the tissue falls under **the hypertrophy stage**, here also results in no injury /dysfunction of tissue. **II. Injury stage**: physical Stress> tissue strength, resulting in **tissue injury**. If physical stress increases relative to the strength of the tissue, the impact of injury is proportionate to relative strength. The impact can vary from micro trauma to macro trauma and further to **tissue death**.

**Note:** The universal unit for the physical stress and tissue strength is calculated as **Stress or strength = force per unit area.**

The area (The knee joint) is common for physical stress applied (knee joint), and the tissue strength of the area (Knee joint) is the same.

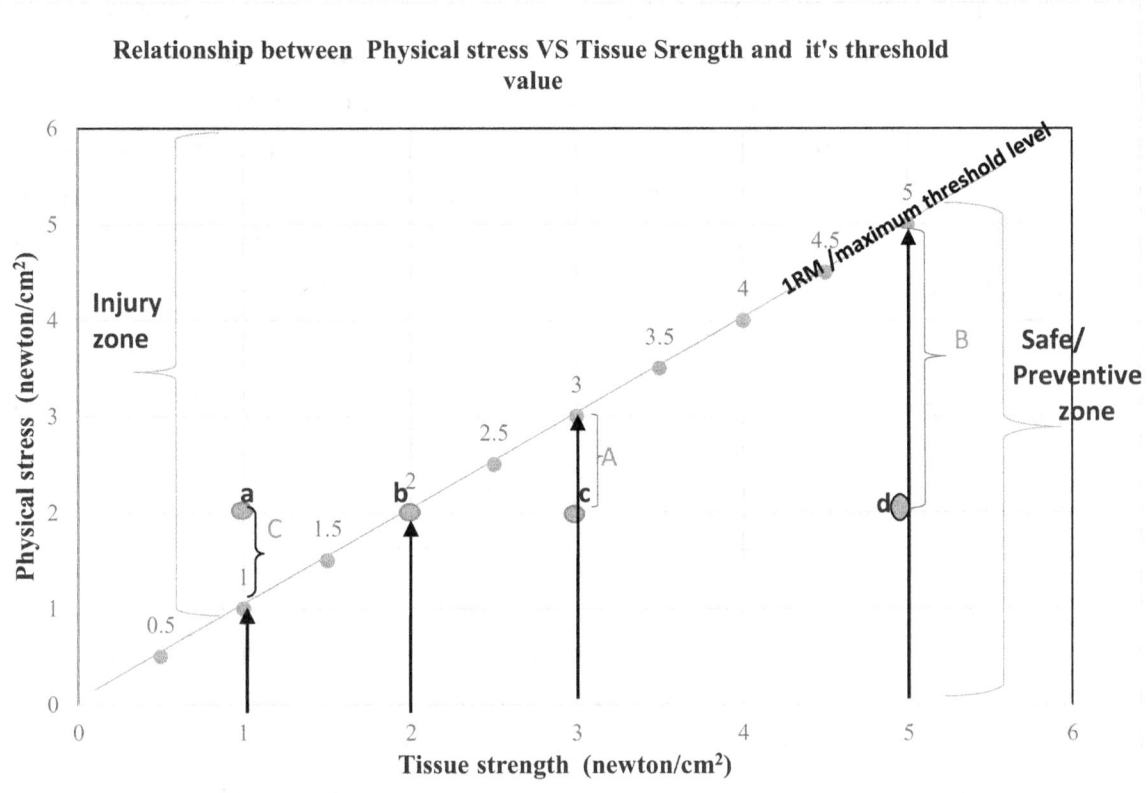

Graph 2: The graph indicates the relative threshold value of tissue. It increases when tissue is strengthened gradually compared to applied physical stress (which remains constant at $2N/cm^2$) on the tissue. Initially, at point "a", the relative threshold value of the tissue is negative, represented as bracket **C**, as the physical stress applied to the tissue was $2N/cm^2$ compared to $1N/cm^2$ of tissue strength. When the tissue is gradually strengthened, tissue strength reaches $2N/cm^2$ at point b, which is equal to physical stress applied ($2N/cm^2$) on the tissue. That is, at this stage, tissue falls at the maximum threshold level. Then, as the tissue is further strengthened, it gradually reaches point "c" ($3N/cm2$ strength) and even further, it reaches point "d" ($5N/cm^2$ strength). So, the threshold level of the tissue also becomes more positive, which is represented by brackets as **A** and **B,** respectively. Therefore, upon increasing the tissue strength as compared to physical stress acting upon the tissue, which remains constant, tissue can be shifted from the injury zone to the preventive /safe zone as the tissue threshold level increases.

As shown in Graph 1&2, the Horizontal X-axis shows the strength of the tissue; the Vertical Y-axis shows the physical Stress acted upon the tissue. Between the X and Y axis, a 45-degree oblique line shows the maximum threshold level/near 1RM level (where physical Stress is equal to the strength of the tissue). Below the oblique line of the maximum threshold level is a preventive/safe zone where tissue injury will not occur. The Hypertrophy stage falls under this zone. If physical stress acting upon the tissue remains constant and the strength of the tissue gradually increases, the threshold value or strength of the tissue increases, thereby indicating there will not be any injury.

The injury zone is above the maximum threshold level in the graph. That is, relatively, the strength of the tissue becomes weaker compared to the stress applied to it. As the strength of the tissue remains constant, relative physical stress acting upon the tissue increases, leading to a decrease in the tissue's threshold value and may become negative.

The points in Graph 1 **a, b & c** are the relationship between the physical Stress acting upon the tissue and the tissue strength. As the physical Stress acted upon the tissue (2 Newton/cm$^2$) exceeds the strength (1Newton/cm$^2$) of the tissue, it is at point "**a**" where tissue falls under the **injury zone.** At point "**b**", **the** tissue will be on **a maximum threshold level**, as the physical Stress acted upon the tissue (2 Newton/cm$^2$) is equal to the strength of the tissue (2 Newton/cm$^2$). At point "**c**", the tissue will fall under the **Safe /Prevention zone** as the physical Stress acted upon the tissue (2 Newton/cm$^2$) is less than the strength of the tissue (3 Newton/cm$^2$). On observation of the pattern [a, b, c, in Graph **1** and a, b, c and d in Graph **2],** where physical Stress remains constant, the strength of the tissue is increased, and the tissue moves from the injury zone to maximum threshold level progressing to preventive/safe zone. Additionally, a tissue threshold value or the tissue's relative strength increases compared to physical Stress.

The two **main stages** in relation to physical Stress acted upon the tissue and the strength of the tissue are as follows: - (Refer: flowchart 1 and Graph 1 and 2)

**A. Prevention**: Relative physical Stress acted upon the tissue is (less or equal to) ≤ the strength of the tissue. Therefore, there will be no tissue injury[11].

**B. Injury[12]/Dysfunction:** Physical Stress acted upon the tissue through activity > strength of the tissue, resulting in tissue injury/dysfunction.

Graphs 1 and 2 depict that if physical stress applied over the tissue remains constant and tissue strength increases, the threshold value of the tissue increases, which will be in the safe/preventive zone. When tissue becomes stronger with progressive strengthening, even though physical Stress acted upon the tissue increases, there is a chance that the tissue will still be in the preventive zone, or at least the impact of injury will be less. If tissue strength remains constant and physical Stress acted upon the tissue increases, the tissue will fall under the injury zone. Another possibility is that if relative Stress is proportionate to (or) equal to the strength of the tissue, then there will not be any injury, and the tissue will reach the maximum threshold level (safe/preventive zone).

**A. Prevention**: Relative physical Stress acted upon the tissue is (less or equal to) ≤ the strength of the tissue. Therefore, there will not be any tissue injury. This stage is further divided into two sub-stages.
  **a) Hypertrophy** - Relative physical Stress acted upon the tissue (less than) < the strength of the tissue.
  **b) Maximum threshold zone** - Relative physical Stress acted upon the tissue (proportion to) / = the strength of the tissue.

**a) Hypertrophy:** physical Stress acted upon the tissue (less than) < the strength of the tissue.

At this stage, in a given activity, if physical stress acting on tissue is less than the strength of the tissue. Or suppose it falls below the maximum threshold of tissue (i.e., the maximum stress threshold is defined as the amount of stress the tissue can bear just before it fails). In that case, there won't be an injury, as the tissue is strong enough to take the physical stress.

Another important point is that one should analyze which particular tissue is stressed more in a given activity. Therefore, it can be strengthened until it becomes stronger/hypertrophy relative to physical Stress. Therefore, to prevent any dysfunction /injury, tissue should always be under hypertrophy. Based on this explanation, a physical therapist can advise patients about how this theory can be applied in day-to-day activities of life[10]. That is the importance of doing specific exercises for the tissues that are under more stress. Patients can be educated on the importance of daily exercise so that tissue is always under the hypertrophy stage, preventing injury/recurrence of dysfunction.

Recent research suggests that the knee is stressed in ascending order in the following activities of daily life (ADL).

Standing < walking < stairs-ascending < stairs-descending < squatting-rise < squatting-down. [13-14]

**Example 1-** The common activity of daily life, squatting down and rising, is physical Stress, where the maximum stress falls on the knee[13,14], and the targeted tissue to be strengthened will be the knee joint. Suppose a person's capacity (strength/endurance of the knee/1RM) of squatting down and rising at a stretch in one day is ten times on a particular surface with an 'X' speed and 'Y' duration. If he does it five times, then there will be no injury or dysfunction of the joint. That indicates that the knee joint strength (i.e., Strength of ligaments, tendons, bones, and muscles surrounding the joint) is more than the physical Stress caused by five times squatting down and rising.

In this stage, the strength of the knee tissue is more than the Stress on the tissue caused by squatting down and rising, and it will be safe as long as the person does not cross the limit of ten times Squatting down and rising with the same speed and duration on the same surface. Therefore, the tissue surrounding the knee joint is relatively stronger than the physical stress of squatting down and rising five times. Based on this, it can be said that tissue strength is relatively **hypertrophied** compared to the physical stress that acted on it.

b) **Maximum threshold zone**: Relative Physical Stress acted upon the tissue is equal to (=)the strength of the tissue.

This stage also does not result in any injury/dysfunction. The tissue undergoing physical stress is relatively strong enough to take the stress or is just equal to the maximum threshold level of the tissue.

**Example 2-** (Same person as in example 1) Strength of the knee tissues has the capacity (strength/endurance of the knee or 1RM) of squatting down and rising at a stretch in one day ten times on a particular surface with an 'X'speed and 'Y'duration without any injury or dysfunction. If he does ten squats, there won't be injury or dysfunction. Indicating the knee joint strength (i.e., Strength provided by ligaments, tendons, bone, and muscles surrounding the joint) is **just enough** to take the physical stress caused by ten times of squatting down and rising. If the person does it more than ten times in one day, he might have had an injury.

Here, the key is to know the strength of the targeted tissue, that is, the knee, in the form of 1Repetition Maximum[24,25] or maximum threshold level. So that we know not to overuse it and, at the same time, strengthen particular tissues without injury.

**B. INJURY:** Physical Stress acted upon the tissue through activity (greater than) > tissue strength.

This stage is subdivided into two.

**(a) INJURY**

**(b) DEATH**

**a) INJURY:** Physical Stress acted upon the tissue through activity (**excessively high**) > tissue strength.

Physical Stress acting upon the tissue through activity is **excessively higher** than the strength of the tissue, resulting in injury/dysfunction. Tissue damage is caused by excessive Stress resulting in pain or discomfort, impairment of function, or both. The maximum threshold level is defined as the amount of Stress the tissue can bear just before it fails. Stress levels that exceed the maximum stress threshold are considered excessive and result in tissue injury.

-McGill[26] proposed - Injury or "failure of a tissue" occurs when the applied load exceeds the failure tolerance of the tissue, and structures of the lower back are influenced by the history of recent physical stresses so that the accumulation of individual stresses can cause injury. Further, he added the character of the load (load rate, mode of load compression, bending, torsion, and shear), and the properties of the tissue determine the type and extent of the tissue damage.

McGill[26] described the three mechanisms of injury to the lower back tissues. One mechanism of injury to the lower back tissues is a single application of a relatively high load or stress. McGill provided the example of a person riding a snowmobile thrown from the machine, landing on a flexed spine, and experiencing a sudden posterior disc herniation. The second mechanism of injury to the lower back tissues is multiple moderate loads or stresses applied to the lower back structures. In this case, the injury is the result of accumulated trauma. McGill provided the example of a worker lifting boxes in which lower back tissues are loaded repeatedly, causing a slow degradation of tissue tolerance. The third mechanism of injury is low loads sustained by the lower back over a long period. An example of this mechanism of injury is construction workers who install rods on the floors of a new building and remain in a flexed posture for prolonged periods.

Ligaments can tear with one bout of a high-magnitude force (e.g., injury of the medial collateral ligament from a tackle to the lateral knee). Increasing evidence suggests that ligaments also can fail from repeated bouts of moderate-magnitude stress. For example, women have a much higher incidence of anterior cruciate ligament injury from non-contact sporting events compared with men[27]. Huston et al. [27] speculated that this finding might be related to anatomical differences, such as a wider pelvis and greater Q angle in women, that result in greater cumulative Stress on the anterior cruciate ligament during typical activities such as walking or running.

- Radin and colleagues[28-31] have described similar mechanisms of injury involved in articular cartilage degeneration and joints.

**Example 3-** (Same person as in example 1&2)
As previously mentioned, the strength of the knee tissue has the capacity to squat down and rise at a stretch in one day 10 times on a particular surface with an 'X' speed and 'Y' duration without any injury or dysfunction. If the person does it 15 times, it results in an injury or dysfunction of the knee joint, indicating the knee joint strength (given by ligaments, tendons, and muscles surrounding the joint) is **not enough** to take the physical Stress caused by 15 times of squatting down and rising. That means the knee surrounding tissue's maximum threshold level can take the Stress of 10 repetitions of squatting down and rising with the same speed and duration on the same surface without causing injury/dysfunction. In this case, the strength of the knee is (less than) < the physical Stress of 15 squatting down and rising. That results in the micro or macro injury of the knee joint.

**b) DEATH**: Physical Stress acted upon the tissue through activity (**extremely high**) > strength of the tissue results in tissue death.

Stress that is **Extreme deviation** from the maximum threshold on the tissue that exceeds the adaptive capacity of the tissue results in **tissue death**.

Tissue death can occur when tissues are exposed to extremely high or extremely low-stress levels (atrophy) and cannot adapt or recover.

When tissues are exposed to an extremely high level of physical stress (>70% of 1RM), where tissue cannot return to a normal level by the natural way of healing, the process is called tissue death. Example: complete tear of the knee joint ACL in a football game.

**Note:** not only extremely high but extremely low physical Stress (< 55% of 1RM), which cannot maintain the tissue maintenance level, also gradually leads to disuse atrophy and death.

## II. RELATIONSHIP BETWEEN PHYSICAL STRESS ACTED UPON THE TISSUE VS TISSUE ADAPTATION.

The change in the relative level of physical Stress causes a predictable and adaptive response in all biological tissues, mainly musculoskeletal tissue. Specific thresholds define each characteristic tissue response's upper and lower stress levels. Other biological tissues are beyond the scope of the book.

Changes in the relative level of physical Stress cause a predictable adaptive response in all biological tissues, like their structure and composition, to meet the mechanical demands of routine loading. Deviation from the routine of steady-state loading provides a stimulus for tissue adaptation that allows tissues to meet the mechanical demands of a novel environment.

Biological tissues exhibit mainly three characteristic responses to physical Stress. Each response is predicted to occur within a defined range along a continuum of stress levels.

**Important Adaptive Responses to Physical Stress**

Mainly, the three tissue adaptive responses to physical stress are as follows.

**A. Atrophy and death-** Decreased stress tolerance
**Atrophy** (decreased stress tolerance): Physical stress levels that are lower than the maintenance range (< 55% of 1**RM**) result in decreased tolerance of tissues to subsequent stresses. Atrophy is one common mechanism by which tissues become less tolerant of subsequent physical stresses. Atrophy occurs when tissue degeneration exceeds tissue production and has been observed in response to reduced stress levels (Graph 3).

Other examples of adaptations that may reduce stress tolerance include hormonal changes, altered cell membrane excitability, and changes in the material properties of tissues.

Graph 3 reveals that at point "**c**," the strength of the tissue (3N/cm$^2$) is greater than the physical Stress acted upon it (2N/cm$^2$) if a tissue is not undergoing the required amount of Stress, which maintains the present strength.

(For example - if initial tissue strength is 3N/cm$^2$ at point "**c**" in graph 3, the tissue is disused or has not undergone minimum stress that is 55% of 3N/cm$^2$ (1RM) for some time, then after a period of time tissue strength decreases to point "**b**" where tissue strength becomes to 2N/cm$^2$. During which physical Stress acted upon remains the same 2N/cm$^2$. If tissue is further disused for a long time, it may go into the injury zone towards point "**a**," where tissue strength further decreases to 1N/cm$^2$. It is shown as the atrophy line in graph 3. In the long run, if tissue is disused or not maintained at the maintenance stress level (around 55% of 1RM), the tissue strength relatively becomes weaker than the physical stress acting on it. Further, it may fall into **"tissue death."**

At point "**a**" on graph 3, the tissue strength is 1N/cm$^2$, and physical stress acted upon is 2N/cm$^2$, which indicates the tissue fall under the injury zone. From here, if tissue undergoes progressive strengthening (55% -70% of 1RM), it will go into the maximum threshold level –i.e., point "**b**", where tissue strength will be 2N/cm$^2$, and stress acted upon remains the same 2N/cm$^2$. Again, further strengthened, it may go into the safe/preventive zone, i.e., point "**c**" (tissue strength has progressed to 3N/cm$^2$ and physical Stress acted on tissue is less than the strength that is 2N/cm$^2$). It is represented as a progressive strengthening line in the graph.

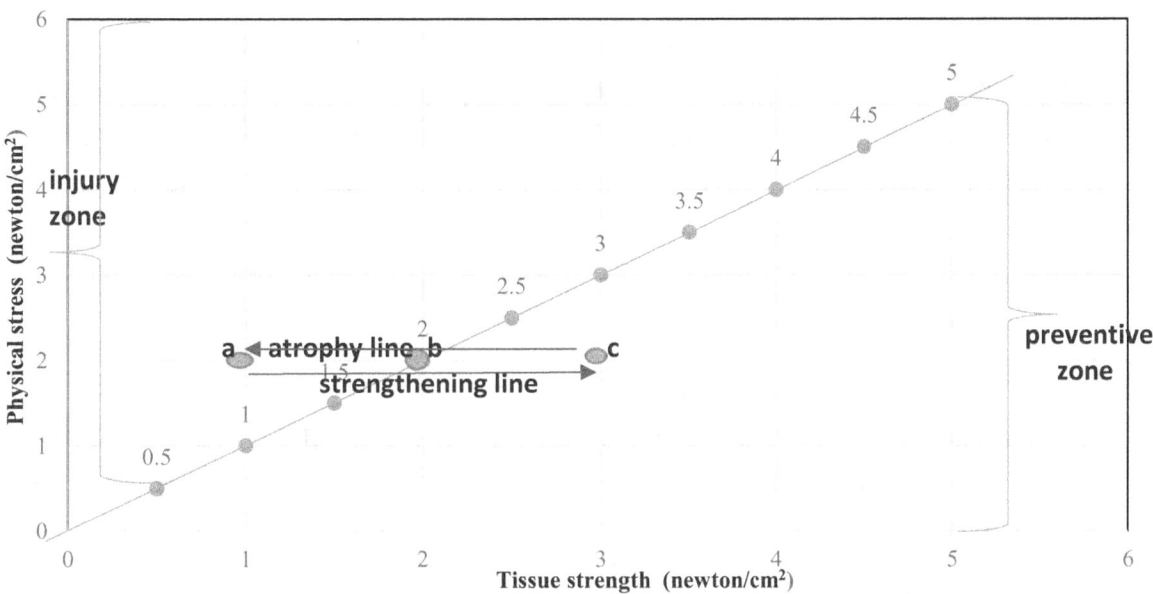

Relationship between physical stress VS tissue atrophy and strengthening

Graph 3: Relative nature of physical Stress, atrophy and tissue strength: physical stress acted upon the tissue remaining constant, which is ($2N/cm^2$). Tissue strength will be decreased in case of tissue disuse/ atrophy from point "c" to point "a" The directed arrow line is called the atrophy line. Tissue strength can be increased from point "a" to "c", indicated by a directed arrow line called a graded strengthening line. As physical stress can be increased or decreased, likewise, the strength of the tissue can be increased or decreased. Therefore, they are termed relative.

Evidence also supports the idea that tissues within the musculoskeletal system atrophy become less tolerant of physical Stress if the Stress on the tissue diminishes below a baseline level[32, 33-36]. Unfortunately, tissues typically atrophy at a faster rate than hypertrophy [32, 33]. Muscles can lose 6% to 40% of their ability to generate force over 4- to 6 weeks of bed rest or immobilization.[34] Bone mineral density is also lost in response to diminished physical Stress. Leblanc et al. [35] found that BMD is reduced by 3% to 4% at the femoral neck and lumbar spine after 17 weeks of bed rest in healthy young men. Holick[36] summarised the current literature by indicating that unloading of the skeleton, either due to strict bed rest or in zero gravity, leads on an average to 1% to 2% reduction in BMD at selected skeletal sites each month.

Likewise, ligaments respond to reduced mechanical stress. Woo and colleagues[35,37] have documented a decline in the mechanical properties of the rabbit medial collateral ligament in response to 9 weeks of immobilization. These researchers reported that the stiffness, the ultimate load before failure, and the energy-absorbing capacity of the immobilized medial collateral ligament-bone complex were approximately one-third of those variables in the contra-lateral, non-immobilized control limb.[37]Strict bed rest or zero gravity leads to a 1% to 2% reduction of BMD at selected skeletal sites each month. Atrophy occurs when tissue degeneration exceeds tissue production. If prolonged for a longer duration, **tissue death** can occur.

**B. Maintenance**: The homeostasis of tissue (Refer to the section - tissue adaptation in maintenance).

**Tissue adaptation in maintenance:** Physical Stress, which is acted upon, will be a stimulus for a tissue adaptation to maintain the available strength; therefore, it is also called the **maintenance stage.**

Physical stress levels in the maintenance range (approximately 55% of 1RM) result in no tissue change[9]. Tissue homeostasis occurs when tissue degeneration equals tissue production, resulting in tissue turnover without net gain or loss.

The stress levels promoting tissue homeostasis are defined as maintenance; the stress range may differ for different people. The steady-state or equilibrium response occurs when tissues are exposed to the same stress levels they have become accustomed to.

Like the bone, tendon and ligament adaptation models predict that deviations from a typical range of strain (change in length relative to original length) stimulus values promote adaptive responses in these tissues. These models require 1.5% to 3.0% strain values to maintain tissue homeostasis[26]. Strain values above this range will increase the cross-sectional area and stiffness of tendons and ligaments (hypertrophy), whereas strain values below this range predict decreases in these parameters (atrophy). If tissue remains in physical stress lower than the maintenance range, it may lead to severe atrophy and **tissue death**.

Recent research suggests that gradual strengthening should be between 55%-70 % of 1RM to strengthen muscle/tissue without injury. That means particular muscle maintenance should require around 55%1RM stress. In the same way, when physical stress >70% of 1RM, it will cause muscle/tissue injury from micro-trauma to macro-trauma or tissue death, depending on the relative increase of stress over the strength of the tissue.

**Physical stress levels that are lower than the maintenance range:** Result in decreased tolerance of tissues to subsequent Stress. In recent research, it is evident that in order to maintain homeostasis, tissue should undergo physical Stress, which should be around 55% of 1RM. If it is less than 55% of 1RM, the tissue becomes gradually atrophied, where tissues become less tolerant of subsequent physical stresses. Atrophy occurs when tissue degeneration exceeds tissue production.
Other adaptations that may reduce stress tolerance include hormonal changes, altered cell membrane excitability, and changes in tissue material properties. This means that tissue strength is lower than the physical stress it acts upon and, therefore, more prone to injury. When tissue becomes more atrophied, it may result in tissue death.

**C. Hypertrophy:** Increased stress tolerance (Refer to tissue adaptation in hypertrophy).
**Tissue adaptation in hypertrophy:** Stress levels that are applied in strengthening to increase hypertrophy of the tissue fall in the range of 55-70% of 1RM. This adaptation falls higher than the maintenance (55%1RM) threshold level yet is lower than the maximum threshold value (70%1RM); first, there will not be tissue injury, and it can positively affect tissue adaptation.
Musculoskeletal tissues subjected to stress levels higher than the maintenance range and lower than the maximum threshold level will become more tolerant to subsequent physical stresses and more resistant to injury (i.e., tissues become stronger). This adaptation occurs when tissues can recover and adapt to previous

bouts of physical stress. Steady increases in physical stress through progressive resistive exercise cause muscle fibres to hypertrophy and become capable of generating greater force. Likewise, higher-than-normal levels of physical stress can promote remodelling in bone[15]. Wolff's Law provides an excellent example of how one specific biological tissue, bone, responds to physical stress by remodelling. Wolff's Law states that the thickness, number, and orientation of trabeculae will correspond to the distribution of mechanical stresses on bone[15]. A consequence of stress-induced bone remodelling is that the strength of bone is most significant in the direction in which loads are most commonly imposed[16]. For example, the maximum stress tolerated by bone just before failure has been found to be higher for compressive loads than for tensile or shear loads, reflecting the predominantly compressive loads experienced by bone during weight bearing[17]. Runners with a documented increase in bone mineral density (BMD) in the leg, but not the arm, compared with non-athletes, provide one example of mechanically induced adaptations in bone. Similarly, contralateral differences in arm BMD have been observed in volleyball, basketball, and tennis players but not in swimmers. [18, 19]

Other research has demonstrated that tendons and ligaments respond to exercise-induced stress with increases in cross-sectional area, stiffness, and tensile strength. [20-23]

## III. RELATIONSHIP BETWEEN PHYSICAL STRESS ACTED UPON THE TISSUE VS TISSUE STRENGTHENING.

Tissue strengthening is tissue adaptation, which falls under "**tissue adaptation in hypertrophy**"[48]. In order to make tissue strong, it has to undergo stress. As we mentioned, physical stress could cause three main tissue adaptations. Those are: 1. Tissue injury (Physical stress > Tissue strength). 2. Tissue maintenance (physical stress is just enough to maintain/homeostasis of tissue). 3. Increase in tissue strength (hypertrophy).

Therefore, without causing any injury to tissue, the required strength of tissue can be achieved with the knowledge of tissue adaptation to physical stress.

Stress levels that are higher than the maintenance (>55% of 1RM) ranges yet are lower than the threshold value for injury (< 70% of 1RM) can have positive effects on tissue adaptation. Musculoskeletal tissues subjected to levels of stress (55%-70% of 1RM) that are higher than normal become more tolerant to subsequent physical stresses and are more resistant to injury (i.e., tissues become stronger). This type of adaptation occurs when tissues can recover and adapt to previous bouts of physical stress. Steady increases in physical stress through progressive resistive exercise cause muscle fibres to hypertrophy and become capable of generating greater force. Likewise, higher-than-normal levels of physical stress can promote remodelling in bone.[15] Wolff's Law provides an excellent example of how one specific biological tissue, bone, responds to physical stress by remodelling. Wolff's Law states that the thickness, number, and orientation of trabeculae will correspond to the distribution of mechanical stresses on bone.[15] A consequence of stress-induced bone remodelling is that the strength of bone is greatest in the direction in which loads are most commonly imposed.[16] For example, the maximum stress tolerated by bone just before failure has been higher for compressive loads than for tensile or shear loads, reflecting the predominantly compressive loads experienced by bone during weight-bearing.[17] Runners have documented an increase in bone mineral density (BMD) in the leg, but not the arm, compared with non-athletes who provide one example of mechanically induced adaptations in bone.[51] Similarly, contralateral differences in arm BMD have been observed in volleyball, basketball, and tennis players but not in swimmers.[18,19]

# CHAPTER 2
## Progressive strengthening and fitness of desired tissue: Knee joint-specific

One should understand the in-depth meaning of tissue fitness, strength, and endurance to understand the principles of progressive strengthening and fitness. Recent research assessing tissue strength and endurance makes it possible to estimate the relative threshold value required to promote the desired tissue response for each circumstance. Following tissue strength and endurance assessment, rehabilitation programs can be tailored to enhance the factors contributing to tissue strengthening and repair and minimize factors contributing to tissue injury.

**Muscle strength** is a muscle's ability to contract with maximal force. It will become relative if compared to physical stress acted upon the muscle. When muscle strength is constant and physical stress acts upon the muscle increases, it can be seen that muscle strength becomes lesser relative to physical stress and vice versa. Suppose physical stress acted upon the tissue is constant, and the strength of the tissue gradually increases. In that case, it can be seen that tissue strength relatively becomes stronger than physical stress acting on it. Muscle strength describes how strong a muscle is or how much force it can exert. Physiotherapists often measure tissue strength by determining the maximum weight a person can lift at one time, i.e. **1 Repetition Maximum** [24, 25, 38]

**Muscle endurance**[24]- Tissue endurance is the ability of a tissue to contract repeatedly over an extended period. It describes how long one can sustain a given type of tissue exertion. By determining the maximum weight a person can lift 20 times consecutively, fitness professionals measure muscle endurance.

**Fitness** - The ability of one's Neuro-musculoskeletal system to perform daily and recreational activities without undue fatigue and injury.

**Graded resistance strengthening** - Controlled and progressively stressed the body's musculoskeletal system using resistance (i.e., weights, resistance bands, body-weight) exercise to build and maintain desired tissue fitness. Tissue fitness involves having adequate muscular strength and endurance.

Better tissue strength and endurance can be built through resistance exercises. Resistance training is also referred to as weight training or strength training and can be done with measured weights, body weight, or other resistance equipment (i.e., exercise bands or exercise balls). Resistance exercises stress the body's musculoskeletal system, enlarging muscle fibers and improving neural control of muscle function, resulting in greater muscle strength and endurance.

Resistance training offers varied benefits that physiotherapist recommends for nearly all musculoskeletal rehabilitation programs. Regular resistance training can make daily activities easier[54]-such; carrying around a backpack full of heavy textbooks will not tire as much; bringing in a bag of groceries will be less taxing, and taking the stairs will seem natural and feel better than riding in an elevator. No matter what health and fitness goals, resistance training can be an important and rewarding wellness tool throughout life[55].

Muscles, tendons, and ligaments require stimulation to contract. For a voluntary skeletal muscle to contract, the nervous system must send a signal directly to the muscle. When it is required to move any portion of the torso - for example, if one desires to strike a right-hand finger, the brain will send a sign down the spinal cord through the motor nerves to the skeletal muscle fibers of the finger. One motor nerve will stimulate many skeletal muscle fibers, creating a functional unit called a motor unit. Therefore, a motor unit is a motor nerve, and all the muscle fibers it controls[56].

The strength of a muscle contraction depends upon the intensity of the nervous system stimulus, the number and size of motor units activated, and the types of stimulated muscle fibers. A motor unit can be small or large, depending on the number of muscle fibers it stimulates[57]. Small motor units are comprised of slow-twitch fibers; large motor units are comprised of fast-twitch fibers.

For example, suppose a person is getting ready to lift a heavy weight. In that case, the central nervous system sends a stronger signal, activating a greater number of large, fast motor units, resulting in more forceful muscle contraction than merely picking up an apple. Strengthening the tissue benefits increased fitness level and specific physiological changes that have significant fitness and wellness benefits, which are listed in Table 1.

**Health Benefits of Resistance Training**[39]: Resistance training can effectively develop muscular strength, muscular endurance, and muscle mass in a broad range of people, including women and older adults. Older adults lose muscle mass and quality (less strength for the same muscle mass), a condition known as Sarcopenia. Resistance training can help slow down the loss of muscle mass[2]. Resistance training also enhances muscle strength, which protects joints and improves stability and balance, thus reducing the risk of falls. Resistance training can be a great tool to help older people prevent fractures from occurring due to falls. Regular resistance training will increase muscle, bone strength, and bone density, leading to strong bones and more protection against fall fractures. Resistance training programs designed for older adults, such as Stay Strong Stay Healthy (the University of Missouri, Extension), also support a better quality of life by promoting independence and maintaining functional abilities[62]. Research demonstrates that resistance training may decrease the risk of heart disease by lowering body fat, decreasing blood pressure, and improving cholesterol levels[63]. The American Heart Association recommends resistance training as a component of a comprehensive exercise program (not a replacement for aerobic exercise in a program) designed to help meet the health and fitness goals of people with and without heart disease[40].

TABLE 1. Physiological Changes from Resistance training

| Increased | Decreased |
| --- | --- |
| Muscle mass | |
| Muscular strength and/or Muscular endurance | Percentage of body fat |
| Bone mineral density | Time required for muscle contraction |
| Basal metabolic rate | Blood pressure (if high) |
| Intra-muscular fuel stores (ATP, Phosphocreatine, glycogen) | Blood cholesterol (if high) |
| Tendon, ligament, and joint strength | |
| Coordination of motor units | |
| Insulin sensitivity | |

Injury prevention tips are often specific to chosen activity[44] and the specific tissue under stress[45]. However, strong muscles, bones, and connective tissues are the common denominators for preventing injury in any activity. Regular resistance training improves muscular strength and endurance and the strength of tendons, ligaments, and other supporting structures around the joint. As the joint becomes stronger than stress, it is protected better from injury. A stronger body can handle the physical stresses of everyday life (carrying heavy books or groceries, lifting laundry baskets, moving furniture, etc.) with less chance of injury. A strong, pain-free back and proper posture are crucial to daily functioning without injury. Individuals who participate in regular strengthening exercises have stronger postural muscles and report less low back pain.

Men and women begin to lose muscle mass as they age. They lose up to one-third of their muscle mass due to changes in hormones, activity, nutrition and chronic or acute illnesses. Sarcopenia, literally "poverty of flesh", is the term applied to the age-related loss of skeletal muscle. Sarcopenia[46] reduces overall physical functioning by decreasing muscular strength and endurance, causing a loss in muscle power or the capacity to exert force rapidly. Regular resistance training helps maintain physical function with aging[43,51], starting between the ages of 25 and 30. While no one is immune from ageing, resistance training throughout life can significantly slow natural muscle loss. In fact, an older individual who does progressive strengthening shows a rate of improvement equal to younger people. An increase in Neuro-musculoskeletal system fitness and the improvements it brings to everyday physical functioning help individuals live independently for a longer period of time[46, 47].

**Assessment of Muscular Strength and Endurance:**

Before planning an appropriate progressive strengthening program, assessing current Muscle strength and endurance is important. Furthermore, compare the results with the norm table provided in this chapter for age and gender or use it as a starting point for designing a program. After following the program for a few weeks, follow-up assessments will help evaluate the progress and make adjustments to stay on track.

**Test for Muscle strength:** Tests of Muscle strength gauge the maximum amount of force generated in a muscle.

**TEST: One RM**[24,41] test is the most common tool fitness instructors and physiotherapists use to assess their patients' muscular/tissue strength. To participate in the tests safely, patients should have detailed instructions for the test procedure, know general weight-training guidelines, and have qualified physiotherapists standing nearby to watch and assist if necessary. **One RM** test is performed by discovering the maximum amount of weight a patient can lift one time on a particular exercise. To accurately determine 1RM within three to five trials, muscle fatigue from repetitions does not change the result.

In general health and fitness classes or at the beginning of weight-training programs, physiotherapists often tell patients to predict their 1RM instead of attempting a maximum lift. This is particularly true when patients are new to resistance training and are unfamiliar with weight-training guidelines.

The next step is determining 1RM of knee tissue through a particular exercise targeting specific tissue. To predict 1RM, the patient will lift, press, or pull a weight that fully fatigues his upper- or lower-body muscles in 2 to 10 repetitions. Use a formula that converts the actual weight lifted and the real number of repetitions to predict 1 RM (refer to tables 5 & 6). Tables 2 and 4, Flowchart can be used to design knee tissue fitness program. Targeted knee tissues to be strengthened mainly are quadriceps, hamstrings, and other surrounding soft tissue like tendons and ligaments. As targeted knee tissues are mainly the quadriceps and hamstrings, the exercise selected will be squatting down and raising. In the same way, patients can perform these tests for any weight-training exercise and then convert them to the predicted **1RM** value of the targeted tissue. Many weight-training programs use a percentage (55% to 75%) of **1RM**[47] to determine a safe starting level for progressive strengthening programmes [49-50].

In this context, the maximum threshold level can be defined as the maximum tissue strength, which can take the maximum stress without injury or is nearly equal to **1 RM**. (Refer to TABLE 3, Graph 4, and ACSM's Resistance-Training Guidelines for starting a safe percentage of 1RM for tissue strength and endurance). A maintenance level is a level which falls around 55% of 1RM, which is the lower line of the progressive strengthening range represented in graph 4.

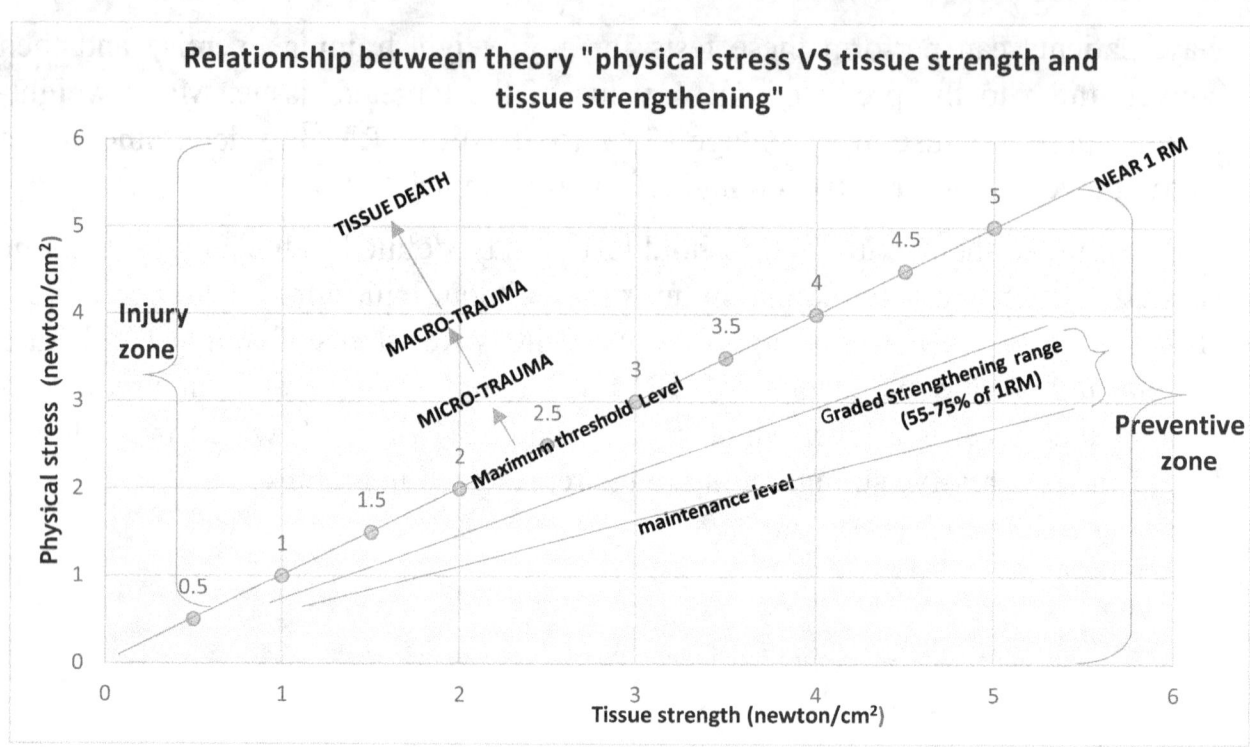

Graph 4: Maximum threshold level is nearly equal to 1RM. Safe resistance/stress for Strengthening is 55-75% of 1RM. That is, resistance should not be lower than or higher than the range 55-75% of 1RM. Minimum stress of around 55% of 1RM is needed to maintain the tissue maintenance level. Tissue needs bouts of rest and time for adaptation to accommodate resistance and increase its threshold/strength.

**Test for muscular endurance:** Muscular endurance tests evaluate a muscle's ability to contract for an extended period. Some tests must be performed in a weight room, whereas others require only body weight for resistance and can be performed anywhere.

**20RM Tests** - Any weight-training exercises can be used to find 20 repetitions maximum (20 RM). The test determines the maximal amount of weight the body can lift exactly 20 times in a row before the muscle becomes too fatigued to continue.

20RM tests are particularly useful for setting tissue endurance goals and tracking progress. Try to discover 20RM within 1-3 trials to avoid tissue fatigue and alteration in results. (Table 8)

**Calisthenic Tests:** Calisthenics is a conditioning exercise that uses body weight for resistance. Calisthenic tests use sit-ups, curl-ups, pull-ups, pushups, and flexed arm support/hang exercises to assess muscular endurance.

## Relationship between tissue strength and endurance in strengthening: Strength VS Endurance Exercises

Endurance training comes in two forms. Strength training targets tissue/muscles to improve mobility strength by potentially yielding visible muscle development. i. Tissue/ Muscular endurance helps muscles sustain their activity over a long period of time, ii. Cardiovascular endurance measures the ability to keep working when the heart is racing, and breathing is elevated.

Few repetitions with higher resistance will produce an increase in **Muscle Strength**. More repetitions with lower resistance will produce an increase in **Muscle Endurance**. The strength and endurance continuum reflects an overlap between the two kinds of development. **(Refer to Graph 5)**

**According to the requirement of ADL-Activity of** daily life, we can choose strength and/or endurance training.

There can not be a perfect exercise focusing on one fitness area at the expense of another that will not favour health. Strength and endurance training are needed for the physical condition to be at its peak. Incorporating strength and endurance into a workout routine requires no special skill or equipment.

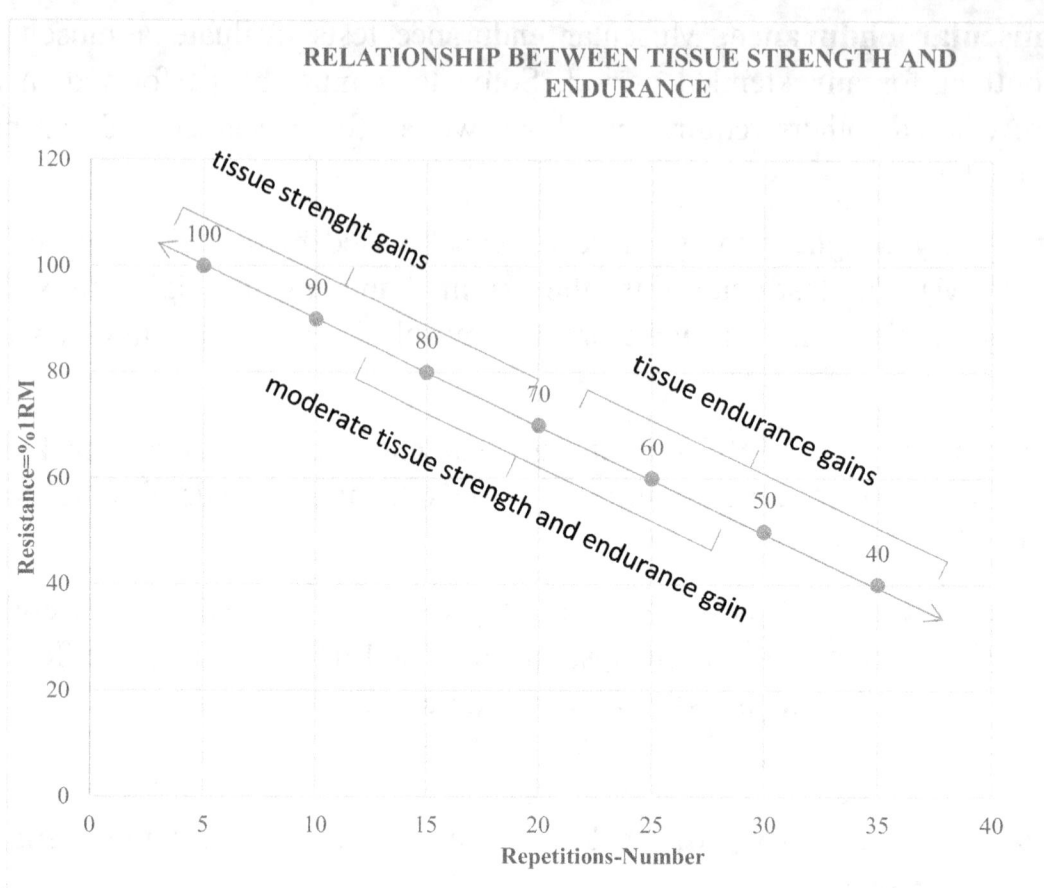

Graph 5: Few repetitions with higher resistance will produce gains in **Muscle Strength**. More repetitions with lower resistance will increase **Muscle Endurance**. The strength and endurance continuum overlaps the two kinds of development.

**Design a progressive strengthening program:** Designing an effective resistance-training program requires knowledge about the relationship between physical stress versus tissue strength, adaptation, and strengthening. Based on this theory, we can plan a safe and effective tissue fitness program. The following are the three important steps for designing an effective strengthening program.

**1. Set appropriate tissue functional fitness goals:** Include some specific goals for improving tissue function in a fitness plan. Function-based goals focus on tissue capabilities, including gaining better tissue strength, greater tissue endurance, or both. Setting knee tissue fitness goals (table 9) will guide setting goals for realistic changes in muscle function and then help assess improvements.

**2. Explore equipment options**: A progressive strengthening program is used to decide whether to go with weight machines, equipment or no equipment. This is an important decision, and it depends on the fitness goals, type of equipment available, experience with weight-training exercises, and preferences.

**MACHINES -** If there is no experience with resistance training, weight machines can be very useful; systems such as Cybex, Nautilus, Life Fitness, and many others allow isolating and strengthening specific muscle groups to train without a spotting partner. Exercise physiotherapists consider free-weight exercises a more advanced approach to weight training than machine-weight exercises[59]. Free-weight exercises use dumbbells, barbells- benches [incline, flat, or decline], squat hack and related equipment. Free-weight exercises allow the body to move through its natural range of motion instead of the path predetermined by a weight machine. Both require and promote the development of more muscle control. Some athletes prefer free-weight exercises because the balance and movement patterns needed to lift free weights successfully are closer to their sport/activity, such as tossing a football, putting a shot, or doing the breaststroke. As workout facilities often have both free weights and weight machines, many people start their resistance-training program exclusively with machine-weight exercises and then progress to free weights within the first few months.

**Alternate Equipment** –Resistance can be increased with equipment other than machines or free weights. Resistance bands made of tubing or flat strips of rubber simultaneously increase resistance throughout the range of motion and improve muscular endurance. Different exercises can be performed with resistance bands, and they are easy to fold up and pack perfectly in a suitcase or gym bag for a portable workout. Stability balls (also called Swiss, fitness, or exercise balls) are

18–30 inch diameter [vinyl balls that] have various uses for muscular fitness, endurance, and balance. Ball routines involve performing exercises while sitting, lying, and/or balancing on the ball. The ball exerciser must use core trunk muscles to counteract the natural instability of the ball, which enhances overall body function. People sometimes use heavy-weight balls called medicine balls to increase resistance, individually, with a partner, or in a group. A Medicine ball can be held during calisthenic or free-weight exercises or pass a ball from partner to partner for a functional increase in muscle endurance.

**No-Equipment Training-** Calisthenics such as push-ups, pull-ups, lunges, squats, leg lifts, and clips do not involve equipment. Instead, they use body weight to provide resistance, like resistance bands, perfect for maintaining muscular strength and endurance while travelling.

**3. Learn and apply the FITT principle[58]- FITT** stands for frequency, intensity, time, and type. The acronym represents a checklist for determining how often, how hard, and how long to exercise, and what types of exercise to choose at the current level of muscular fitness. (Refer to tables 3 and 7.)

**Frequency of Training**: The training frequency to reach the goal and the schedule will determine how often the training will be each week. At a minimum, each muscle group should be worked twice per week if the workout involves the whole [upper limb, lower limb, etc.]; it requires two sessions in the gym each week. If the muscle workouts are split (for example, in the upper / lower limb), four times per week is required. Table 3 represents the American College of Sports Medicine (ACSM) guidelines for muscle strength and endurance programs. Let each muscle group rest for 48 hours before taxing it again with resistance training[52]. Therefore, schedule workouts to have at least two days' break when it is just beginning. Microdamage occurs within the muscle cells when performing an intense weight-training session, and rest time is needed for muscle repair and adaptation. Muscles will adapt by constructing new actin and myosin contractile proteins and other supporting structures. Over time, this adaptation results in stronger, leaner, larger muscles. Intense workouts of the same muscle group on subsequent days will disrupt the repair and adaptation process. Rather than faster muscle development, overtraining is more likely to cause injuries, muscle fatigue, and weakening. An exception can be made for lower-intensity muscular fitness classes or callisthenics, which can be done daily as long as they are not fatigued. Muscle soreness that sets within a day or two is called delayed onset Muscle Soreness (DOMS) and is a sign that the body is not ready for the amount of overload applied. Contrary to popular belief, it is not lactic acid that causes DOMS; accumulated lactic acid is cleared from the muscle cells within hours of exercise[52]. If weight amounts are selected correctly, the muscles will sustain small amounts of microdamage and will not result in soreness, and the body can repair itself within 48 hours after the workout.

**The intensity of Training** -The intensity of a weight-training program refers to the amount of resistance applied through any given exercise. Resistance here means the weight that one is moving. For each exercise, the intensity will depend on one's fitness goals for that particular muscle group or one's body as a whole. The ACSM guidelines in Table 3 for muscle strength and endurance can help you choose weight-training intensities (shown as a percentage of your 1RM).

The choice of each exercise should be enough to overload the muscle group working. (One should feel slight discomfort or muscle fatigue at the end of the exercise set). If fatigue is not felt during the entire set of repetitions and feels like lifting the weight another 3 to 10 times is feasible, then the intensity is too low. If the intensity selected is correct for building muscular strength, it will be almost completely fatigued by each set of repetitions. The correct intensity for building muscle endurance will leave the muscle group fatigued but not the maximal exhaustion as with strength building. Resting between sets will affect weight training intensity and performance on subsequent exercises. The greater the weight lifted for strength building, the longer the rest period is needed between sets. Resting periods should be shorter for muscular endurance-building exercises. In fact, shorter rest will help build better muscular endurance. (Table 3 Provides guidelines for determining appropriate rest periods between sets.)

**Time (Sets[53] and Repetitions)**: Choosing the appropriate number of repetitions or lifts within each set is another essential part of setting up a resistance-training program. Once again, fitness goals help determine the number of sets and repetitions to execute for each exercise. Weight-training experience and the time available to work out will also affect the planning. ACSM recommends performing one set of each exercise during a given workout session (See Tables 3 and 7). If there is no experience in resistance training, progress can be observed with just one set per muscle group. Although additional benefits are gained from extra sets, two sets will not translate into double the benefits of one. If there is a lack of time, one is sufficient. As the resistance-training program progresses, increase the sets from one to two, eventually to three or more. Evidence suggests that three sets will produce twice the strength gains of one set.[53] patients can execute one, two, or three sets of all exercises or perform one set of specific exercises, two of others, and so on. Remember, overtraining one particular muscle group can lead to muscle imbalance and injury. If the muscular fitness goals include improvement in muscular strength and endurance, choose a number of sets and repetitions that fall between the ACSM recommendations for strength and endurance (Table 3). Intensity and repetitions have an inverse relationship relative to muscular strength and endurance (refer to graph 5); for muscular strength development - lift heavy weights with few repetitions. For muscular endurance - lift lighter weights with more repetitions. A good starting point for a balanced strength/endurance program is 1-2 sets of 10 repetitions per exercise. (Table 2- Outlines sample resistance-training programs for the knee.)

**Type:** Choosing Appropriate Exercises plays an important role. (Which exercises should be started during each session?) The final part of designing a muscular fitness program is deciding on appropriate exercises, remembering to work toward muscle balance within all major muscle groups, creating one's own muscular fitness goals, as shown in Table 9 and using Table 3 to start planning resistance-training program. The next step is deciding which exercises will help attain muscular fitness goals. As this book focuses on the knee, the targeted tissue will be the quadriceps, hamstrings, and other soft tissues like tendons and ligaments surrounding the knee. Therefore, the best exercise for progressive strengthening would be squatting down and standing. For a starting program, choose between 1 or 2 exercises, remembering that each additional exercise will increase the time of the exercise session; too many exercises may lead to splitting the workout into alternating selections of exercises on different days. In choosing exercises, the client may select weight machines, free weights, callisthenics, or a combination of all three. Most weight training programs will include all three depending on the available equipment.

## Table 2: Flowchart to design knee tissue fitness program:

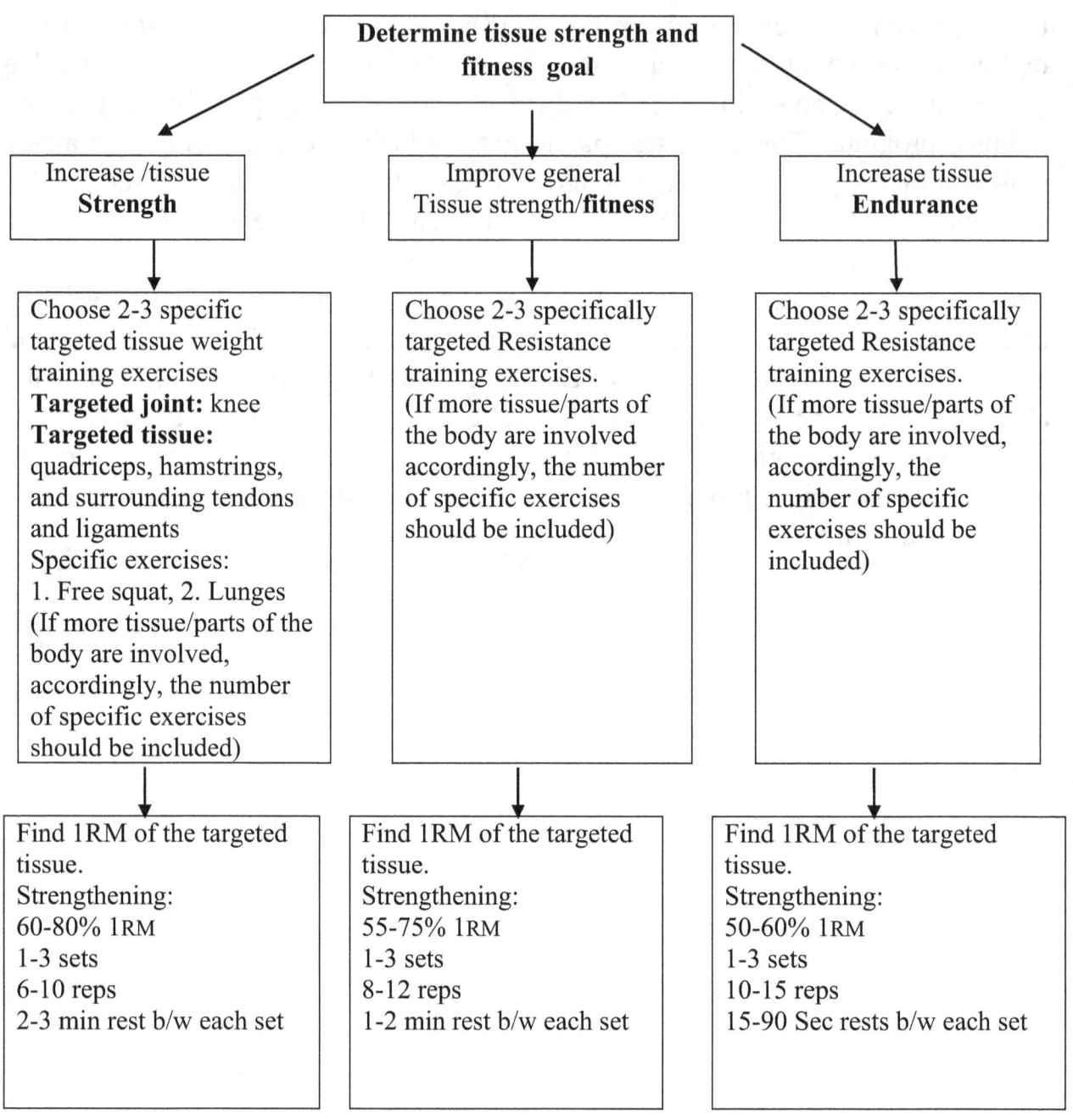

TABLE 3: ACSM'S Resistance training guidelines for tissue Strength and Endurance.

## Recommendations for the General Adult Population

| Frequency (days/week) | 2–3 |
|---|---|
| Intensity (how hard) | Lift to fatigue |
| Time (sets/reps) | 1 set; 3–20 repetitions |
| Type (exercises) | Machines, free weights, and/or callisthenics; 2-3 exercises for the targeted tissue. |

## Strength, Endurance and Progression Guidelines for Healthy Adults

| Muscular Strength | Frequency | Intensity | Time (sets/reps) (1–3 min rest between sets) |
|---|---|---|---|
| Novice | 2–3 days/week | 60%–70% 1 RM | 1–3 sets, 8–12 reps |
| Intermediate | 2–4 days/week | 70%–80% 1 RM | Multiple sets, 6–12 reps |
| Advanced | 4–6 days/week | 80%–100% 1 RM | Multiple sets, 1–12 reps |

| Muscular Endurance | Frequency | Intensity | Time (sets/reps) (30 Sec–2 min rest between sets) |
|---|---|---|---|
| Novice | 2–3 days/week | 50%–70% 1 RM | 1–3 sets, 10–15 reps |
| Intermediate | 2–4 days/week | 50%–70% 1 RM | Multiple sets, 10–15+reps |
| Advanced | 4–6 days/week | 30%–80% 1 RM | Multiple sets, 10–25+reps |

Sources: American College of Sports Medicine(ACSM), Guidelines for Exercise Testing and Prescription, the 7th Edition. Baltimore, MD: Lippincott Williams & Wilkins, 2006; Kraemer W. J., Adams K., Cafarelli E., et al. "Writing Group for the ACSM Position Stand. Progression Models in Resistance Training for Healthy Adults," Medicine and Science in Sports and Exercise 34, no. 2 (2002): 364–380.

**TABLE 4: Sample Designs for Knee Tissue Strengthening Program, including sections I and II.**

As the book deals mainly with the knee joint and its exercises to develop knee strength and endurance without injury, this will be an example for designing any other targeted tissue in the body. As it is known, if strengthening and endurance exercises are not done scientifically, applying theory - "physical stress on the tissue VS tissue strength as well as the principles of tissue adaptation in strengthening", tissue may become prone to injury.

The first step in strengthening is to note the targeted tissue/joint and choose a specific exercise. Therefore, the targeted tissue that needs to be strengthened here is the knee joint, so one should choose specific knee exercises that will strengthen the knee joint. Finally, a strengthening protocol needs to be followed.

Choosing appropriate tissue for knee strengthening, i.e., major muscle/tissue groups that have to be worked on are the quadriceps, hamstrings, and associated ligaments and tendons of the knee joint. The second step is choosing the appropriate targeted tissue to be strengthened in the form of exercise. The strength of squat exercise is assessed; in a way, the strength of the targeted muscles is assessed. Hence, the targeted knee tissue strengthening in the form of exercise is squatting down and rising. Therefore, increase the 1RM of the squat to strengthen the targeted knee tissue as required.

**Assessing knee tissue strength and tissue endurance through "squat" exercise**

Name: _____ Date: _____
Physiotherapist/Instructor: _____

**Purpose:** To assess the present strength and endurance of knee tissue through the squat exercise.

**Directions:** Complete Sections I–II according to the physiotherapist's direction. If you are completing this with weights, you must have proper supervision. You can complete calisthenic assessments safely if you follow the procedures carefully.

## Section I: Knee tissue strength assessment:

### One Repetition Maximum (1RM) Prediction Assessment of squat

The "gold standard" for measuring muscular strength is using a one-repetition maximum (1RM) to determine the maximum amount of weight you can lift once. Table 5 will estimate 1RM for the squats; by finding the weight, you can maximally lift 2 to 10 times.

**1. Warm-up.** Complete 3 to 10 minutes of light cardio-respiratory activity to warm the tissue. Perform range-of-motion exercises and light stretches for the joints and muscles to be used.
- Targeted tissue: Quadriceps, hamstrings, tendons, and ligaments of the knee
- Targeted exercise: squatting down and standing
- Cardiorespiratory activity: spot jogging for 2 min
- Knee range of motion exercises: knee flexion and extension exercises, sitting for 1 minute and lying supine 1 minute.
- Knee tissue stretching: a. Quadriceps, b. Calf, c. Hamstrings. Stretch for 30 Sec and repeat 2-3 times.

**2. Important knee exercises are: (a) Free weight squats**
                                      **(b) Machine squats,**
                                       **(c) Lunges**

**(a) Free weight squat**[42,51]

**Muscles targeted** - quadriceps, hamstrings, other soft tissues like tendons and ligaments of the knee.

i. As shown in Figures 1 and 2 below, stand with feet placed shoulder-width apart, toes pointed out slightly, and hands-on-hips or across the chest, head neutral, and back straight. Centre your weight over your arches or slightly behind.

ii. Squat down, keeping weight centred over the arches and actively flexing (bending) hips until your legs break parallel. During the movement, the back should be straight, shoulders back, and chest out, and let your thighs part to the Side so that you are "squatting between your legs."

iii. Push back up to the starting position, hinging at the hips and not with the spine, maximizing the use of the rear hip and thigh muscles, and maintaining a straight back and neutral head position.

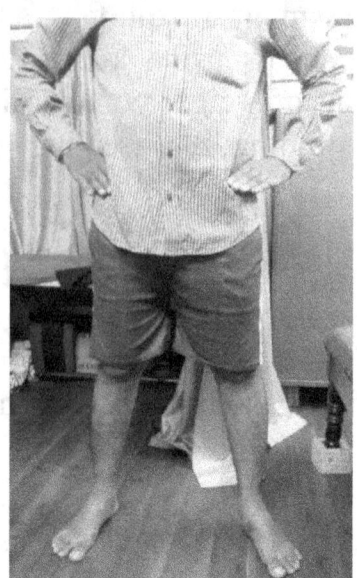
Figure 1: Starting position for squatting

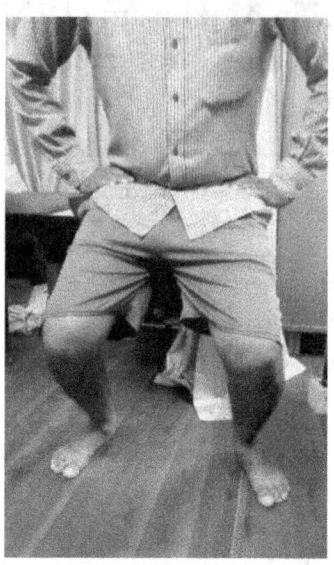
Figure 2: Knee flexed position of squatting

**(b) Hack squats:** The figure below shows the squats performed on an inclined platform (hack squat machine) using weights; this allows controlled movements to build the lower body while reducing the risk of damaging or injuring the knee.

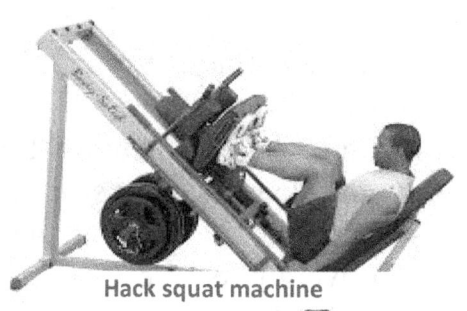
Hack squat machine

**(c) Lunges:** Muscles targeted - quadriceps, hamstrings, and surrounding tendons and ligaments of the knee. Figures 3 and 4 show that they stand with feet shoulder-width apart. Step forward and transfer weight to the forward leg. Lower the body straight down with weight evenly distributed between the front and back legs. Keep the front knee in line with the ankle by striding out far enough. Return to the starting stance and repeat with the other leg.

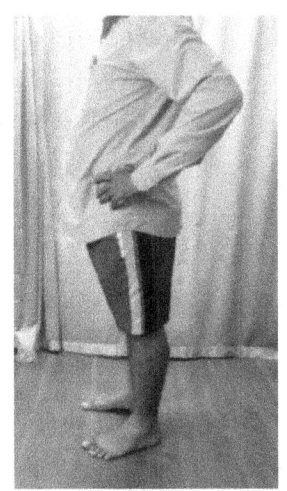

Figure 3: Starting position for lunges

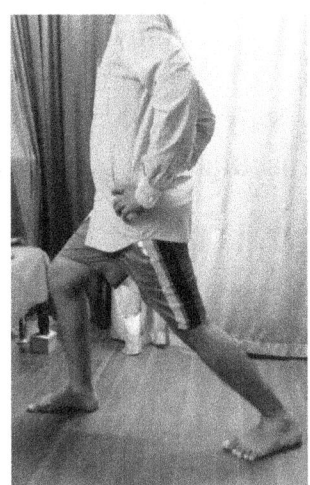

Figure 4: Standing to one leg step forward

**3. Find the appropriate strength assessment weight and the number of repetitions.** Set a weight that can be lifted at least 2 times but not more than 10 times. Perform the lift as many times as possible (to complete fatigue) up to 10 repetitions. If lifting more than 10 repetitions is possible, try using heavier weights that are difficult to lift more than 2 -10 times. To prevent muscle fatigue from altering the results, attempt the assessment not more than 3 times to find the proper weight and number of repetitions. Suppose the level of muscle fatigue is reached; rest and perform the test again the next day by recording the results.

**4. Find predicted 1RM.** Predict 1RM based on the number of repetitions performed. If the weight lifted was between 20 and 250 pounds, use the 1RM Prediction Table 5 to find your predicted 1RM. If the weight is lifted over (with repetitions) 250 pounds, use the Multiplication Factor Table 6 to find the predicted 1RM.

**Muscular Strength Results:**
**Squat:** Weight lifted _____ Repetitions _____

Weight lifted (lb)            Multiplication factor*            Predicted 1 RM (lb)

\-\-\-\-\-\-\-\-\-\-\-\-\-\-\-\-\-\-\-\-\-\-\-\-\-\-× \-\-\-\-\-\-\-\-\-\-\-\-\-\-\-\-\-\-\-\-\-\-\-\-\-\-\-\-   =   \-\-\-\-\-\-\-\-\-\-\-\-\-\-\-\-\-\-\-\-\-\-\-\-\-\-\-\-

*Multiplication factor from the Multiplication Factor Table 6.

Section II: Muscular endurance assessment: Squat with weight

**Twenty Repetition Maximum (20RM) Assessments**

The 20RM assessment is a weight-lifting assessment of muscular endurance. You can measure your improvement by performing the assessments before and after completing 8 to 12 weeks of muscular fitness exercises. This assessment will help to plan a muscular fitness program.

**1. Prepare for the muscle endurance assessments.** Check if the muscular strength assessment is completed and if the warm-up is already done. If not, perform a warm-up similar to the one described in Section I.

**2. Find your 20RM for squatting** by setting a weight that can be lifted a maximum of 20 times. Perform the lifting, increase or decrease the weight and try again until you find your 20RM. In order to make sure that muscle fatigue does not alter your results, try to find your 20 RM within three tries. If it takes longer, rest and perform the test again the next day. Record your results on the next page.

Muscular Endurance Weight Lifting Results
Squat: 20RM, weight lifted _____

**The Free Weight Squat[42] Endurance Test**

Instructions: as shown in figure 5 and 6

1. Stand with feet placed shoulder-width apart, toes pointed out slightly, and hands on hips or across your chest, head neutral, and back straight. Centre your weight over your arches or slightly behind.

2. Squat down, keeping weight-centred overarches until thighs are parallel with the floor. Push back up to the starting position, maintaining a straight back and neutral head position.

3. Perform as many squats as you can without stopping.
   Number of squats: _____

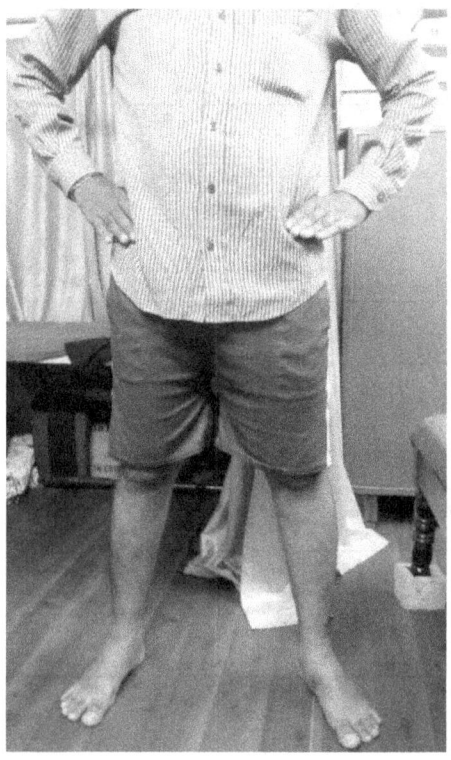

Figure 5: Standing, starting position of the squat.

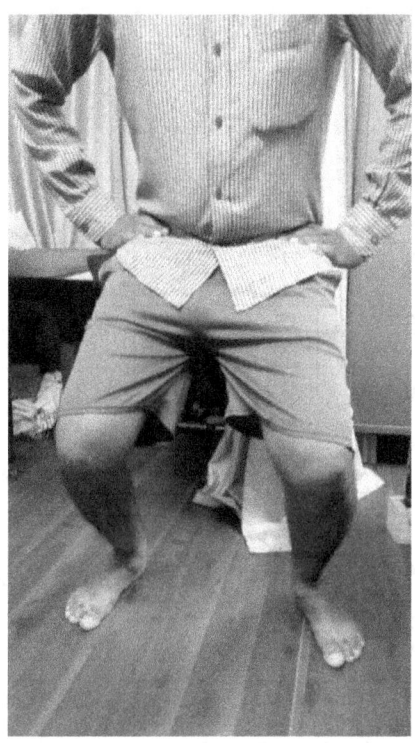

Figure 6: Squatting down.

**Rating free Squat Endurance Test Result:**

The total score is the number of completed squats. Refer to the appropriate portion of Table 8 for a rating of leg muscular endurance. Record the rating below and in summary at the end of Table 8.

Rating: _____

**TABLE 5: 1RM Prediction: Showing weight lifted and the number of repetitions performed till fatigue**

| Wt lb | REPETITIONS | | | | | | | | | |
|---|---|---|---|---|---|---|---|---|---|---|
| | 1 | 2 | 3 | 4 | 5 | 6 | 7 | 8 | 9 | 10 |
| 20 | 20 | 21 | 21 | 22 | 23 | 23 | 24 | 25 | 26 | 27 |
| 25 | 25 | 26 | 26 | 27 | 28 | 29 | 30 | 31 | 32 | 33 |
| 30 | 30 | 31 | 32 | 33 | 34 | 35 | 36 | 37 | 39 | 40 |
| 35 | 35 | 36 | 37 | 38 | 39 | 41 | 42 | 43 | 45 | 47 |
| 40 | 40 | 41 | 42 | 44 | 45 | 46 | 48 | 50 | 51 | 53 |
| 45 | 45 | 46 | 48 | 49 | 51 | 52 | 54 | 56 | 58 | 60 |
| 50 | 50 | 51 | 53 | 55 | 56 | 58 | 60 | 62 | 64 | 67 |
| 55 | 55 | 57 | 58 | 60 | 62 | 64 | 66 | 68 | 71 | 73 |
| 60 | 60 | 62 | 64 | 65 | 68 | 70 | 72 | 74 | 77 | 80 |
| 65 | 65 | 67 | 69 | 71 | 73 | 75 | 78 | 81 | 84 | 87 |
| 70 | 70 | 72 | 74 | 76 | 79 | 81 | 84 | 87 | 90 | 93 |
| 75 | 75 | 77 | 79 | 82 | 84 | 87 | 90 | 93 | 96 | 100 |
| 80 | 80 | 82 | 85 | 87 | 90 | 93 | 96 | 99 | 103 | 107 |
| 85 | 85 | 87 | 90 | 93 | 96 | 99 | 102 | 106 | 109 | 113 |
| 90 | 90 | 90 | 93 | 95 | 98 | 101 | 108 | 112 | 116 | 120 |
| 95 | 95 | 98 | 101 | 104 | 107 | 110 | 114 | 118 | 122 | 127 |
| 100 | 100 | 103 | 106 | 109 | 113 | 116 | 120 | 124 | 129 | 133 |
| 105 | 105 | 108 | 111 | 115 | 118 | 122 | 126 | 130 | 135 | 140 |
| 110 | 110 | 113 | 116 | 120 | 124 | 128 | 132 | 137 | 141 | 147 |
| 115 | 115 | 118 | 122 | 125 | 129 | 134 | 138 | 143 | 148 | 153 |
| 120 | 120 | 123 | 127 | 131 | 135 | 139 | 144 | 149 | 154 | 160 |
| 125 | 125 | 129 | 132 | 136 | 141 | 145 | 150 | 155 | 161 | 167 |
| 130 | 130 | 134 | 138 | 142 | 146 | 151 | 156 | 161 | 167 | 173 |

| | | | | | | | | | |
|---|---|---|---|---|---|---|---|---|---|
| **135** | 135 | 139 | 143 | 147 | 152 | 157 | 162 | 168 | 174 | 180 |
| **140** | 140 | 144 | 148 | 153 | 158 | 163 | 168 | 174 | 180 | 187 |
| **145** | 145 | 149 | 154 | 158 | 163 | 168 | 174 | 180 | 186 | 193 |
| **150** | 150 | 154 | 159 | 164 | 169 | 174 | 180 | 186 | 193 | 200 |
| **155** | 155 | 159 | 164 | 169 | 174 | 180 | 186 | 192 | 199 | 207 |
| **160** | 160 | 165 | 169 | 180 | 175 | 186 | 192 | 199 | 206 | 213 |
| **165** | 165 | 170 | 175 | 180 | 186 | 192 | 198 | 205 | 212 | 220 |
| **170** | 170 | 175 | 180 | 185 | 191 | 197 | 204 | 211 | 219 | 227 |
| **175** | 175 | 180 | 185 | 191 | 197 | 203 | 210 | 217 | 225 | 233 |
| **180** | 180 | 185 | 191 | 196 | 203 | 209 | 216 | 223 | 231 | 240 |
| **185** | 185 | 190 | 196 | 202 | 208 | 215 | 222 | 230 | 238 | 247 |
| **190** | 190 | 195 | 201 | 207 | 214 | 221 | 228 | 236 | 244 | 253 |
| **195** | 195 | 201 | 206 | 213 | 219 | 226 | 234 | 242 | 251 | 260 |
| **200** | 200 | 206 | 212 | 218 | 225 | 232 | 240 | 248 | 257 | 267 |
| **205** | 205 | 211 | 217 | 224 | 231 | 238 | 246 | 255 | 264 | 273 |
| **210** | 210 | 216 | 222 | 229 | 236 | 244 | 252 | 261 | 270 | 280 |
| **215** | 215 | 221 | 228 | 235 | 242 | 250 | 258 | 267 | 276 | 287 |
| **220** | 220 | 226 | 233 | 240 | 248 | 256 | 264 | 273 | 283 | 293 |
| **225** | 225 | 231 | 238 | 245 | 253 | 261 | 270 | 279 | 289 | 300 |
| **230** | 230 | 237 | 244 | 251 | 259 | 267 | 276 | 286 | 296 | 307 |
| **235** | 235 | 242 | 249 | 256 | 264 | 273 | 282 | 292 | 302 | 313 |
| **240** | 240 | 247 | 254 | 262 | 270 | 279 | 288 | 298 | 309 | 320 |
| **245** | 245 | 252 | 259 | 267 | 276 | 285 | 294 | 304 | 315 | 327 |
| **250** | 250 | 257 | 265 | 273 | 281 | 290 | 300 | 310 | 322 | 333 |

**TABLE 6: Multiplication factor table for predicting 1RM:**

| Repetitions | 1 | 2 | 3 | 4 | 5 | 6 | 7 | 8 | 9 | 10 |
|---|---|---|---|---|---|---|---|---|---|---|
| Multiplication Factor | 1.0 | 1.07 | 1.11 | 1.13 | 1.16 | 1.20 | 1.23 | 1.27 | 1.32 | 1.36 |

Table and multiplication factors generated using the Bryzcki equation: **1 RM = weight (kg) / [1.0278-(0.0278 ×repetitions)].**

*Source:* Adapted from Bryzcki, M. "Strength Testing: Predicting a One-Rep Max from a Reps-to-Fatigue," *J Phys EducRecreation Dance* 64 (1993): 88–90.

**TABLE 7: Workout plan design with FIIT principle under the guidelines of ACSM's Resistance-Training Guidelines for tissue Strength and Endurance (Table 3)**

| Frequency | Intensity | Time | Exercises for knee |
|---|---|---|---|
| Beginner: 2 days/week | 55%–65% 1RM | 1 set, 10 reps (1–2 min rest) | 1. Squat, 2. Lunges |
| Intermediate: 4 days/week | 70%–80% 1RM2 | 3 sets, 5–12 reps (2–3 min rest) | 1. Squat, 2. Lunges |

The above program is designed for healthy individuals with normal knees who want to increase their fitness level according to daily activity. Therefore, it is useful in the prevention of injury/dysfunction.

**Note:** an individual who had injury/dysfunction of any part of the body, e.g., knee (as the book is specifically for the knee joint), requires assessment and treatment, which is mentioned in chapters 9, 11 &12. Simultaneously, according to the patient's recovery, gradual fitness of desired tissue can be achieved with progressive strengthening. In these cases, progressive strengthening depends on phases of injury: acute, sub-acute, and chronic, as it is known. The acute injury requires rest, icing, immobilization, electrotherapy (to reduce inflammation), and anti-inflammatory drugs. Sub-acute phase strengthening can be progressed from isometrics and passive movements to active assisted to active. The chronic phase additionally requires active resistance to resistance movements.

## TABLE 8: Ratings of the Squat Endurance Test

Number of Squats Performed

| Men | Very Poor | Poor | Below Average | Average | Above Average | Good | Excellent |
|---|---|---|---|---|---|---|---|
| Age: 18–25, | ‹25 | 25–30 | 31–34 | 35–38 | 39–43 | 44–49 | ›49 |
| 26–35, | ‹22 | 22–28 | 29–30 | 31–34 | 35–39 | 40–45 | ›45 |
| 36–45, | ‹17 | 17–22 | 23–26 | 27–29 | 30–34 | 35–41 | ›41 |
| 46–55, | ‹9 | 13–17 | 18–21 | 22–24 | 25–38 | 29–35 | ›35 |
| 56–65, | ‹9 | 9–12 | 13–16 | 17–20 | 21–24 | 25–31 | ›31 |
| 65 +, | ‹7 | 7–10 | 11–14 | 15–18 | 19–21 | 22–28 | ›28 |
| **Women** | Very Poor | Poor | Below Average | Average | Above Average | Good | Excellent |
| Age: 18–25, | ‹18 | 18–24 | 25–28 | 29–32 | 33–36 | 37-43 | ›43 |
| 26–35, | ‹20 | 13–20 | 21–24 | 25–28 | 29–31 | 33–39 | ›39 |
| 36–45, | ‹7 | 7–14 | 15–18 | 19–22 | 23–26. | 27–33 | ›33 |
| 46–55, | ‹5 | 5–9 | 10–13 | 14–17 | 18–21 | 22–27 | ›27 |
| 56–65, | ‹3 | 3–6 | 7–9 | 10–12 | 13–17. | 18–24 | ›24 |
| 65 +, | ‹2 | 2–4 | 5–10 | 11–13 | 14–16. | 17-23 | ›23 |

SOURCE: www.topendsports.com/testing/tests/home-squat.htm

Summary of Results:
Squat endurance test: Number of squats: _____,
Rating: _____

**Note:** Muscular endurance is specific. Rating may vary considerably with different parts of the body. Rating of the targeted tissue strength and endurance may not be accurate, as every person's lifestyle or daily ADL activity varies over time. Therefore, the amount of stress on targeted tissue also varies occasionally. Indicating physical stress becomes relative to tissue strength. Based on the relative nature of the physical stress, strength and endurance of the tissue should be targeted. At the end of the progressive strengthening program, targeted tissue strength and endurance should always be greater than the relative physical stress acted upon it.

**TABLE 9: Setting knee tissue fitness goals:**

Name: _____ Date: _____
Physiotherapist: _____ Section: _____

**Materials:** Results from tissue fitness assessments, calculator, etc.

**Purpose:** To learn how to set appropriate tissue fitness goals (short- and long-term). One should critically evaluate the obstacles, overcome them, and the resources needed to reach the goals successfully.

**Directions:** Write out your personal goals and reflections in the following sections.

**Short and long-term goals**

**(i) Short-term Goals (3–6 months)**

1. Muscular Strength Goal: _____

    Target Date: _____

2. Muscular Endurance goal: _____

    Target Date: _____

3. Functional task/ADL achieved with ease: e.g. targeted progressive strengthening would be squatting down and standing 50 times/day at a stretch in order to achieve the functional task of jogging 5 km /day at a stretch without causing knee injury.

**(ii) Long-term Goals (12months)**

1. Muscular Strength Goal: _____

    Target Date: _____

2. Muscular Endurance Goal: _____

    Target Date: _____

3. Functional task/ADL achieved with ease: e.g., targeted progressive strengthening would be squatting down and standing 100 times/day at a stretch to achieve the functional task of jogging 10 km /day at a stretch without causing knee injury.

According to recent scientific studies, the Knee is stressed in ascending order following daily life activities (ADL).

Standing < walking < stairs -ascending < stairs-descending < squatting-rise < squatting-down.[13-14]

After assessing the present strength and endurance by predicting 1RM, it can be correlated to the functional capacity of ADL (Activities of daily life). E.g., the present functional capacity of squatting down and rising is 10 repetitions. Furthermore, suppose the targeted squatting down and rising activity of daily life needs to be 20 repetitions. The strength can be increased with progressive strengthening (%55 – 75 of 1RM); at a point where the strength of knee tissue is 1RM, it will be sufficient for 20 repetitions of squatting down and rising in a day; this point is the goal is accomplished.

However, suppose one keeps on strengthening the tissue. In that case, everyday knee tissue gets stronger, and not only our functional capacity of ADL, like walking, stairs ascending and descending, jogging, and running capacity will become easier, but also one will be less prone to injury. One will be on the safer side even when there is a sudden increase in ADL. As it is known from the analysis of **"physical stress VS tissue strength theory**," knee tissue will always be in the preventive zone, and tissue threshold value gradually increases.

Specific Functional goals/task[60] can be targeted with an assessment like 1RM, and gradually, one can increase the required 1RM to achieve the targeted functional goals. Therefore, strength and endurance results can be correlated to functional goals. In fact, recent research shows that functional task training is better than traditional strengthening or that a combination of both strengthening and functional training together can achieve better results[61].

These above-mentioned progressive strengthening program principles could be applied to any part of the body tissue to achieve required tissue strength and functional goals.

# CHAPTER 3
## Variable factors affecting the level of the physical stress on the tissue or the adaptive response of tissues to physical stress: knee joint-specific

The previous chapters focused on the knowledge about the relationship between the physical stress acted on the tissue vs the strength of the tissue; the following chapter deals with the variable factors affecting the level of Physical Stress on tissues and the Adaptive Response of tissues to Physical Stress. This knowledge will guide in dealing with injury prevention and rehabilitation of various Neuro-muscular-skeletal problems.

The stress threshold required to achieve a given tissue response may vary among individuals depending on the presence or absence of several modulating variables. There are four categories of variables (Tab. 1) that can modulate either:

(1) **The level of stress on tissues** or
(2) **The response of tissues to a given level of physical stress** (I.e., threshold values for tissue adaptation and injury).

Because of the complex interaction among variables, these variables can be used to construct models that predict the relative influence of stress-related and non-mechanical variables on tissue adaptation and injury. Factors that can change the stress level on tissues or the threshold values for tissue adaptation and injury are summarized in Table 1, including movement and alignment and extrinsic, psychosocial, and physiological factors. As the book focuses on the perspective of knee joint tissue, the four categories of variables regarding knee joint tissue are elaborated.

**Variable factors affecting the level of Physical Stress on knee tissues and the adaptive response of knee tissues to physical stress:**

In order to analyze the effect of variable factors on the knee joint (tissue), one should know the activities in which the knee is stressed more.

In recent research, an electronic knee prosthesis was designed to measure tibia forces in vivo during activities of daily living after total knee arthroplasty was done. The ascending order of compressive loads in the activities has been noted. They are as follows- cycling < walking < stairs ascending < stairs descending < jogging < squatting to standing < standing to squat < jump[13-14].

**Table 1.** Variables: factors affecting the level of Physical Stress on knee tissues or the adaptive response of knee tissues to Physical Stress: source from "Physical Stress Theory."

1. **Movement and Alignment Factors**

    Muscle performance (force generation, length)

    Motor control

    Posture and alignment

    Physical activity

    Occupational, leisure, and self-care activities

2. **Extrinsic Factors**

    Orthotic devices, taping, assistive devices

    Footwear

    Ergonomic environment

    Modalities

    Gravity

3. **Psychosocial Factors**

4. **Physiological Factors**

    Medication

    Age

    Systemic pathology

    Obesity

Example: Specific activities involving knee stress in full extension landing result in an enormous amount of pressure on the knee joint as a result of the body's inability to utilize the lower extremity muscle and other soft tissue to stabilise the knee, thereby maximizing the threat of injury when the load exceeds the highest safety threshold[64].

Knowing the activities of daily life in which the knee is stressed, variable factors that contribute to excessive stress on the knee tissue can be analysed, and some variable factors can be modified to reduce stress on the knee tissue.

**1. Movement and alignment factor:** more from the point of view of the knee. Other than the knee, it is beyond the scope of the book.

**a) Muscle performance** - Tissue strength, endurance, and length /flexibility are required for different activities. Muscle performance Includes force generation muscle length, a critical aspect of movement influencing tissue stress. Any stress placed on a joint first passes through the surrounding tissue, and if it is strong, it acts as a shock absorber.

Tissue strength and endurance:
For example- if the surrounding tissues of the knee joint, i.e., muscles, ligaments, and tendons, are strong and flexible enough to take the physical stress acted upon it, there will not be any injury, or the impact of the injury will be less.

Decreased tissue length:
For example, tight hamstrings result in knee extension loss, leading to knee mal-alignment. The response of knee tissue strength to a given activity (physical stress acted upon the tissue) becomes less, which means the threshold value of the knee tissue is decreased by the knee extension loss, but the primary dysfunction is hamstring tightness. Therefore, less physical stress will make the tissue more prone to injury /dysfunction.

**b) Motor control** - is defined as the study of the nature and cause of movement, [65] representing a major component of physical therapists' expertise[67]. Evaluating how people control their movements to accomplish tasks provides insight into how stress is applied to the body's tissues during movement.

Examples: A person's activity demands continuous standing for 5 hours, but the strength of knee tissue can withstand the physical stress for only 3 hours, which will become prone to a knee injury. A physiotherapist can advise the patient to modify long-standing to avoid knee dysfunction/injury; that pattern of long-standing can be modified by bouts of rest/sitting every 1 hour for 5 minutes to recoup the continuous tissue stress. Long-term point of view: knee joint tissue can be strengthened by setting a goal to withstand the stress of long, continuous standing. The goal can be achieved by applying the step-by-step principle of knee strengthening, as mentioned in the previous chapter.

Assistive devices/orthotics like knee braces can be advised while standing for passive support until tissue gets progressively strengthened. Sometimes, a combination of rest, strengthening, and orthotic support is beneficial.

In another example, Maluf et al. [66] have proposed that the daily repetition of similar movements and posture may result in excessive stress on the lower back tissues. These authors suggest that physical therapists can identify and modify motor recruitment patterns potentially contributing to patients' low back pain during daily activities. Maluf et al. [66] contend that an important role of physical therapists is to identify patterns of movement that contribute to excessive tissue stress and teach patient-appropriate movement strategies to prevent tissue injury and pain.

### c) Posture and alignment

Kendall et al.[68] have emphasized the relationship between posture, impairments, and pain. Based on their clinical observations, Kendall's basic premise was a standard or "ideal" posture, and deviation from this ideal posture leads to characteristic patterns of musculoskeletal impairments and pain[68 (p5)]. For example, Kendalls predicts that a person with excessive lumbar lordosis would have weak abdominal and hamstring muscles, with short, strong low-back and hip flexor muscles. [68 (p126)]

Deviation from normal posture and alignment leads to a decrease in the strength of the tissue. Any dysfunction of the joint or tightness/contracture of soft tissue or any combination leads to abnormal posture and misalignment.

**Example:** Straight landing from a height on the legs exerts enormous pressure on the knee joint due to the body's inability to utilize the lower extremity muscles, thereby maximizing the threat of injury when the load exceeds the height-safety threshold[14].The researchers conclude that extended-knee landing results in serious deformation of the meniscus and cartilage and increases the risk of bone-to-bone contact and serious knee injury when the load exceeds the threshold safety height. This risk is considerably more significant than the risk of injury associated with walking downhill or flexion landing activities[69].

For patients with chronic deficiency of the postero-lateral structures, using gait analysis techniques and retraining can change the kinetics and kinematics of the hip, knee, and ankle to more normal levels. The abnormal knee hyperextension can be significantly reduced by encouraging adduction and extension moments about the knee and taking loads on the medial tibiofemoral compartment[70].

Loss of dorsiflexion could be because of the anterior talus and/or tight calf of the foot, which in turn exerts genu recurvatum force (i.e., Hyper-extension of the knee). Therefore, the ankle's normal dorsiflexion must be restored to reduce abnormal stress on the knee.

Knowledge about the knee's normal gait patterns and joint deformities, i.e., genu varum, valgum, and recurvatum is necessary so that extrinsic or intrinsic (arthrokinematic dysfunctions) factors that exert abnormal forces at the knee can be diagnosed and treated early.

Some extrinsic factors like worn-out lateral footwear lead to varus force -abnormal compression at the medial compartment and gapping at the lateral compartment of the knee.
In the long run, it might end with varus knee deformity. Vice versa if medial side worn-out footwear leads to the valgus knee.

We commonly observe people with "poor" postures, which are pain-free and those with "good" postures with pain. People's activities vary widely, resulting in different stress demands on the body's tissues. Therefore, the therapist's examination should focus on the postures and movements (physical stress) that cause pain[66,71-73] so that one can treat both.

Kendall's theory proposes that postural deviations are one of the essential components of musculoskeletal pain; however, pain patterns should be evaluated in a broader context to consider other potential sources of tissue stress. Postural deviations become one of many potential factors that may place stress on tissues within this context. Postural deviation may be the primary factor contributing to excessive tissue stress in some people.

**d) Physical activity** - Physical activity is another component of movement resulting in tissue stress. It is defined as "bodily movement produced by skeletal muscle contraction that substantially increases energy expenditure."[74] Physical activities may be divided into the specific subcategories of **occupational, leisure, and self-care activities**. Physical activity improves health by increasing stress in a broad range of tissues, making the tissues more tolerant of subsequent physical activity. Because the tissues are more tolerant of physical stress, they are less likely to be injured.

Increased physical activity has been linked to many positive health benefits, including lower risk for non-insulin-dependent diabetes mellitus,[75] strokes,[76] and obesity[77]. This reduction in the likelihood of injury occurs regardless of whether the tissue is part of the cardiovascular/pulmonary, integumentary, musculoskeletal, or neuromuscular system. Physical therapists should use their expertise to instruct how people can increase overall physical activity without injuring specific structures (i.e., Back or knee).

A physiotherapist should analyze a specific part of the body structure, like joint or soft tissue and their stress levels, according to the lifestyle of the person/physical activities. A specific activity like squatting has different stress levels on various joints of the body because of the centre of gravity, position, leverage, ground reaction force, and strength of the surrounding tissue of the joint. By knowing the activities that cause stress on specific tissues, a physiotherapist can prescribe progressive strengthening that is proportional to physical activities. Therefore, one can always be in a preventive zone and prevent injury/dysfunction of the tissue.

**Example:** physical activity from the point of view of the knee. One needs to know the activities in which the knee is stressed more.

In research, an electronic knee prosthesis is placed to measure tibia forces in vivo during activities of daily living after total knee arthroplasty was done. The ascending order of compressive loads in the activities is as follows – cycling < walking < stairs ascending < stairs-descending < jogging < squatting to standing < standing to squat < jump[13].

Specific activities involving knee stress in full extension landing result in enormous pressure on the knee joint due to the body's inability to utilize the lower extremity muscle, thereby maximizing the threat of injury when the load exceeds the highest safety threshold[64, 65].

By applying the above knowledge to the patient's daily life or lifestyle activities, one can advise the patient to do progressive strengthening in proportion to the stress level. Sometimes, stressful activities can be reduced, and the strength of the tissue can be increased. Alternatively, reducing the unnecessary stressful activities in which tissue is stressed more so that tissue will be in the preventive zone.

**2. Extrinsic factors** - Extrinsic factors are factors outside the body that can influence either the stress level on tissues or the threshold for tissue adaptation and can cause injury. Therefore, some of the extrinsic factors that can be modified or utilized by physiotherapists are emphasized.

**a) Orthotics** - Orthotic devices can be used to modify physical stress on biological tissues and can be used as an adjunct to other interventions in several phases of tissue adaptation. An orthotic device can be used to relieve stress from injured tissue.

In the context of the knee, knee braces[78] or caps can be used during the acute phase of knee injury or whenever activities involve more stress on the knee. So that physical stress on the knee can be reduced, and there will be additional passive support on the knee tissue during the activities, which will assist in natural healing by stabilizing the knee joint in various activities of daily life.

Weight cuffs, dumbbells, or barbells can be used to strengthen the knee's surrounding tissue progressively.

A component of orthotic devices should be chosen to achieve the desired stress level on the tissue. Knee logs (refer to knee treatment chapter 9) can assist in sustained gliding of the desired bone of the joint to achieve a range of motion of the knee joint and a sustained stretch of soft tissue. Likewise, taping[79] can restore normal alignment, immobilization, and stability of the affected part in the acute phase of injury and assist in natural healing, thereby reducing pain and inflammation. Assistive devices (e.g., Crutches, walkers, canes) may be practical adjuncts to help modify stress on injured knee tissue.

**b) Footwear** is another extrinsic factor that can influence stress, primarily on the foot, which goes up the chain to the knee, hip, and then ileum. By analyzing the biomechanics of the foot, one can diagnose the abnormal forces acting on it and can advise footwear modification to correct foot, knee, and body alignment.
Example: Medially worn-out footwear leads to gradual foot deformity (pronated foot). The pronated foot leads to internal tibial rotation and proximal tibia medial glide/shift. That, in turn, forces the knee into the valgus knee. Likewise, laterally worn-out footwear leads to supinated foot. The supinated foot leads to external tibial rotation, and the proximal tibia shifts laterally. That, in turn, forces the knee into a varus knee. The same can be corrected by medial raise[80] of footwear for valgus knee and lateral raise for varus knee[80, 81].

**c) Ergonomics environment** - is another factor that can be modified to influence tissue stress. Changes can be achieved by redesigning the job site or tools to reduce the demands of jobs requiring high force, high repetition, and bad posture[82]. As we know, frequent stair climbing is stressful to the knee. In ascending the stairs, the knee tissue has to work against gravity, and while descending, the knee tissue needs to control gravity. Therefore a house/office with stairs can be replaced with an escalator or lift, reducing stress on knee tissue. Knee braces can be used during the peak hours of the job, where activities such as continuous standing and walking, etc., will reduce the stress on the knee tissue.

Another important occupation where knee joint ergonomics plays an important role in the construction field[83]- extension to tools can be added while working at waist height instead of kneeling. If one has to kneel, one should be advised to wear knee pads and take micro-breaks of 10-20sec to extend the legs and allow the knee to return to the resting position. Raising the work from the ground at a construction site, for example, will help maintain the knees' health by limiting kneeling, squatting, and contact stress (kneeling on a hard floor). Excessive kneeling can cause the bursa to become irritated, leading to pain, inflammation, and a limited range of motion.

**d) Modalities** - e.g., Heat, cold, electrotherapy; some modalities can be used to modify the stress level or the response of biological tissue to stress application. Modalities have a secondary role in treatment but may be indicated to augment the body's adaptive capabilities. Heat is an example of a modality that can be used to modify the response of tissues to physical stress. For example, the elevation of muscle temperature is thought to help prevent strain injuries (i.e., raise the threshold for muscle injury) by allowing muscles to stretch more and tolerate higher loads before failure[84]. For instance, electrical stimulation can be used to augment short and long-term muscle force production, especially in the presence of pathology that limits the normal force-generating capacity of muscle, especially after ligament injury[85] or spinal cord injury.[86]Warm water assists in chronic stiffness and dull pains, whereas cold water assists in reducing inflammation in acute pain.

**e) Gravity** is an extrinsic factor used by physical therapists to modify the external load on the body. By modifying the orientation of the body or limbs with respect to the ground, physical therapists can increase or decrease forces exerted on the body during movement and consequently alter the forces that must be generated internally to produce movement[87]. Modalities or devices, such as aquatic therapy[88] or weight-supported walking devices [89,] may also be used to modify tissue stress by altering the effects of gravity.

Example: hydrotherapy[90]- water allows movements and exercises to be done while limiting the effect of gravity and pressure on weak areas of the body. The viscosity nature of water resists movement by friction, allowing strengthening and conditioning injury while reducing the risk of further injury due to loss of balance. Water exercises allow hydrostatic pressure nature to process the forces perpendicular to the body surface at every point, increasing kinesthetic (body motion or position) and proprioception (posture, self-regulating) awareness.

According to acute, sub-acute, and chronic cases, we can choose gravity-eliminated, assisted, or resisted planes, depending on the patient's capabilities during progressive strengthening.

**3. The psychological factors** are unique to each person's lifestyle and potentially can be modified. Psychosocial factors can profoundly influence healing and tissue adaptation, especially related to tissue injury. Logically, these factors are related to a thought level. Feeling good and confident can release endorphins into the blood, positively affecting tissue adaptation, injury, and healing. Psychological stress[91] leads to clinically relevant delays in wound healing.

**4. Physiological factors** - influence the ability of the tissue to respond to physical stress. Physicians are better placed to modify or treat physiological imbalances. However, the physiotherapist should be aware of the influence of physiological imbalances that can affect the prognosis of tissue adaptation and recovery from injury.

Physical therapists should also know some of the mechanical factors that can profoundly affect the physiology of synovial fluid in the joint. Regular Range of motion of the knee has to be maintained as normal human knee motion causes intra-articular joint space pressure changes that subserve the regulation of synovial fluid inside the joint, condylar cartilage nutrition, Joint stability, and Vascular flow. Refer to Chapter 4

**Deficiency** - calcium[92] deficiency can cause osteoporosis or osteopenia. Because calcium plays an important role in the functioning of muscles and nerves, its deficiency causes problems in the muscular and nervous systems. People without sufficient vitamin D are also at risk for calcium absorption, as vitamin D helps the body use calcium[93]. Lack of it may cause rickets, a disease where the bones become soft and weak, causing the bones in the legs of the infants to bend. Taking calcium and vitamin D supplements plays an important role in regulating the normal neuro-musculoskeletal system.

Sometimes, medicine causes side effects, and regular exercise may yield good results. For example, corticosteroid use is having a complex impact on tissue.

Corticosteroids can simultaneously cause a decrease in inflammation in one tissue (positive effect on stress tolerance) and cause atrophy in other tissues such as skin, bone, and muscle (negative effect of stress tolerance)[94]. Exercise may help to offset muscle atrophy from medications such as glucocorticoids[95].

**Age** - is another important physiological factor. Ageing has a negative effect on tissue adaptation. Kohrt[96] believes that a considerable portion of the negative effects attributed to ageing may be due to an age-associated decrease in inactivity. Ageing lowers the ability of tissues to tolerate stress and has a general tendency to lower the threshold for injury. The stress level required to promote tissue hypertrophy and increase stress tolerance is generally greater for healthy young subjects than for older subjects. Young people can exercise and stress their tissues more aggressively with less fear of injury than older people. The negative effects of ageing can be modified through increased stress on the tissue. Increased stress, applied through a progressive increase in activity or exercise, theoretically, can help prevent or reverse some of the negative effects of ageing. Increasing evidence suggests that tissues remain responsive to physical stress well into old age, and positive adaptations to increased activity and exercise can decrease functional limitations and disability.[97-99]

**Systemic pathology** includes the many diseases that can affect tissues' ability to adapt to physical stress. Physical therapists often encounter systemic pathologies such as diabetes mellitus and rheumatoid arthritis. Like the effects of ageing, many forms of systemic pathology lower the ability of the tissue to tolerate stress and have a general tendency to lower the threshold for injury. One example of this is the effect of peripheral neuropathy on cortical bone mass in the feet and hands of patients with diabetes. Although systemic pathology has a negative impact on tissue adaptation, carefully applied physical stresses can positively affect people with chronic diseases. However, systemic pathology may lower the threshold for tissue injury; many people with systemic pathology respond positively to exercise, both in terms of increased stress tolerance and reduction of disease complications. Growing evidence supports this prediction[100-104]. Traditionally, people with rheumatoid arthritis have been excluded from vigorous activities that might exacerbate joint inflammation[100]. However, studies have shown that progressive resistive exercises and aerobic exercise programs can increase muscle performance, fitness levels, and bone mineral density with no exacerbation of disease activity in patients with rheumatoid arthritis.[100-103] The positive effects of aerobic exercise for patients with cardiovascular disease have been well documented.101 Likewise; evidence indicates that increased activity in small increments can positively reduce the burden of hyperinsulinemia and diabetes.

**Obesity** is defined as an increase in body weight beyond the limitation of skeletal and physical requirements due to excessive fat accumulation[105]. Bodyweight is the physical stress that tissues of the body must bear during physical activity. Obesity is a risk factor for certain types of injury and a negative factor for recovery from injury. In addition, obesity has been linked with low activity levels.[106] People who are obese may be at greater risk of injury than those who are not obese because high-stress, low-repetition activities are more damaging than low-stress, high-repetition activities[108-111]. Evidence exists to support this prediction. For example, a population-based (n350, 95 men and 255 women, 55 years of age or older) longitudinal study (mean follow-up duration 5.1 years) reported that the risk of incident radiographic knee osteoarthritis was significantly increased among subjects with higher baseline body mass index (odds ratio18. 3, 95% confidence interval 5.1–65.1).[112]

Suppose a person cannot reduce his weight for any reason. In that case, the impact of the additional stress of body weight and the physical stress can be taken by additional progressive strengthening. Therefore, an additional strength of the tissue has to be always greater than physical stress plus the stress of the body weight.

Principles of variable factors affecting the level of physical stress on the tissue or the adaptive response of tissues to physical stress can be applied to any part of the body tissue. This chapter applies the above principles to the Knee joint for better understanding.

**Note:** Chapters 1, 2, and 3 are related; references to these chapters are clubbed as one for the convenience and better understanding of the reader.

## References: (Chapters 1, 2, and 3)

1. Tipler PA.Physics.2nd Ed. New York, NY: WorthPublishersInc; 1982. 7 Brown M, Holloszy JO. Effects of alow intensity exercise program on selected physical performance characteristics of 60- to 71-year old. Ageing (Milano). 1991; 3:129–139.

2. Brown M, Holloszy JO. Effects of a low-intensity exercise program on selected physical performance characteristics of 60 to 71year old. Ageing (Milano).1991; 3:129–139.

3. Fiatarone MA, O'Neill EF, Ryan ND, et al. Exercise training and nutritional supplementation for physical frailty in very elderly people. N Engl J Med. 1994; 330:1769–1775. Physical Therapy. Volume 82. Number 4. April 2002 Mueller and Maluf.399by guest on October 12, 2014http://ptjournal.apta.org/Downloaded from

4. Minor MA, Hewett JE, Webel RR, et al. Efficacy of physical conditioning exercises in patients with rheumatoid arthritis and osteoarthritis. Arthritis Rheum. 1989; 32:1396–1405.

5. Frontera WR, Meredith CN, O'Reilly KP, et al. Strength conditioning in older men: skeletal muscle hypertrophy and improved function. J Appl Physiol. 1988; 64:1038–1044.

6. Kohrt WM, Ehsani AA, Birge SJ Jr. Effects of exercise involving predominantly either joint-reaction or ground-reaction forces on bone mineral density in older women. J Bone Miner Res. 1997;12:1253–1261.

7. Herman WH. Diabetes and exercise [commentary]. Clin Diabetes. 1999;17:156.

8. McArdle WM, Katch FI, Katch VL. Exercise Physiology: Energy, Nutrition, andHumanPerformance.4thed.Baltimore, Md: Williams&Wilkins Co; 1996. 14 Guide to Physical Therapist Practice. 2nd ed. Alexandria, Va: American Physical Therapy Association; 2001.

9. Michael j mueller and Katrina S Maluf et al. Tissue adaptation to physical stress: a proposed "physical stress theory" to guide physical therapist practice, education, and research. Physio Thor. 2002; 82:383-403.

10. Warren l.Hammer.Functional soft tissue examination and treatment by manual methods. 2007;23

11. Gail A. Shafer-Crane. Repetitive Stress and Strain Injuries: Preventive Exercises for the Musician, Phys Med Rehabil Clin N Am 17 (2006) 827–842

12. Slobounov SM (2008). Injuries in Athletics, Causes and Consequences, Springer, 25-43.

13. D'Lima DD, Steklov N, Fregly BJ, etal. In vivo contact stresses during activities of daily living after knee arthroplasty. J Orthop Res. 2008 Dec; 26 (12): 1549-55. Doi: 10.1002/jor.20670.

14. Markus S. Kuster, Graemea. Wood, et al. Joint load considerations in total knee replacements From the University of Western Australia, Australia VOL. 79-B, NO. 1, JANUARY 1997

15. Turner CH. Three rules for bone adaptation to mechanical stimuli. Bone. 1998;23:399–407.

16. Frankel VH, Nordin M. Basic Biomechanics of the Skeletal System. Philadelphia, Pa: Lea and Febiger; 1980.

77. Weiner S, Traub W, Wagner HD. Lamellar bone: structure-function relations. J Structural Biol. 1999;126:241–255.

18. CalbetJA, MoysiJS, DoradoC, RodriguezLP. Bone mineral content and density in professional tennis players. Calcif Tissue Int. 1998;62: 491–496.

19. Lee EJ, Long KA, Risser WL, et al. Variations in the bone status of contralateral and regional sites in young athletic women.Med Sci Sports Exerc. 1995;27:1354–1361.

20. Cabaud HE, Chatty A, Gildengorin V, Feltman RJ. Exercise effects on the strength of the rat anterior cruciate ligament. Am J Sports Med. 1980;8:79–86.

21. Tipton CM, Matthes RD, Vailas AC, et al. The response of the Galago senegalensis to physical training. Comp Biochem Physiol A. 1979;63:29–36.

22. Woo SL, Gomez MA, Sites TJ et al. The biomechanical and morphological changes in the medial collateral ligament of the rabbit after immobilization and remobilization. J Bone Joint Surg Am. 1987;69: 1200–1211.

23. Woo SL, Ritter MA, Amiel D, et al. The biomechanical and biochemical properties of swine tendons: long term effects of exercise on the digital extensors. Connect Tissue Res. 1980; 7:177–183.

24. Janet L Hopson, Rebecca J, et al., get fit, stay well, 3rd edition), chapter 5. Building muscular strength and endurance, 2014, p (10)

25. ACSM, resistance training for health and fitness, 21 June 2007,https://www.acsm.org/docs/brochures/resistance-training.pdf

26. McGill SM. The biomechanics of low back injury: implications on current practice in the industry and the clinic. J Biomech.1997; 30:465–475.

27. Huston LJ, Greenfield ML, Wojtys EM.Anterior cruciate ligament injuries in the female athlete: potential risk factors. Clin Orthop. 2000;372:50–63.

28. Radin EL. Osteoarthritis: what is known about prevention. Clin Orthop. 1987;222:60–65.

29. Radin EL, Parker HG, Pugh JW, et al. Response of joints to impact loading, III: the relationship between trabecular microfractures and cartilage degeneration. J Biomech. 1973;6:51–57.

30. Radin EL, Paul IL. Response of joints to impact loading, I: in vitro wear. Arthritis Rheum. 1971;14:356–362.

31. Simon SR, Radin EL, Paul IL, Rose RM. The response of joints to impact loading, II: in vivo behavior of subchondral bone. J Biomech.1972; 5:267–272.

32. Kohrt W. Physical activity plays a leading role in skeletal health. Biomech. April 1999:57–64.

33. Woo SL, Gomez MA, Akeson WH. Mechanical behaviors of soft tissues: measurements, modifications, injuries, and treatments. In: NahumAM, MelvinJ, Eds. TheBiomechanicsofTrauma. East Norwalk, Conn: Appleton Century Croft; 1985:109–133.

34. Bloomfield SA. Changes in musculoskeletal structure and function with prolonged bed rest. Med Sci Sports Exerc. 1997;29:197–206.

35. Leblanc AD, Schneider VS, Evans HJ, et al. Bone mineral loss and recovery after 17 weeks of bed rest. J Bone Miner Res. 1990;5:843–850.

36. Holick MF.Perspective on the impact of weightlessness on calcium and bone metabolism.Bone. 1998;22 (Suppl 5): 105S–111S.

37. Woo SL, Gomez MA, Woo YK, Akeson WH. Mechanical properties of tendons and ligaments, II: the relationships of immobilization and exercise on tissue remodelling. Biorheology.1982; 19:397–408.

38. Jeff M. Reynold, Toryanno J, et al. Prediction of one repetition maximum strength from multiple repetition maximum testing and anthropometry, Journal of Strength and Conditioning Research, 2006, 20 (3), 584–592

39. Nobuko Hongu, Michael J, et al., Resistance training: health benefits and recommendations, The University of Arizona Cooperative Extension, April

2015, https://extension.arizona.edu/sites/extension.arizona.edu/files/pubs/az1659-2015.pdf

40. Williams MA et al. (2007) Resistance exercise in individuals with and without cardiovascular disease: 2007 update: a scientific statement from the American Heart Association Council on Clinical Cardiology and Council on Nutrition, Physical Activity, and Metabolism. Circulation. 2007 Jul 31; 116(5):572-584.

41. Dong-il Seo 1, Eonho Kim, et al.Reliability of the one-repetition maximum test based on a muscle group and gender, Journal of Sports Science and Medicine (2012) 11, 221-225.

42. Dale A. lesuer et al. The accuracy of prediction equations for estimating 1 RM performance in the bench press, squat, and deadlift. Journal of strength and conditioning research, 1997, 11(4), 211-213

43. Todd M Manini, Marco Pahor. Physical activity and maintaining physical function in older adults, Br J Sports MED. 2009 Jan; 43(1): 28–31.

44. Jennifer Gatz, Golf Specific Strengthening and Stretching Exercises J. https://www.bnl.gov/bera/activities/golf/golf/golf_exercises.pdf

45. AAOS, knee conditioning program, http://orthoinfo.aaos.org/PDFs/Rehab_Knee_6.pdf

46. Alfonso j. Cruz-Jentoft1, Jean Pierre Baeyens2, et al., Sarcopenia: European consensus on the definition and diagnosis, Report of the European Working Group on Sarcopenia in Older People, Age and Ageing 2010; 39: 412–423

47. Lustosa, Gomes Pereira et al., Impact of Aerobic Training Associated with Muscle Strengthening in Elderly Individuals at Risk of Sarcopenia: A Clinical Trial, Lustosa, J Gerontol Geriatr Res 2015, 4:2

48. Campos, G.; Luecke, T.; Wendeln, H.; Toma, K.; Hagerman, F.; Murray, T.; Ragg, K.; Ratamess, N.; Kraemer, W.; Staron, R. (2002). "Muscular adaptations in response to three different resistance-training regimens: Specificity of repetition maximum training zones".European Journal of Applied Physiology 88 (1–2): 50–60. doi:10.1007/s00421-002-0681-6. PMID 12436270.

49. Rhea MR; Ball SD; Phillips WT; Burkett LN (2002). "A comparison of linear and daily undulating periodized programs with equated volume and intensity for strength". J Strength Cond Res 16 (2): 250–5. Do:10.1519/1533-4287 (2002)016<0250: ACOLAD>2.0.CO;2.PMID 11991778.

50. Buford TW; Rossi SJ; Smith DB; Warren AJ (2007). "A comparison of periodization models during nine weeks with equated volume and intensity for strength". J Strength Cond Res 21 (4): 1245–50. Doi: 10.1519/R-20446.1. PMID 18076234.

51. Werner W.K. Hoeger, Sharon A hoger; chapter 4, fitness and wellness; 2012,336

52. Gina kolata, Lactic Acid Is Not Muscles' Foe; Its Fuel, May 16, 2006, http://www.nytimes.com/2006/05/16/health/nutrition/16run.html?fta=y

53. J. Munn, et al., "Resistance Training for Strength: Effect of Number of Sets and Contraction Speed," Medicine and Science in Sports and Exercise 37, no. 9 (2005): 1622–26.

54. LJ White, SC McCoy et al., Resistance training improves strength and functional capacity in persons with multiple sclerosis, Multiple Sclerosis 2004; 10: 668/674

55. Shannon L. Mihalko and Edward McAuley, Strength Training Effects on Subjective Well-Being and Physical Function in the Elderly, Journal of Aging and Physical Activity, 1996, 4, 56-68

56. Neurological Physiotherapy 2nd Edition. Susan Edwards. 2002, Churchill Livingstone, UK

57. Sunderland, neuroscience, 2nd edition: motor unit, http://www.ncbi.nlm.nih.gov/books/NBK10874/

58. National Association for Sport, Physical Education For Lifelong Fitness 3rd Edition: chapter 6,2010,352

59. Jeffrey M. McBride, Machine versus Free Weights, the National Strength and Conditioning Association (NSCA)

    http://www.elitesc.co.uk/files/machine_versus_free_weights.pdf

60. Stutz-Doyle, Christine M., "The Effects of Traditional Strengthening Exercises Versus Functional Task Training on Pain, Strength, and Functional Mobility in the 45-65-Year-Old Adult with Knee Osteoarthritis" (2011). Seton Hall University, Dissertations and Theses (ETDs). Paper 98.

61. Robert Graham, Karen Sullivan, Functional Strength Training for Amputees, Exercise for Optimum Function;

    http://www.amputee-coalition.org/inmotion/nov_dec_10/strength_training.pdf

62. Ball S et al. (2013) Outcomes of Stay Strong, Stay Healthy in community settings. Journal of Aging and Health; 25 (8): 1388- 1397

63. Cornelissen VA, Fagard RH, Coeckelberghs E, Vanhees L. (2011) Impact of resistance training on blood pressure and other cardiovascular risk factors: a meta-analysis of randomized, controlled trials. Hypertension. 58(5):950-958.

64. Majid Davoodi Makinejad, [1]Noor Azuan Abu Osman, et al., Preliminary analysis of knee stress in Full Extension Landing, Clinics (Sao Paulo). 2013 Sep; 68(9): 1180–1188.

65. Shumway-Cook A, Woollacott MH. Motor Control: Theory and Practical Applications. Baltimore, Md: Williams & Wilkins Co; 1995.

66. Maluf KS, Sahrmann SA, Van Dillen LR. Use of a classification system to guide nonsurgical management of a patient with chronic low back pain. Phys Ther. 2000;80:1097–1111.

67. PhilosophicalStatementonPhysicalTherapy.HOD06-83-03-05, 17. Alexandria, Va: American Physical Therapy Association; 1987. Applicable House of Delegates Policies.

68. Kendall HO, Kendall FP, Boynton DA. Posture and Pain. Malabar, Fla: Robert E Krieger Publishing Co Inc; 1985.

69. Majid Davoodi Makinejad, Preliminary analysis of knee stress in Full Extension Landing, Clinics vol.68 no.9 São Paulo 2013

70. Timothy P. Heckmann, Frank R. Noyes, Chapter 29. Correction of Hyperextension Gait Abnormalities: Preoperative and Postoperative Techniques, In print, Noyes' Knee Disorders: Surgery, Rehabilitation, And and Clinical Outcomes. 2nd Edition. Elsevier, Philadelphia, PA, 2016.

71. Delitto A, Erhard RE, Bowling RW. A treatment-based classification approach to the low back syndrome: identifying and staging patients for conservative treatment. Phys Ther. 1995;75:470–485.

72. McKenzie R. The Lumbar Spine: Mechanical Diagnosis and Therapy. Waikanae, New Zealand: Spinal Publication Ltd; 1989

73. Van Dillen LR, Sahrmann SA, Norton BJ, et al. Reliability of physical examination items used for classification of patients with low back pain. Phys Ther. 1998;78:979–988.

74. ACSM's Guidelines for Exercise Testing and Prescription. Franklin BA, Whaley MH, Howley ET, eds. 6th ed. Philadelphia, Pa: Lippincott Williams & Wilkins; 2000.

75. Helmrich SP, Ragland DR, Leung RW, Pattenbarger RS Jr. Physical activity and reduced occurrence of non-insulin-dependent diabetes mellitus. N Engl J Med. 1991;325:147–152.

76. Hu FB, Stampfer MJ, Colditz GA, et al. Physical activity and risk of stroke in women. JAMA. 2000;283:2961–2967.

77. Schrauwen P, Westerterp KR. The role of high-fat diets and physical activity in the regulation of body weight.Br J Nutr. 2000;84:417–427. 44 Bonutti PM, Windau JE, Ables BA, Miller BG. Static progressive stretch to reestablish elbow range of motion. Clin Orthop. 1994;303: 128–134.

78. Duivenvoorden T, Brouwer RW, et al., Braces and orthosis for osteoarthritis of the knee, 16 March 2015 ttp://www.cochrane.org/CD004020/MUSKEL_braces-and-orthosis-for-osteoarthritis-of-the-knee

79. Afp Diagnostic challenges, October 2013, Taping for knee osteoarthritis, Volume 42, No.10, October 2013, Pages 725-726 http://www.racgp.org.au/afp/2013/october/taping-for-knee-osteoarthritis/

80. Seema Malvankar, Wasim S Khan, et al., how Effective are Lateral Wedge Orthotics in Treating Medial Compartment Osteoarthritis of the Knee? A Systematic Review of the Recent Literature, Open Orthop J. 2012; 6: 544–547.

81. Russel Rubin, Hylton, Use of Laterally Wedged Custom Foot Orthosis to Reduce Pain Associated with Medial Knee Ostcoarthritis a Preliminary Investigation, July/August 2005 • Vol 95 • No 4 • Journal of the American Podiatric Medical Association

82. Cumulative Trauma Disorders: A Manual for Musculoskeletal Diseases of the Upper Limbs. Putz-Anderson V, ed. New York, NY: Taylor and Francis; 1988.

83. DCBS, Protect your knees and your future, Construction, Ergonomics, http://www.cbs.state.or.us/osha/pdf/pubs/4844c.pdf

84. Garrett WE Jr. Muscle strain injuries. Am J Sports Med. 1996;24 (Suppl 6): S2–S8. 400. Mueller and Maluf Physical Therapy. Volume 82. Number 4. April 2002 by guest on October 12, 2014

http://ptjournal.apta.org/Downloaded from

85. Snyder-Mackler L, Delitto A, Bailey SL, Stralka SW. The strength of the quadriceps femoris muscle and functional recovery after reconstruction of the anterior cruciate ligament: a prospective, randomized clinical trial of electrical stimulation. J Bone Joint Surg Am. 1995;77: 1166–1173.

86. Belanger M, Stein RB, Wheeler GD, et al. Electrical stimulation: can it increase muscle strength and reverse osteopenia in spinal cord injured individuals? Arch Phys Med Rehabil. 2000;81:1090–1098

87. Kendall FP, McCreary EK.Muscles: Testing and Function. 3rd ed. Baltimore, Md: Williams & Wilkins Co; 1983.

88. Prins J, Cutner D. Aquatic therapy in the rehabilitation of athletic injuries. Clin Sports Med. 1901;18:447–461.

89. Warning, Muller S. Laufbandlocomotionwithbodyweightsupport improved walking in persons with severe spinal cord injuries. Paraplegia. 1992;30:229–238.

90. Dr. Craig W. Martin, HYDROTHERAPY, Review on the effectiveness of its application in physiotherapy and occupational therapy. Kukuh Noertjojo, Health Care Analyst (May 2004).http://www.worksafebc.com/health_care_providers/Assets/PDF/hydrotherapy_application_physiotherapy.pdf

91. Jean-Philippe, Janice, et al., The Impact of Psychological Stress on Wound Healing: Methods and Mechanisms, ImmunolAllergyClinNorthAm. 2011 Feb; 31 (1): 81–93.

92. Dr. Lawrence Wilson CALCIUM: November 2014, the centre for development.

    http://drlwilson.com/Articles/calcium.htm

93. Holick MF; Vitamin D deficiency. N Engl J Med. 2007 Jul 19;357 (3): 266-81. Scientific Advisory Committee on Nutrition; Update on Vitamin D, February 2007.

94. Craig CR, Stitzel RE.Modern Pharmacology. 4th ed. Boston, Mass: Little Brown & Co; 1994.

95. Czerwinski SM, Kurowski TG, O'Neil TM, Hickson RC. Initiating regular exercise protects against muscle atrophy from glucocorticoids. J Appl Physiol. 1987;63:1504–1510.

96. Kohrt W. Physical activity plays a leading role in skeletal health. *Biomech.* April 1999:57–64.

97. Brown M, Holloszy JO. Effects of a low-intensity exercise program on selected physical performance characteristics of 60- to 71-year old. Ageing (Milano). 1991;3:129–139.

98. Fiatarone MA, O'Neill EF, Ryan ND, et al. Exercise training and nutritional supplementation for physical frailty in very elderly people. N Engl J Med. 1994;330:1769–1775. Physical Therapy. Volume 82. Number 4. April 2002 Mueller and Maluf. 399by guest on October 12, 2014.

http://ptjournal.apta.org/Downloaded from

99. Frontera WR, Meredith CN, O'Reilly KP, et al. Strength conditioning in older men: skeletal muscle hypertrophy and improved function. J Appl Physiol. 1988;64:1038–1044.

100. Minor MA, Hewett JE, Webel RR, et al. Efficacy of physical conditioning exercises in patients with rheumatoid arthritis and osteoarthritis. Arthritis Rheum. 1989;32:1396–1405.

101. McArdle WM, Katch FI, Katch VL. Exercise Physiology: Energy, Nutrition, andHumanPerformance.4thed.Baltimore, Md: Williams&Wilkins Co; 1996. 14 Guide to Physical Therapist Practice. 2nd ed. Alexandria, Va: American Physical Therapy Association; 2001.

102. van de Ende CH, Breedveld FC, le Cessie S, et al. Effect of intensive exercise on patients with active rheumatoid arthritis: a randomized clinical trial. Ann Rheum Dis. 2000;59:615 621.

103. Westby MD, Wade JP, Rangno KK, Berkowitz J. A randomized controlled trial to evaluate the effectiveness of an exercise program in women with rheumatoid arthritis taking low dose prednisone. J Rheumatol. 2000;27:1674–1680.

104. Irwin ML, Mayer-Davis EJ, Addy CL, et al. Moderate-intensity physical activity and fasting insulin levels in women: the Cross-Cultural Activity Participation Study. Diabetes Care. 2000;23:449–454.

105. Anderson DM, Patwell JM, Plaut K, McCullough K, eds. Dorland's Medical Dictionary. 27th ed. Philadelphia, Pa: WB Saunders Co; 1988.

106. Schrauwen P, Westerterp KR. The role of high-fat diets and physical activity in the regulation of body weight. Br J Nutr. 2000;84:417–427. 44 Bonutti PM,

Windau JE, Ables BA, Miller BG. Static progressive stretch to reestablish elbow range of motion. Clin Orthop. 1994;303: 128–134.

107. Cumulative Trauma Disorders: A Manual for Musculoskeletal Diseases of the Upper Limbs. Putz-Anderson V, ed. New York, NY: Taylor and Francis; 1988.

108. Radin EL. Osteoarthritis: what is known about prevention. Clin Orthop. 1987;222:60–65.

109. Radin EL, Parker HG, Pugh JW, et al. Response of joints to impact loading, III: the relationship between trabecular micro-fractures and cartilage degeneration. J Biomech. 1973;6:51–57.

110. Radin EL, Paul IL. Response of joints to impact loading, I: in vitro wear. Arthritis Rheum. 1971;14:356–362.

111. Simon SR, Radin EL, Paul IL, Rose RM. The response of joints to impact loading, II: in vivo behavior of subchondral bone. J Biomech. 1972;5:267–272.

112. Cooper C, Snow S, McAlindon TE, et al. Risk factors for the incidence and progression of radiographic knee osteoarthritis. Arthritis Rheum. 2000;43:995–1000.

# CHAPTER 4
## Synovial Mechanics: Concepts of etiologies and effects of normal human Knee pressure variations with movement

This chapter is distinctive research done by the eminent scholar William O Irvine, MD, Department of Orthopaedics, Orthopaedics Indianapolis, USA[25]. As the research is relevant to the content of this book, it is included to provide insight into the importance of having a complete range of motion of the joint and guided usage of the achieved movement and then reversing the process of arthritis/dysfunction.

Normal human knee motion causes intra-articular joint space pressure changes that subserve the

1. **Regulation of synovial fluid inside the joint: mechanics of synovial fluid influx and outflux**
2. **Condylar cartilage nutrition,**
3. **Joint stability and**
4. **Vascular flow.**

Human knee pressure variations during motion are fundamental. They are caused by macro-anatomic changes in the knee while functioning. The knee is closed except for the arterial blood enters, and venous blood and lymph exit in response to intrinsic pressure-volume changes with motion. In addition to experiencing motion and load transfer, the knee is a hydraulic pump moving fluids in and out, and within itself, movement and pressure variation of the knee joint primarily causes condylar cartilage nutrition. The physiological benefits of knee pressure variation are condylar cartilage nutrition, joint stability and vascular flow.

**Abbreviations:** MCL: Medial Collateral Ligament; SMCL: Superficial Medial Collateral Ligament; DMCL: Deep Medial Collateral Ligament; MM: Medial Meniscus; FTPTA: Femoral-Tibial to Patellar Tendon Area; FTPTV: Femoral-Tibial to Patellar Tendon Volume; MRI: Magnetic Resonance Imaging; P: Pressure of FTPTV; V2: FTPTV Fat Pad Volume + Synovial Fluid Volume; C: Constant; SF: Synovial Fluid; ROI: Region Of Importance.

Research by Alexander et al. on live humans documented positive gauge pressures in the intra-articular knee joint space during terminal arcs of active extension and flexion. In contrast, between these two extremes, gauge pressures were negative[1]. Etiologies of these pressure variations have not been established.

Intra-articular knee joint space negative pressure aetiology studies by others have considered micro-structure transfer processes such as plasma and lymph colloid osmotic pressures [2,3]. These micro-structure processes have not been proven significant in the causation of diarthrodial joint negative pressure.

Normal human knee motion causes intra-articular joint space pressure changes that subserve fluid movement into and out of the intra-articular joint space[2,4].

Essential in knee pressure-volume causation is the articular space[16]. The articular space has central and peripheral boundaries. Centrally, they are the proximal tibia and distal femur, including its metaphysis. Peripherally, circumferentially disposed soft tissues, including the patella with its horizontal retinacula and the quadriceps femoris tendon, all enclosed in the deep fascia, constitute its external boundary. These tissues form a nearly closed sleeve. The articular space within these boundaries includes the mobile amalgam of soft tissues, intra-articular knee joint, and popliteal space. The mobile amalgam is comprised of no calcified condylar-cartilage of the proximal tibia, distal femur, and patella plus cruciate ligaments, popliteus tendon, menisci, synovium, and associated fat. The intra-articular knee joint space, containing only synovial fluid, is bordered by condylar and meniscal cartilage plus synovium. The popliteal space contains Neuro-vascular structures that service the knee, leg, and foot.

This chapter aims to reveal how motion may cause supra-atmospheric (positive) and sub-atmospheric (negative) pressures in the knee articular space. However, the analytical portion of this study, magnetic resonance imaging (MRI), concentrates on FTPTV, a subset of the articular space, and projects these pressures/volume changes to similarly apply to the remainder of the articular space. The following concepts indicate how these pressures support condylar cartilage nutrition, meniscal load-bearing and joint stability, and popliteal artery and venous flow.

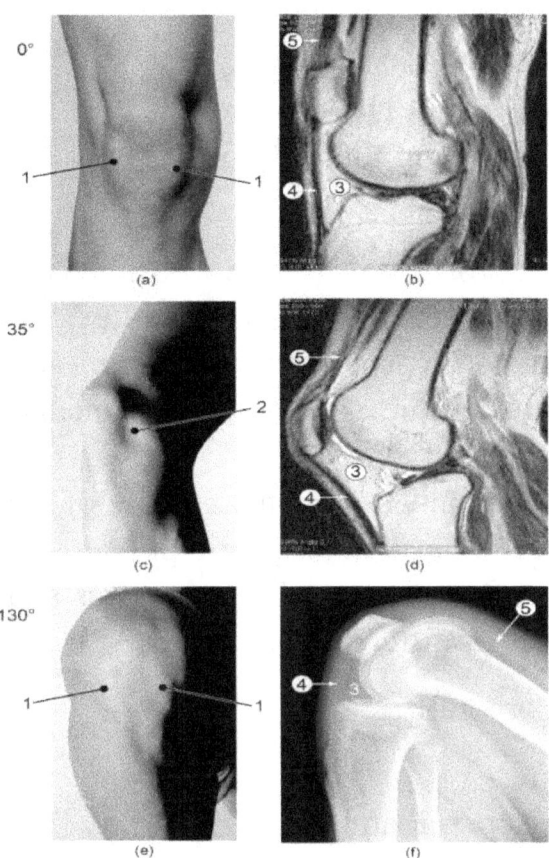

Figure 1: Right knee topographical, MRI @ 0° and 35°, and X-ray @ 130°. (a) Frontal view photograph at 0°. (b) MRI sagittal image at 0°. (c) Frontal medial oblique view photograph at 35°. (d) MRI sagittal image through femoral condyle at 35°. (e) Frontal view photograph at 130°. (f) Lateral view X-ray at 130°. 1 bulging medial and lateral parapatellar tendon, fat pads; 2 depressed medial parapatellar tendon area; 3 FTPTA; 4 patellar tendon; 5 quadriceps femoris tendon.

**Supportive evidence:**

1. **External topographic anatomy**
2. **Internal gross anatomy**

**1. External topographic anatomy: from Figure 1**

**Tool:** Observation anteriorly and palpation medially of the right knee at 0°, 35°, and 130°.

**The results**: Bulgings are evidence of articular space positive pressure, which occurs about the knee during advanced arcs of extension and flexion. Most evident is the bulging of parapatellar tendon fat pads beneath the skin and deep fascia. These bulgings are positioned between the patellar tendon, medial, lateral, and vertical patellar retinacula (Figures 1a and e).

Less obvious visually, yet evident on palpation, is the bulging of the medial joint line at 0° and 130°. In these advanced arcs, atmospheric pressure is less than the articular space pressure[1]. The difference between these pressures and atmospheric pressure is mathematically expressed as differential pressure ($\Delta P$):

**$\Delta P$ = P** [extra corporal] – **P** [intra corporal]

Where
**P** extra corporal = atmospheric pressure = **P** atm
**P** intracorporal = articular space pressure = **P** articular space

Therefore

**$\Delta P$ = Patm – P** articular space

$\Delta P$ was negative in advanced extension and advanced flexion, indicating positive gauge pressure within the knee articular space [1].

As evidence of articular space negative pressure, depressions about the knee occur during mid-flexion. The most evident depressions are in the parapatellar tendon, the anterior medial (Figure 1c), and anterior lateral retro-patellar tendon plane regions. Less obvious visually, yet evident on palpation, is depression of the medial joint line at 35°. Because atmospheric pressure is greater than articular space pressure in mid-flexion, $\Delta P$ is positive, indicating negative gauge pressure within the knee articular space[1].

## 2. Internal gross anatomy:

**Tools:**

**i. Magnetic resonance imaging:** MRI is performed on the subject. Scans are performed every 0.4 cm at 0° and 35° in both sagittal and axial planes. Imaging is undertaken to determine the change in volume of the infra-patellar fat pad in moving from 0° to 35°.

Considering any sagittal plane, the portion of the articular space that specifically defines the femoral-tibial to the patellar tendon area (FTPTA) anteriorly is the patellar tendon mechanism plus deep fascia and posteriorly the; (1) anterior non-load-bearing infra-patellar-calcified femoral and tibial condylar surfaces; (2) anterior margins of the menisci; and (3) inter-condylar notch synovium. FTPTA, principally infra-patellar fat pad, includes its associated synovium and synovial fluid.

**ii. Radiograph:** A lateral radiograph of the subject's weight-bearing right knee was taken at 130°, instead of MRI because available MRI chamber space was insufficient to accommodate the 130° exam.

**Results:**

**i. MRI:** Axial images reveal the popliteal artery and vein enlarged when moving the knee from 0° to 35°, indicating increased flow capacity at 35° (Figures 2b and d). At 0°, synovial fluid and infra-patellar fat pad venous engorgement are absent; however, at 35°, gross synovial fluid and infra-patellar fat pad venous engorgement are discovered (Figure 2a and c). A single sagittal image is selected to illustrate the relative sizes of FTPTA and gross synovial fluid portions of FTPTA at 35° per ROI (region of interest) in Figures 2e and f.

FTPTA synovial fluid collections are discovered in the infra-patellar and inter-condylar notch spaces only in the 35° exam (Figure 2a through d). It is observed that when it approaches 350 degrees of knee flexion, either from full flexion or from extension synovial fluid collection /volume is optimum.

**ii. Radiograph:** At 130°, the anterior femoral and patellar cams are disengaged while the extensor mechanism and hamstring tendons are in close proximity to the femur. Because the quadriceps tendon rides deep in the anterior inter-condylar groove, the supracondylar space between the quadriceps tendon and anterior distal femoral metaphysis is markedly diminished over 35° per MRI (Figure 1, f and d, respectively). These anatomic configurations are compatible with compression of the articular space, including the supra-patellar pouch. The above-mentioned evidence-based study revealed that MRI with an extensor mechanism under tension demonstrates gross synovial fluid production and enlargement of the popliteal artery and vein under negative pressure at 35°. It offers an explanation for the enigma of condylar cartilage nutrition, ΔPs effect on meniscal load-bearing, and joint stability. Finally, it offers additional consideration regarding the transfer of popliteal venous blood (knee, leg, and foot) to the femoral vein.

Cyclical positive and negative intra-articular knee joint space pressures relate to joint angle during motion. The rate of intra-articular knee joint pressure changes is related to anatomic features of the joint capsule with surrounding soft tissues plus those of the femur and tibia[4]. The relationship between joint angle and synovial fluid pressure is of considerable physiologic significance because the rate of fluid absorption from an intra-articular joint space varies with pressure[1,2].

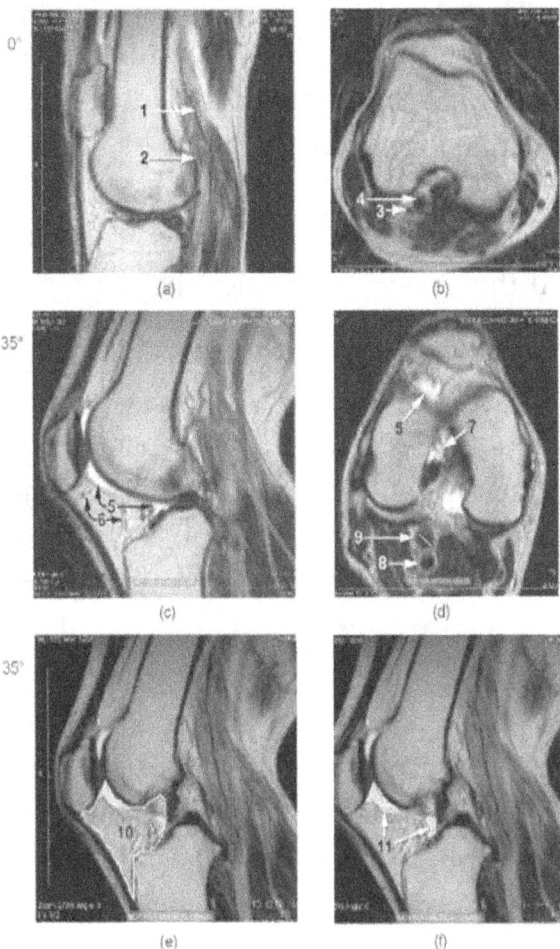

Figure 2: Right knee MRI. (a) Sagittal view through the medial aspect of lateral femoral condyle at 0°. (b) Axial view through femoral condyles at 0°. (c) Sagittal view through the medial aspect of lateral femoral condyle at 35°. (d) Axial view through femoral condyles at 35°. (e) Sagittal view through the inter-condylar notch at 35° with FTPTA ROI (region of importance). (f) Sagittal view through the inter-condylar notch at 35° with synovial fluid ROI. 1 popliteal vein; 2 popliteal artery; 3 stenosed popliteal vein; 4 narrowed popliteal artery, intraluminal diameter = 0.33 cm; 5 patellar fat pad, associated synovial fluid loculations; 6 grossly dilated patellar fat pad venous structures; 7 peri-anterior cruciate synovial fluid loculation; 8 engorged popliteal vein; 9 distended popliteal artery, intraluminal diameter = 0.45 cm; 10 ROI is FTPTA at 35°; 11 ROIs are gross synovial fluid portions of FTPTA at 35°.

## Etiologies of pressure variations:

Ventilation, the process of alternating movement of anabolic-laden atmospheric gas into catabolic-laden gas out of the lungs, is a function of the thoracic cage that creates pressure-volume variations. Conceptually, providing nutrition for knee condylar cartilage similarly involves the movement of anabolic-laden fluids into catabolic-laden fluids out of the intra-articular joint space portion of the articular space. These fluid movements are generated by pressures resulting from potential volume changes with motion. Potency volume is the volume of the articular space or any portion thereof at any arc position if that space is at atmospheric pressure.

The articular space is nearly closed. The exception is that the vascular system has ingress and egress. Since content volume is nearly fixed, pressure variation with motion means motion is associated with articular space volume capacity changes. During advanced flexion or extension, the volume of the contents within the articular space is greater than the articular space volume capacity at atmospheric pressure. Thereby, gauge pressure becomes positive. During mid-flexion, the volume of the articular space contents is insufficient to fill the articular space volume capacity at atmospheric pressure, resulting in negative gauge pressure. However, since the articular space is nearly closed, it is partially open. As a result, both pressures and content volume adjust in response to the motion. Negative gauge pressures of mid-flexion enlarge FTPTV by causing infra-patellar fat pad, venous and interstitial tissue engorgement, plus increasing SF. Positive gauge pressures of advanced arcs decrease FTPTV by minimizing infra-patellar fat pad, venous and interstitial fluid volumes, and decreasing SF.

Condyles of the femur each have two distinct, nearly circular cams, one anterior and the other posterior. The central portion between these cams has a greater radius of curvature (flatter) than either the anterior or posterior cam[5]. The central flatter portions of the femoral condyles, load-bearing through most of the superior medial and lateral tibial articular surfaces (tibial plateaus) at 0°, are non-load-bearing at 35°. Synchronously, when moving from 0° to 35°, the posterior cams move from posterior and non-load-bearing to mid-tibial plateaus and load-bearing, substantially decreasing femoral-tibial contact areas and increasing non-contact femoral-tibial space. The previously non-articulating anterior femoral cams engage the patella, pushing it forward, pulling its tendon and vertical retinacula anteriorly; this enlarges the potential space between the anterior patellar tendon mechanism plus deep fascia and the posterior: (1) non-load-bearing infra-patellar calcified cartilage of the femur and tibia, (2) menisci and (3) inter-condylar notch synovium (FTPTA). The product of FTPTA and mediolateral boundaries of this anatomy defines FTPTV. At 35°, the volume of the infra-patellar fat pad is less than the maximum potential FTPTV capacity at atmospheric pressure, resulting in negative pressure. A plastic model demonstrates negative pressure production (Supplementary Data, Items 4 and 5)[1]. When moving from 0° to 35°, as the inferior patellar-pole moves anteriorly, the extensor mechanism angulates about the superior patellar-pole quadriceps tendon and inferior patellar-pole patellar tendon attachment sites. The patella, supported by the prominent anterior condylar cams, is then positioned to separate the quadriceps femoris tendon from the distal femoral metaphysis.

Consequently, the interposed suprapatellar pouch experiences decompression. A positive value for ΔP is associated with the incurving of the quadriceps tendon. This incurving is consistent with negative gauge pressure between the quadriceps femoris tendon and the distal femoral metaphysis (Figure 1d).

During advanced extension, the anterior femoral and patellar articular cams have dwelled, which decreases the potential FTPTV capacity from that during mid-flexion. This occurs by bringing the patellar tendon-retinacular structures closer to the anterior infra-patellar femoral-tibial non-load bearing calcified cartilage as well as menisci and inter-condylar notch synovium. Concomitantly, the hamstrings and gastrocnemius tendons move nearer to the posterior femoral and tibial condyles. These events result in decreased non-contact femoral-tibial space and compression. The posterior capsule-oblique popliteal ligament complex compresses the mobile soft tissues postero-centrally.

Additionally, tough horizontal fibres of the popliteal fascia, through their attachment to fibres of the fascia lata, compress the posterior knee, including the popliteal space; this occurs because fascia lata fibres attach directly and indirectly to the proximal tibia anteriorly and are taut at 0°. This spatial configuration causes compression of the articular space positioned between central rigid osseous structures and the peripheral circumferentially disposed of musculotendinous, ligamentous, and deep fascial structures. As a result, positive pressures develop in the articular space, which includes structures within FTPTV as evidenced by out curving of the patellar tendon (Figure 1b). Also, bulging occurs at more elastic sites, especially where the only deep fascia covers the mobile articular space fat.

This is most evident in the medial and lateral parapatellar tendon regions (Figure 1a).

Again, the cams dwell during advanced flexion, even though the anatomic configuration is different from that during advanced extension. In advanced flexion and extension, FTPTV capacity is insufficient to contain the volume of the intra-patellar tendon, fat pad, plus synovial fluid at atmospheric pressure. This causes positive pressure within FTPTV-contained structures, bulging the parapatellar tendon regions during advanced flexion and extension (Figure 1e and a, respectively).

Gross synovial fluid and grossly dilated infra-patellar fat pad veins are discovered on MRI during mid-flexion but not during advanced extension (Figure 2c and a, respectively). It is proposed that an increase in FTPTV from advanced flexion and extension to mid-flexion is due to the influx of plasma dialysate as synovial fluid and as the infra-patellar fat pad, venous, and venous interstitial tissue engorgement. Efflux of these fluids occurs when the pressures become positive during advanced flexion and extension.

An inverse relationship exists between soft tissue-synovial fluid pressure and FTPTV capacity. Relatively high FTPTV capacity during mid-flexion corresponds to negative gauge pressure, and relatively low FTPTV during advanced extension corresponds to positive gauge pressure on a continuum basis during motion[1]. Assessment of FTPTV with MRI during advanced flexion of 130° was not obtained due to insufficient chamber space at 130°. However, the bulging of positive pressure at 0° was similar to bulging at 130°.

**Effects of pressure variations:**

The benefits of positive and negative pressures in the articular space include:

**1. Condylar cartilage nutrition,**
**2. Joint stability and**
**3. Vascular flow.**

**1. Condylar cartilage nutrition:**

Mechanics: When the articular space pressure is positive at 0°, the three anterior and two posterior cams are non-load-bearing and contiguous with a thin film of synovial fluid backed by synovium (Figure 1b). When the articular space pressure is negative during mid-flexion, these cams are load-bearing and mostly not contiguous with synovial fluid backed by synovium (Figure 1d). During the negative pressure phase of load-bearing motion, cam condylar interstitial catabolite loaded fluid is forced into the intra-articular joint space at and near load-bearing sites. This is evidenced by synovial fluid accumulations[12, 13], especially in the patella-femoral articulation (Figure 2c). Simultaneously, the hydrokinetic active transport influx of anabolite-loaded plasma dialysate into the intra-articular joint space occurs, promoting the mixing of their respective metabolites; these fluid transfer processes associated with mid-flexion reverse during arcs of advanced extension and advanced flexion. During these advanced states, articular space pressures are positive, and all three cams are mostly non-load-bearing and contiguous with synovial fluid backed by the synovium.

Three mechanisms that allow condylar interstitial fluid reconstitution are as follows.

1st- The electrical disparity between negatively charged compressed condylar cartilage aggregans and positively charged interstitial and synovial fluid counterions such as calcium ($Ca^{++}$) and sodium ($Na^+$) force synovial fluid to flow into condylar interstitial spaces via osmosis, obtaining overall electro-neutrality as condylar cartilage decompression occurs.

2ed- Mechanical memory during elastic compression deformation of condylar collagen and large proteoglycan fibrils during load-bearing assists in reconfiguring condylar tissues to their non-compressed state as load-bearing diminishes. This force causes the expanding condylar cartilage to imbibe synovial fluid [9, 11,19].

3rd - Positive intra-articular joint space pressure facilitates synovial fluid movement into expanding non-load-bearing cartilaginous tissues and through synovium to the sub-synovium peri-capillary interstitial spaces.

During motion, non-load-bearing and load-bearing states transfer fluid from sub-synovium micro-vasculature to condylar cartilage and back. Condylar load-bearing alternating with non-load bearing is a determinant of fluid movement out of and into condylar tissue; condylar interstitial efflux is due to load-bearing compression deformation. As condylar cartilage unloads, it expands from a previously compressed state associated with the anabolic-rich synovial fluid influx from intraarticular joint space into the condylar cartilage [9-11, 18, 19].

Conceptually, these events provide sufficient non-vascular condylar cartilage nutrition during a period of high demand.

## 2. Joint stability

Menisci bear the load and provide knee joint stability and shock absorption while evenly dispersing synovial fluid [20]. The deep medial collateral ligament (DMCL) attaches to the periphery of the middle one-third of the medial meniscus (MM). The descending distal oblique ligament (posterior oblique ligament) and the ascending distal oblique ligament fibres of the superficial medial collateral ligament (SMCL) attach to the posterior one-third of the MM. The semimembranosus tendon partially inserts directly into and indirectly through the descending distal oblique ligament into the posterior MM[21-24].

In extension, the MM is partially forced medially out of the space between the femoral and tibial condyles, pushing and tensing the DMCL, providing meniscal load-bearing and stability. This is evident by the palpable bulging of the anterior two-thirds of the MM and MCL at full extension. However, when the knee moves from full extension to mid-flexion, the previously bulging MM and associated DMCL become palpably recessed due to net forces related to positive $\Delta P$. One explanation is positive $\Delta P$ is associated with increased non-load-bearing femoral and tibial space during mid-flexion. $\Delta P$ would force the MM laterally into the interstices created by the femoral condyles, changing from large to small load-bearing areas of the medial tibial plateau, creating more non-contact femoral-tibial space. This would cause load-bearing through the anterior two-thirds of the MM, providing stability by increasing the load-bearing area and maintaining tension in the DMCL. When the knee moves from mid-flexion to advanced flexion, the MM is forced medially, maintaining tension in the DMCL.

Pressures in the articular space change from positive to negative as the knee actively moves from advanced flexion to mid-flexion. At this time, the medial posterior femoral condyle translates anteriorly and rotates superiorly away from the posterior medial tibial condyle. These simultaneous events enlarge the non-load-bearing femoral and tibial space between the posterior medial femoral and tibial condyles (Figures 1, f, and d, respectively). Accordingly, net forces related to positive ΔP push the posterior MM inward to fill the impending femoral-tibial void, resulting in meniscal load-bearing, which provides stability.

The lateral femoral-tibial articulation is somewhat different from the medial in form and function condylar articulation. However, from the perspective of pressure-volume, they are similar.

## 3. Vascular flow

The popliteal space's diamond-shaped perimeter borders are the hamstrings (semimembranosus and semitendinosus) proximo-medially and the biceps femoris proximo-laterally. Distally, the diverging gastrocnemius musculo-tendon heads complete the perimeter borders. The floor consists of the planum popliteal femoral proximally, fascia of the popliteus muscle distally and the posterior capsule-oblique popliteal ligament complex in the middle. The roof comprises the strong, mostly transverse fibres of the popliteal fascia, which attach to and are continuous with the fascia lata. This space contains major Neuro-vascular structures; the most significant in this study is the popliteal artery and vein [24].

The popliteal space is unique in that during the negative pressure phase, an additional separate dynamic from that of the extensor mechanism and femoral cams causes this space to experience negative pressure. The additional cause of negative pressure is a function of the hamstrings and gastrocnemius tendons-popliteal fascia mechanics (Figure 3).

During extension, the popliteal fascia is taut from its anterior attachments to the extensor mechanism and proximal tibia via the fascia lata, thereby creating compression posteriorly. As a result of this compression, positive pressure develops in the popliteal space, which compresses the popliteal vein, producing stenosis (Figures 2b and 4a). This explains why an individual, such as a soldier, standing at attention with knees locked in full extension may experience venous pooling in knees, legs, and feet sufficient to decrease circulating volume, contributing to syncope.

When the knee is flexed to near 35°, the popliteal fascia is pushed posteriorly on the medial and lateral sides, which is dynamized principally by bowstringing hamstring tendons and secondarily by the head gastrocnemius tendons, creating the centrally recessed popliteal fossa. Accordingly, this produces tension in the popliteal fascia, leading to the formation of the dome of the popliteal fossa (roof of the popliteal space)[24]. Simultaneously, the posterior femoral condyles, which are prominent posteriorly at 0°, vacate their posterior positions by translating anteriorly to 35°. These events facilitate decompression by increasing potential space and, therefore, negative pressure in the popliteal space, causing popliteal vein dilatation and blood aspiration from the knee, leg, and foot. This occurs because the closure of the femoral vein, one-way valves, prevents backflow (Figure 4b). Positive pressures result when moving from 35° to advanced arcs, causing the engorged popliteal vein column of blood to be compressed, ejecting its contents through the adductor Magnus muscle-tendon hiatus into the femoral vein. This is facilitated by the closure of the calf and popliteal vein one-way valves (Figure 4a). As a result, catabolic nutrition of the knee, leg, and foot is served. Such venous flow assistance explains why prolonged sitting should be avoided, as it promotes stasis, which impedes coagulation factors from being diluted by flushing, which may predispose to deep vein thrombosis and pulmonary embolism.

# Chapter 4: Synovial mechanics – Concepts of etiologies and effects of normal human knee pressure variations with movements

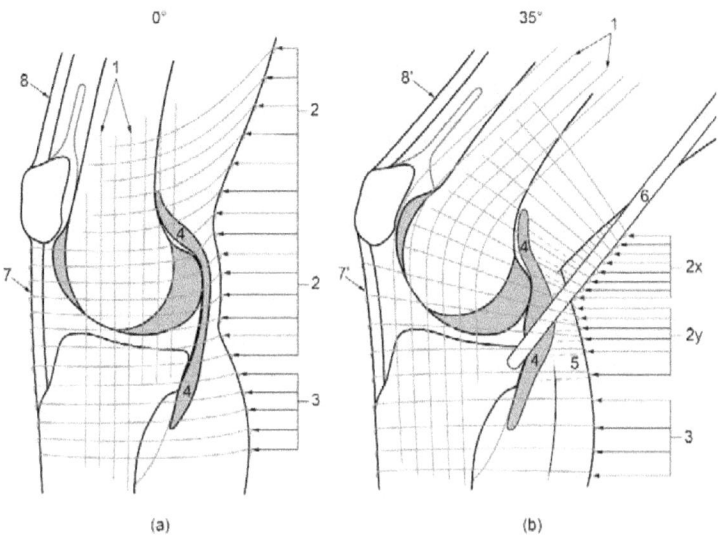

Figure 3: Illustration of right knee medial views fascia lata and popliteal fascia. (a) At 0°, compression of popliteal space by popliteal fascia. (b) At 35°, medial popliteal fascia is pushed posteriorly, dynamized by bowstringing hamstring and gastrocnemius tendons decompressing popliteal space. 1 vertical fibre of fascia lata; 2 horizontal fibres of popliteal fascia; 2x popliteal fascia fibres wrapping 180° around medial hamstring tendons becoming the roof of popliteal space; 2y popliteal fascia fibres wrapping 180° around medial gastrocnemius musculotendon becoming the roof of popliteal space; 3 crural fascia fibres; 4 popliteal space; 5 gastrocnemius medial musculo-tendon; 6 medial hamstring tendons; 7 out curving patellar tendon; 7' incurving patellar tendon; 8 out curving quadriceps tendon; 8' incurving quadriceps tendon.

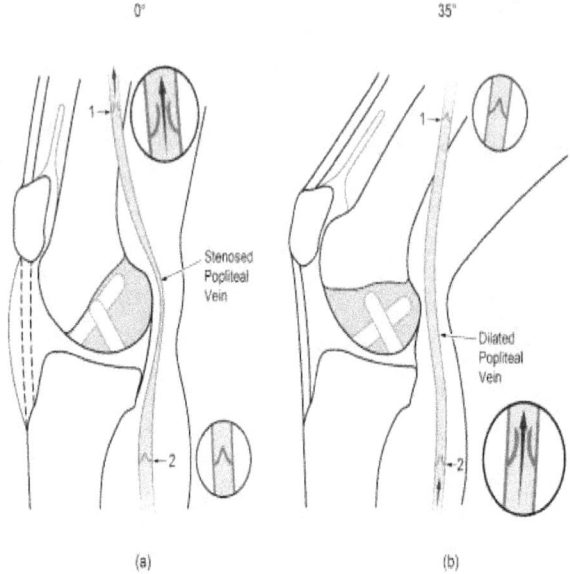

Figure 4: Illustration of Right knee sagittal views stenotic and dilated popliteal vein. (a) At 0°, stenosis occurs with compression of popliteal space. (b) At 35°, dilatation occurs with decompression of popliteal space. 1 femoral vein one-way valve; 2 popliteal vein one-way valve.

## Conclusion

While performing as a bellows, alternating gross anatomic configurations of the moving knee cause pressure changes that physiologically facilitate condylar cartilage nutrition, knee joint stability, and vascular flow. Rhythmical pressure variations in the articular space function of alternating engagement and disengagement of femoral condylar and patellar cams while being encased in a tough, circumferentially disposed soft tissue sleeve. These pressure variations have an inverse relationship with FTPTV. Relatively low articular space pressure during mid-flexion corresponds to relatively high FTPTV, whereas relatively high articular space pressure during advanced extension and advanced flexion corresponds to relatively low FTPTV on a continuum basis during motion. During the negative pressure phase of mid-flexion, capillary plasma as a dialysate and load-bearing condylar interstitial fluid is forced into the intra-articular joint space. These conditions reverse during the positive gauge pressure phases of advanced flexion and advanced extension. Under all these conditions, nutrition is enhanced by metabolite exchange. During motion, pressure variations in the popliteal space, directed by one-way valves, promote blood flow through the popliteal and femoral veins, simulating the mechanical action of a peristaltic pump.

As it is known from the clinical conditions of knee arthritis[14,15], the joints' terminal extension /and terminal flexion are generally lost. That leads to loss of movement. Applying the above research concepts indicates that joints with loss of range will not get sufficient cartilage nutrition, stability, and vascular flow. Once the pathomechanics of the knee dysfunctions are known, the physiotherapist can accurately diagnose and accordingly treat them by restoring the joint's normal range of motion and alignment. Once the normal biomechanics of the joint is restored, normal joint physiology is maintained. Therefore, it can be stated that arthritis can be improved or reversed to normal if diagnosed early with three planar spring test and treated with multi-model conservative interventions designed based on underlying pathomechanics.

**References:**

1. Alexander C, Caughey D, Withy S, Van Puymbroeck E, Munoz D (1996) Relation between flexion angle and intraarticular pressure during active and passive movement of the normal knee. J Rheumatol 23: 889.
2. Levick JR (1979) an investigation into the validity of subatmospheric pressure recordings from synovial fluid and their dependence on the joint angle. J Physiol289: 55, 64, 66.
3. Guyton C, Granger HJ, Taylor AE (1971) Interstitial fluid pressure. Physiological Reviews 51: 552-553.
4. Nade S, Newbold PJ (1983) Factors determining the level and changes in intraarticular pressure in the knee joint of the dog. J Physiol 338: 22.
5. Simon SR (2000) Structure and function of the knee: Orthopaedic BasicScience: Biology and Biomechanics of the Musculoskeletal System. ($2^{nd}$edn), American Academy of Orthopaedic Surgeons, Rosemont, Illinois.
6. Mankin HJ, Mow VC, Buckwalter JA, Iannotti JP, Ratcliffe A (2000) Articular cartilage structure, composition, and function: Orthopaedic Basic Science: Biology and Biomechanics of the Musculoskeletal System. (2ndedn), AmericanAcademy of Orthopaedic Surgeons, Rosemont, Illinois, pp: 452.
7. Mankin HJ, Mow VC, Buckwalter JA, Iannotti JP, Racliffe A (2000) Articular cartilage structure, composition, and function: Orthopaedic Basic Science: Biology and Biomechanics of the Musculoskeletal System. (2ndedn), AmericanAcademy of Orthopaedic Surgeons, Rosemont, Illinois, pp: 452.
8. Miltner O, Schneider U, Graf J, and Niethard FU (1997) Influence of isokinetic and ergometric exercises on oxygen partial pressure measurement in the human knee joint. AdvExp Med Biol 411: 183-184.
9. O'Hara BP, Urban JP, Maroudas A (1990) Influence of cyclic loading on the nutrition of articular cartilage. Ann Rheum Dis 49: 536-539.
10. Ekholm R, Norback B (1951) On the relationship between articular changes and function. Acta Orthop Scand 21: 95.
11. Couchman JR (2001) Structure, function, and biology of joint proteoglycans: Arthritis and Allied Conditions: A Textbook of Rheumatology. (14thedn), Lippincott Williams & Wilkins, Philadelphia, Pennsylvania, pp: 213.

12. McDonald JN, Levick JR (1993) Effect of extravascular plasma protein on pressure-flow relations across synovium in anesthetized rabbits. J Physiol 465: 539,557,540.
13. Levick JR (1987) Synovial fluid and trans-synovial flow in stationary and moving normal joints: Joint Loading Biology and Health of Articular Structures. Bristol, Wright, pp: 162.
14. Recklies AD, Poole AD, Banerjee S, Bogoch E, DiBattista J, et al. (2000) Pathophysiologic aspects of inflammation in diarthrodial joints: OrthopaedicBasic Science: Biology and Biomechanics of the Musculoskeletal System. ($2^{nd}$edn), American Academy of Orthopaedic Surgeons, Rosemont, Illinois, pp: 495.
15. Hale LP, Haynes BF (2001) Pathology of rheumatoid arthritis and associated disorders: Arthritis and Allied Conditions. A Textbook of Rheumatology.(14thedn), Lippincott Williams & Wilkins, Philadelphia, Pennsylvania, pp: 1103.
16. Levick JR (1983) Joint pressure- volume studies: their importance, design and interpretation. J Rheumatol 10: 357.
17. Smith M, Campbell JR (1929) Observations on the lymphatic drainage of joint cavities. ExpBiol Med 26: 397.
18. Mow VC, Flatow EL, Ateshian GA (2000) Biomechanics: Biotribology of diarthrodial joints: Orthopaedic Basic Science: Biology and Biomechanics of the Musculoskeletal System. (2ndedn), American Academy of Orthopaedic Surgeons, Rosemont, Illinois, pp: 174-176.
19. Mow VC, Flatow EL, Ateshian GA (2000) Biomechanics: Biotribology of diarthrodial joints: Orthopaedic Basic Science: Biology and Biomechanics of the Musculoskeletal System. (2ndedn), American Academy of Orthopaedic Surgeons, Rosemont, Illinois, pp: 458-462, 467.
20. Arnoczky SP, McDevitt CA (2000) The meniscus: Structure, function, repair and replacement: Orthopaedic Basic Science: Biology and Biomechanics of the Musculoskeletal System. (2ndedn), American Academy of Orthopaedic Surgeons, Rosemont, Illinois, pp: 536-537.
21. Last RJ (1948) Some anatomical details of the knee joint. J Bone Joint Surg Br 30B: 684-686.
22. Robinson JR, Sanchez-Ballester J, Bull AMJ, Thomas R de WM, Amis AA (2004) The posteromedial corner, revisited: an anatomical description of the

passive restraining structures of the medial aspect of the human knee. J Bone Joint Surgery Br 86B: 674-681.

23. Müller W (1983) The knee: Form, function, and ligament reconstruction. Springer-Verlag, Berlin, Heidelberg, New York, pp: 66-72.

24. Terry RJ, Trotter M (1953) The articulations: Morris' Human Anatomy. (11thedn), The McGraw-Hill Book Company, Inc, New York, New York, pp: 367, 370-1, 567.

25. Citation: Irvine WO (2015) Concepts of Etiologies and Effects of Normal Human Knee Pressure Variations. Anat Physiol 5: 172. doi:10.4172/2161-0940.1000172

# CHAPTER 5
## Soft Tissue: Injury, Healing, Tissue Adhesions, Assessment, and Treatment

**INTRODUCTION TO SOFT TISSUE**
Soft tissue generally involves the following structures:
• **Muscle** - Muscles are made up of fibres that shorten and lengthen to produce movement of a joint. Muscles are attached to bone by tendons.

• **Tendon** - Tendons are tough bones of slightly elastic connective tissue that connect muscle to bone.

• **Ligament** - Ligaments are strong inelastic connective tissue bands connecting bone to bone.

**TYPES OF SOFT TISSUE INJURIES**

• **Bruise (contusion, cork)** is caused by a direct force applied to the body, such as being kicked or making contact with a player, resulting in compression and bleeding into the soft tissue (hematoma).
-Signs and symptoms: Swelling and discolouration.

• **Sprain**- Sprains are caused when the joint is forced beyond its normal range of motion, resulting in overstretching and tearing of the ligament that supports the joint.
-Signs and symptoms: Swelling, loss of power or ability to bear weight, possible discolouration, bruising, and sudden onset of pain.

• **Strain**- Strains are caused by muscle over-stretching or contracting too quickly, resulting in a partial or complete tear of the muscle and/or tendon fibres.
-Signs and symptoms: Swelling, possible discolouration, bruising, or pain on movement.

**OTHER TYPES OF SOFT TISSUE INJURY**

• **Acute injury**- Injuries occurring from microtrauma (overuse) or macro trauma (impact-contact), like disuse fascial adhesions, are known as acute injuries.
-Signs and symptoms: Develop rapidly.

- **Overuse Injury**- Overuse injuries occur as a result of repetitive friction, pulling, twisting, or compression that develops over time.
-Signs and symptoms: Will develop slowly or on and off inflammation and pain.

- **Disuse fascial adhesions**- This leads to loss of flexibility and weakness of surrounding muscles, ligaments, and tendons, leading to injury recurrence.

**MECHANISMS OF INJURY** (Refer to table 1- flow chart)
Many factors (Refer to Chapter 1- physical stress vs strength theory) produce mechanical injuries or trauma in day-to-day activities/lifestyle. Soft tissue damage occurs through direct or indirect trauma to Muscles, Ligament and Joint capsules, and fascia. Usually, direct trauma refers to an injury occurring from blunt trauma or sudden overload known as macro trauma, i.e., actual muscle tear or ligament sprain. In contrast, indirect trauma results from repeated submaximal loading, leading to clinical signs and symptoms.

**STAGES OF SOFT TISSUE INJURY**

**I. Acute, II. Subacute/overuse, III. Acute or Chronic**

**I. Acute stage** occurs when direct trauma stems from sudden overloading or macro trauma.
For example, a person suddenly jumps beyond his standard capacity height and has sudden acute pain in the knee joint.

**II. Subacute/overuse stage** occurs when increased load degenerates body tissues due to excessive cumulative loading, leading to microtrauma and accompanying inflammatory response.
For example, let's say a person has the strength of the knee tissue to walk for 3 km on a particular surface with an 'X' speed and a ' Y 'Duration without any injury or dysfunction per day. Suppose he walks for 5 km on the same surface with the same speed and duration, resulting in injury (micro-trauma) or dysfunction of the knee joint soft tissue. In this stage, inflammation and pain of the knee joint are not intense; pain symptoms are on and off, indicating the accumulation of microtrauma and overuse.

**III. Acute/chronic stage**- This stage integrates cumulative loading and sudden overloading (e.g., chronic knee pain for a long). Chronic tendinitis is a degenerative condition without inflammation.

As the connective tissue is deformed, it either stretches or tears, depending on the loading's magnitude, rate, and intensity activity that loads and deforms tissue. It has an effect known as a stress/strain and is described through a load and tissue elongation curve. Collagen deforms under low loads and fails at high loads[1]. When the load is removed from normal tissue during the elastic phase, the material returns to its pre-stretch length. The injury occurs when the tissue is stretched into the plastic phase, causing tissue failure.

The tendon is the least elastic of all the body's tissue. The most frequent site of injury in muscle strains is the myo-tendinous-junction[12] because of increased collagen content at the tendon's transition zone of the muscle sheath. This area has decreased local extensibility as scar tissue and is frequently termed a stress riser. This transition in biologic tissues, which also appears at the tendo-periostial junction, is a point that is more susceptible to stress and injury.

## CHARACTERISTICS OF SOFT TISSUE INJURY AND DYSFUNCTION[15]

**1. Pain:** Injury creates pain from damaged tissue, swelling, and inflammatory chemicals.

**2. Swelling:** Swelling created by injury decreases normal movements of fluids. Swelling reduces the tissue's stability to repair itself. Owing to decreased cellular activity decreased nutrition, and healing.

**3. Soft tissue misalignment:** This dysfunction creates misalignment relative to the neighbouring soft tissue or the joint.

**4. Soft tissue torsion:** Misaligned soft tissue introduces an abnormal tortion[11] or twists into the tissue. The abnormal twist decreases the tissue's water content, leading to adhesions and abnormal soft tissue and associated joint function.

**5. Adhesions:** Abnormal crosslinkings[9] may develop between the fibres, creating adhesions. Adhesions develop if the soft tissues and joints are not adequately mobilised after an injury. If the area adopts the shortened position to avoid pain or because of poor posture, the fibres stick together, losing their ability to glide. This limits the tissue's normal extensibility (length) and creates dysfunction in the soft tissue, joints, and nerves. Adhesions also prevent normal broadening of the soft tissue that occurs during muscle contraction, decreasing their function.

**6. Fluid stagnation:** Sustained muscle contraction and adhesions in chronic dysfunction create fluid stagnation[12,] disrupting the fluid's rhythmic waves that normally circulate through every body region. Stagnation causes decreased cellular activity, nutrition, and waste product accumulation, reducing the tissue's ability to function normally and slowing down the body's constant cellular regeneration.

**7. Neurological dysfunction:** Adhesions and fluid stagnation create abnormal neurological function[10] leading to muscle hypertonicity or inhibition, loss of coordination balance, and postural stability.

**8. Altered muscle performance:** The optimum function of the body comes from good posture and movement that, in turn, requires muscles crossing the joints, which are balanced in strength, extensibility (length), and normal neurological function. This is necessary for fine neurological function, fine motor control, balance, and coordination. Dysfunction leads to patterns of sustained hypertonicity or sustained weakness (inhibition) in the muscle.

**9. Joint restrictions and misalignment:** Loss of normal joint mobility is due to loss of internal and external restrictions. Internal restrictions are due to the loss of glides between joint surfaces. External restrictions may be due to shortened or tightened tissue surrounding the joint, such as adhesions in the ligaments, joint capsule, and short and tight muscles. Joint restriction and misalignment lead to impaired movement.

**10. Emotional and psychological distress:** Patients with chronic pain are often afraid of moving, leading to disused de-conditioning and abnormal function in the muscles and joints, predisposing the area to degeneration.

**PATHOMECHANICS OF SOFT TISSUE DYSFUNCTION**
**(Refer: table 1 flow chart)**
According to the theory "Physical Stress vs Strength of the tissue," soft tissue gets injured when physical stress > soft tissue strength, including inflammation and pain. Soft tissue adhesions and tightness occur as a healing process, leading to the disuse of the terminal range of joints. Accordingly, joint stiffness/dysfunction occurs, and loss of range of motion leads to synovial fluid loss inside the joint as there is no influx and outflux of synovial fluid take place. Cartilage nutrition, joint stability, and vascular flow will be affected by the loss of movement (explained in Chapter 4). Disuse of complete range of motion leads to further tightness and adhesion of soft tissue, again leading to disuse weakness of soft tissue. If this vicious cycle is not diagnosed early and treated, it may lead to arthritic changes.

## Table 1: Flow chart of pathomechanics of soft tissue dysfunction

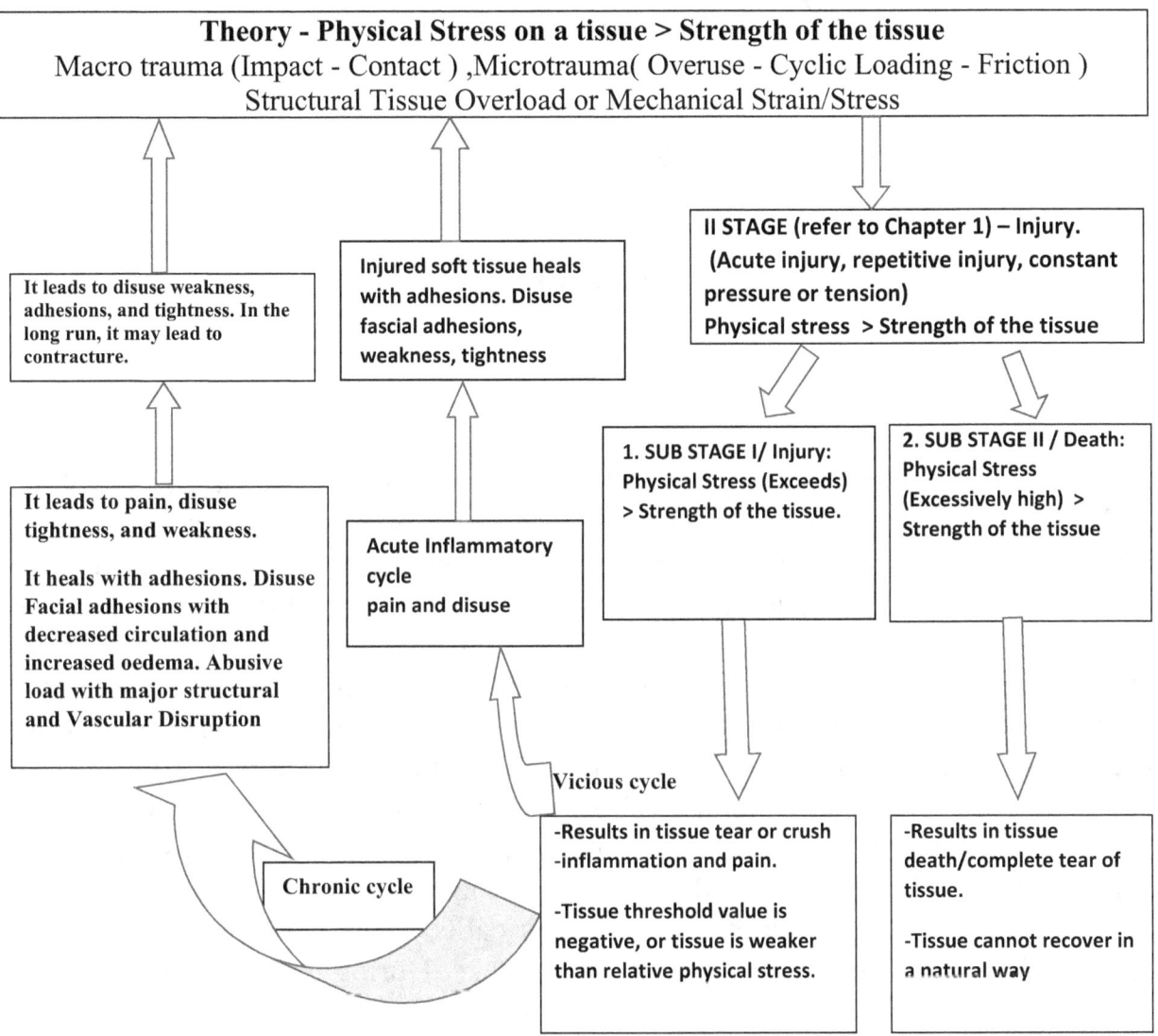

## STAGES OF WOUND HEALING[2]

Acute Inflammation
↓
Regeneration
↓
Remodelling
↓
End of Healing

**A. The Inflammatory Stage**[2, 3]**:** The Inflammatory Stage can last up to 72 hours and involves a number of inflammatory responses, manifested by pain, swelling, redness, and increased local temperature. Accumulation of exudates and oedema begins the process of tissue repair following injury when a blood clot forms and seals the area. In musculotendinous injuries, myofilament reaction and peripheral muscle fibre contraction occur within the first two hours. Oedema and anoxia result in cell damage and death within the first 24 hours, and the release of protein breakdown products from damaged cells leads to further oedema, tissue hypoxia, and cell death. Oedema and joint swelling with or without pain are associated with a reflex inhibition of spinal activation of skeletal muscle. Phagocytosis begins to rid the area of cell debris and oedema, as shown in Figure (A).

**B. Regeneration and Repair:** This stage is called Fibroelastic/collagen-forming phase [4]. This stage lasts from 48 hours to 6 weeks. During this time, structures are rebuilt, and regeneration occurs. Fibroblasts begin to synthesize scar tissue, and these cells produce Type III collagen, which appears in about four days and is random and immature in its fibre organization. Capillary budding occurs, bringing nutrition to the area, and collagen cross-linking begins as the process proceeds; the number of fibroblasts decreases as more collagen is laid down. This stage ends with the beginning of wound contracture and shortening of the margins of the injured area, as shown in Figure (B).

**C. Remodeling Phase:** This stage lasts from 3 weeks to 12 months. It is characterized by the remodelling of collagen to increase the functional capabilities of the muscle, tendon, or other tissues. Gradually cross-linking and shortening of the collagen fibres promote the formation of tight, strong adhesions. Final aggregation, orientation, and collagen fibres occur during this phase, as shown in Figure 1 (C).

Regeneration of the injured muscle does not fully restore muscle tissue to its prior levels, as cross-linking adhesion tissue slows muscle healing. The two processes, Healing and adhesions, compete with each other and impair complete regeneration. Restoration4of normal function following tissue injury/ laceration requires re-establishment of the continuity of the tissue fibres and the gliding mechanism between the soft tissue and its surrounding structures. Soft tissues heal by deposition of scar tissue at the site of injury. In contrast, the initial formation of scar tissue between the soft tissue ends provides physical continuity at the disruption site. The scar tissue's proliferation between injured and adjacent tissues is undesirable and harmful because these attachments impede tissue gliding, which is critical to function. Adhesions result in loss of motion, contracture formation, and functional disability.

**Note:** Another essential component of soft tissue healing is the formation of fascial adhesions[5].

**FASCIA:** - Fascia is a 3-D spider-web-like structure of soft tissue that holds all of our soft tissue (muscles, ligaments, tendons), bones, and organs in place. We have more fascia (or connective tissue) than anything else in our bodies. Fascial sheaths encapsulate every single nerve ending in our body, every muscle fibre, muscle bundle, and muscle group, and then turn into tendons and ligaments (also fascia), which attach to joints and bones.

Fascia is meant to be elastic, flexible and able to move with us. However, overuse, underuse, and injury to any soft tissue (muscle, tendon, ligament, or even fascia) will cause the fascia to shrink, dry up and adhere to itself. Fascia and the underlying muscle tissue can become stuck together, called adhesion, resulting in restricted muscle/soft tissue movement. It also causes pain, soreness, and reduced flexibility or range of motion[14]. Soft tissue adhesions can change the alignment of the joint complex.

For example, when the quadriceps tendon becomes tight because of the adhesions, it will pull the patella superior, causing patella-femoral dysfunction.
Common Synonyms for Adhesions are knots, trigger points, and myofascial trigger points. Moreover, the pain happens because you're asking this dried-up fascia stuck to itself to move with you, which can't. Suddenly, blood isn't flowing freely to muscles, joints and organs; nerve signals are inhibited, and movement becomes sluggish, difficult or painful[13].

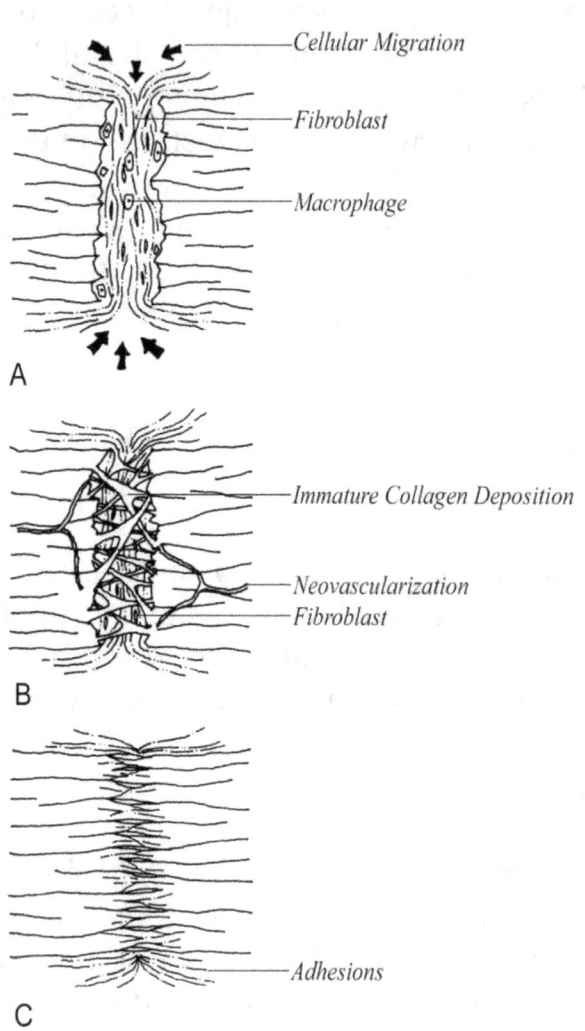

Figure 1:- Shows the step-by-step process of the formation of adhesions.
A. Inflammatory
B. Regeneration, repair/ The Fibro-elastic/Collagen-forming Phase and
C. Remodeling phase

## ASSESSMENT OF SOFT TISSUE INJURIES

Examination of injured soft tissues[20] involves initial muscle palpation with minimal force or compression in the case of acute injuries. And progression to firmer compression or higher loads if increased density has not been distinguished or pain, has not been provoked at the site of the suspected lesion (Refer to Table 2 for examination steps).

One can also have the patient contract the muscle, increasing the tension or passively stretching the myotendinous unit while palpating the area. The pain associated with palpation is secondary to the stimulation of free nerve endings with inflammation, decreased tissue extensibility, or tissue insufficiency.

While palpating muscle tissue, one should carefully search through various layers of tissue to find remnants of injuries and healing. Subtle tissue texture abnormalities may be missed if the tissue is examined erratically. These abnormalities must be considered in formulating an assessment. However, the clinician must avoid going too deep or hard with palpation, using pain as a guideline. The clinician needs to apply pressure and sense the tissue's reactivity. Since scar tissue heals three-dimensionally, it does not fall into place like a brick. Instead, scar tissue reaches in the direction of the fascia and the neighbouring muscle sheaths, binding the tissues together.

For example, if a runner strains a hamstring, the sheath tear heals and binds to the neighbouring muscle sheath. The hamstring muscle group still functions to flex the knee, yet the athlete complains of dull aches or pain in the posterior thigh. The reason may be that the independent movement has been lost, and the area of scar tissue has limited the extensibility of the myotendinous unit. Muscles function, and limbs move, but the normal gliding between neighbouring tissues is lost. As a result, there is a constant low-grade inflammatory process at the site of the decreased mobility. Scar/adhesive tissue has a poor blood supply and is not as strong and more resilient as the primary tissue it replaces. This area will likely be a site of re-injury secondary to the transition zone of normal tissue to scar tissue.

Table 2

Examination of soft tissue injury:

**HISTORY**
- Onset
- Pain location
- Mechanism of injury

**ASSESSMENT**

1. Physical exam
   - Inspection
   - AROM/PROM
   - Palpation
2. Neurological Assessment
   - Myotome, Dermatome, Peripheral nerve tests, Deep tendon reflexes
   - Strength and motor control
3 Special tests
   - Symmetry
   - Palpation of adhesions with deep friction
4. Functional assessment
5. Gait Analysis

**TREATMENT**

1. Treatment goals
2. Treatment plan
3. Treatment Procedures

# TREATMENT FOR STAGES OF SOFT TISSUE WOUND HEALING

## Stage 1:-Acute Inflammatory stage

The first stage of sprain/strain-related injuries is characterized by an inflammatory reaction that involves pain, redness, swelling, and increased local temperature that can last up to 72 hours. Initial treatment of this phase usually includes some form of immobilization or restriction of motion. It should be remembered that immobilization can cause early and significant negative effects on various organs and physiological systems[17].

For example, processes leading to muscle catabolism, atrophy, and quadriceps muscle weakness start as early as 6 hours.

### *Management and Rehabilitation of Stage-1*

Rehabilitation goals during the first phase are as follows:
1) Protect the further injury
2) Control pain
3) Limit swelling
4) Promote normal healing

Therapeutic and rehabilitative strategies appropriate for this stage include pharmacological intervention, physical modalities, immobilization, and therapeutic exercise.

### a. Pharmacological Intervention

The most frequently used drugs include non-steroidal anti-inflammatory medications and analgesics.

### b. Physical Modalities

The most important physical therapy modality used in this stage is cryotherapy (cold therapy), usually accompanied by Protection, Rest, Compression, Elevation, and Support; this combination is commonly called P.R.I.C.E.S Therapy. Cold helps reduce tissue temperature, decrease blood flow and swelling, produce vaso-constriction, and alleviate pain and muscle spasms. In general, crushed ice should be used. Compression using an elastic bandage and elevation of the extremity above the heart level may help control swelling. Another modality used to alleviate pain at this stage is Transcutaneous Electrical Nerve Stimulation (TENS), sometimes applied with ice.

### c. Immobilization

As mentioned above, this stage may require the immobilization of a joint or an extremity. Immobilization accelerates the formation of granulation tissue, limits scar size, and improves penetration of fibres through connective tissue, but as mentioned previously, it also has negative effects. Early mobilization increases tensile tissue strength, improves the orientation of regenerating muscle fibres,

stimulates resorption of connective tissue scar, improves re-capillarization, and decreases muscle atrophy and weakness.
-Taping with biomechanical principles will restore the normal alignment as well as stabilization of desired tissue.

### d. Therapeutic Exercise
Therapeutic exercise may be beneficial during this early stage to minimize deconditioning and promote a rapid transition to the second stage. If symptoms permit, exercises (pain-free passive range movements) to increase range of motion and static (isometric) exercises to minimize strength loss may be started in the injured part and related muscles. Conditioning of the uninjured body parts should be instituted. The transition to this second stage varies with the type and severity of the injury. It is generally desirable to start the second phase as soon as possible to promote faster recovery and return to ADL.

### e. Application of deep transverse friction
Apply low load to affected soft tissue to gradually decrease the tissue density and promote remodelling.

**Stage 2:-Regeneration and Repair** (The Fibro-Elastic/Collagen-Forming stage)
The second stage of any injury is called the repair or fibroblastic phase. This phase lasts from 48 hours to 6 weeks. During this period, structures are rebuilt, and regeneration occurs. Fibroblasts begin to synthesize scar tissue. The nature of the functional loss will determine the selection of therapeutic modalities and exercises needed for this phase. This is a risky period because the absence of pain may tempt the patient to return to the ADL (daily life activity) before the injured tissues are fully rehabilitated.

*Management and Rehabilitation of Stage 2*
The rehabilitation goals in the second stage are to:
a) Allow normal healing (similar to the first phase)
b) Maintain the function of uninjured parts.
c) Increase joint range of motion or flexibility by using graded mobilizations and stretching.
d) Decreasing adhesions/tightness/contracture by soft tissue manipulation such as deep friction (refer to soft tissue mobilization chapter 13). A high, forceful load to break adhesions. This is more applicable to older, dense scar
e) Improve tissue strength and endurance (refer to the theory of tissue strengthening- chapter 2)
f) Improve proprioception, balance, and coordination by including the desired gradual activity of daily life.

## SOFT-TISSUE ADHESIONS AND MANIPULATION

Adhesions generally form due to the body's non-specific attempt to heal a soft tissue injury with a prolonged inflammation process. However, the body will flood the area with collagen when soft tissues are exposed to prostaglandins' "burning" effects (an integral part of the inflammatory process) for too long. This collagen appears in the form of fibrils (strands of collagen) designed to form a scar matrix "to heal the burn." Since there is no real burn to heal and no scar matrix to form, little collagen fibrils start "sticking" tissue layers together instead, sometimes termed fibrosis.[32,33] This becomes a problem because the tissue layers that are supposed to slide past one another no longer can. The tissues then "pull" against one another, causing further stress and pain, extending the inflammation process. Indeed, it is the source of most of the chronic pain conditions seen in the physical medicine, orthopaedic, chiropractic, and rheumatologic fields. These conditions become chronic because most are unaware of the adhesion problem and, quite understandably, fail to treat the condition effectively. These fields continue to successfully treat many of the attending symptoms, often providing temporary relief (especially with pain), but until the adhesions are broken, no real "cure" will be produced. This makes soft tissue manipulation an invaluable technique. Once the adhesions are broken, the tissues have a chance to return to normal, especially if the inflammatory process has also been simultaneously relieved, thus preventing the reformation of the adhesions and ending the vicious cycle.

**Soft tissue manipulation** is defined as the manual manipulation of the body's soft tissues to break adhesions. There are many types of adhesion-breaking techniques, of which the **DTF**- Deep Transverse technique is very effective[6,7].

**Tissue Mobilisation in the Healing Process:** - The goal of mobilising soft tissue in the healing process is to reintroduce controlled stress as the scar matures in an attempt to influence its final form and function[22]. Immobilised scar tissue heals in an irregular form, whereas mobilized tissues with modified stress heal with parallel fibre arrangement. This parallel fibre arrangement demonstrates more elastic qualities whose redundant fold allows mobility without irritation or pain. Examples of good healing are gliding tendons and lengthy, elongated adhesions. Conversely, examples of poor healing are restricted tendons and short, dense adhesions.

Soft tissue mobilisation will not remove scar tissue but will help restore more normal tissue properties. Soft tissue mobilisation is performed like massage, but it is much more specific. The clinician uses his /her fingertips or elbow to identify the lesion, monitor tissue changes, and perform the treatment. When applying soft tissue mobilisation as a treatment choice, the clinician needs to identify the area of increased density, then distinguish the borders and document the feel and density of the tissue. The ability of the tissue to tolerate loading will give the clinician an idea of the level of reactivity and state of healing.

**Approaches to load applications are as follows.**

1. The application of a low load is to change the tissue density and promote remodelling gradually. This can be applied during Stage 1 of soft tissue healing.

2. A high, forceful load is applied to break adhesions. It is applicable to older, dense scars. Therefore, it can be applied mainly during Stage 2 and Stage 3 of soft tissue healing.

-Exercise in early controlled mobilisation has been effective in minimising adhesions during healing, as excess exercise may cause injury. Controlled/progressive strengthening exercises will help resolve and prevent further injury.

**DEEP TRANSVERSE FRICTION MASSAGE AND ITS PRINCIPLES**
The main technique that is more effective in soft tissue mobilisation/manipulation is DTF, or **deep transverse friction massage.**[8, 18]

Deep transverse friction is a specific type of connective tissue massage developed in a practical way by the Late Dr. James Cyriax, an Internist and Orthopedic Surgeon in England[23].

Deep friction massage aims to maintain mobility within the soft tissue structures such as ligament, tendon, muscle, and fascia and prevent adherent scars from forming[26]. (As shown in figure 2) The massage is deep and must be applied transversely to the specific tissue involved, unlike the superficial massage in the longitudinal direction parallel to the vessels, enhancing circulation and return of fluids. Before friction massage can be performed successfully, the correct structure must be found through proper evaluation procedures. The distinction must be made between contractile structures, such as the muscle belly, musculotendinous junction, tendon, tendo-periosteal junction and non-contractile structures, such as the joint capsule, bursae, fascia, dura mater, and ligament. [18]

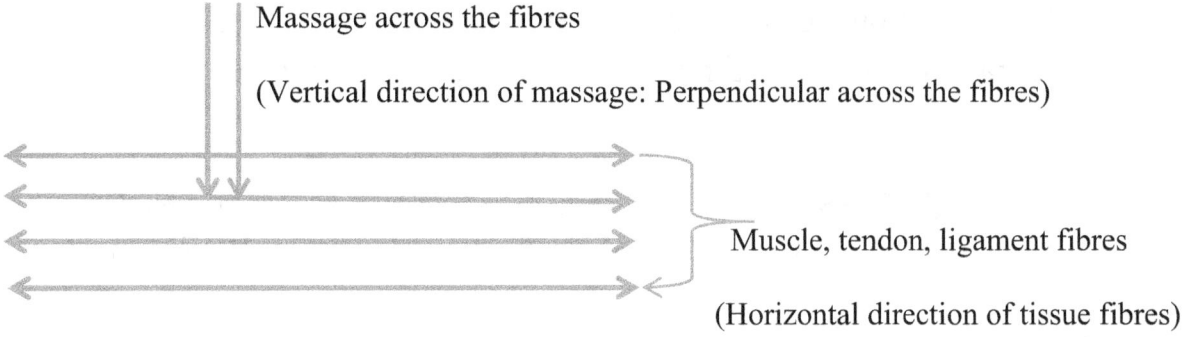

Figure 2: Cross fibre friction massage: Vertical lines represent the deep transverse friction massage given by the therapist. It is perpendicular to the soft tissue's fibres, such as muscles, tendons, and ligaments. Horizontal lines represent soft tissue fibre direction.

**Principles of deep friction massage: -** In addition to finding the right spot, deep friction must also be given most effectively by following the basic principles[27]

1) The proper location must be found through proper evaluation procedures and palpation of the specific tendon, ligament, or muscle.
2) Friction massage must be given across the affected fibres. The thicker and stronger a normal structure, the deeper friction is given strictly across the adhesions.
3) The therapist's finger and the patient's skin must move as one; moving subcutaneous fascia against muscle or ligament could lead to blister formation or subcutaneous bruising.
4) The friction massage must have sufficient sweep and be deep enough[19].
5) The patient must be in a comfortable position.

The frequency and duration of treatment vary with the severity and type of the injury[25]. In a recent injury, i.e., ligament sprain, start with gentle massage to keep mobility. The therapist needs to distinguish between tenderness and pain. Tenderness can be due to deep friction and persist long after the pain disappears. Pain is elicited by clinical assessment and reassessment. Deep friction massage may be given on alternate days or when the excess tenderness has worn off. The duration of the treatment varies. For example, the gentle massage performed may last only 1-2 minutes with an acute ligamentous injury. However, it may take several minutes to get your fingers on the structure, depending on the severity of the pain. Depending on the area and number of structures involved, the treatment duration can be 10-15 minutes with deep friction massage.

## THE MECHANISMS OF MASSAGE AND ITSs EFFECTS ON PERFORMANCE, MUSCLE RECOVERY, AND INJURY PREVENTION[21]

**Biomechanical effects[31]:**
↓ Tissue Adhesion, ↑ Muscle compliance, ↑ Range of joint motion, ↓ Passive stiffness, ↓ Active stiffness

**Physiological effects**: (Changes in tissue or organ)
↑ Muscle blood flow, ↑ Skin blood circulation, ↑ Parasympathetic activity, ↑ Relaxation hormones, ↓ Stress hormones

**Neurological effects[29]:**
↓Reflex stimulation, ↓ neuromuscular excitability, ↓ Pain, ↓ Muscle tension or spasm

**Psychological effects[30]:**
Increased relationship between body and mind, ↑ Relaxation, ↓ Anxiety

## DURATION AND FREQUENCY:
For most lesions, 3 sessions per week is a sufficient frequency with a duration of 10-15 minutes per session. The first session is for 5-10 minutes. In some chronic lesions, the duration of treatment will reach 20 minutes. If more than one spot has to be treated (e.g., Achilles tendinitis), it will be 10 min per localization. If the structure is too tender on palpation, there should be a rest period in the session, and it can be prolonged depending on the patient's condition and tolerance. The treatment can be ended when the patient is symptom-free, and the functional examination has become negative. The remaining local tenderness on palpation can be ignored.

## GOALS
The goals are twofold:
1) To provide movement for the tissue itself and
2) To produce traumatic hyperemia[24].

-In an acute injury, the massage consists of gentle, passive movements that move the structure but will not detach the healing fibrils from properly forming. The transverse movement imitates the structure's normal mobility by broadening but not stretching[28] or tearing the healing fibres. The movement encourages realignment and lengthening of these fibres. Traumatic hyperemia results in the enhancement of blood supply to the area. The hyperemia appears to diminish pain by increasing the speed of destruction of Lewis' P substance, probably due to the release of histamine. Lewis' P factor is an authoritative metabolite that accumulates ischemia. [20]

## PRECAUTIONS:

1) Soft tissue manipulation is contraindicated over the site of acute phlebitis, thrombophlebitis, or phlebothrombosis. Soft tissue manipulation over such a site may cause the dislodgment of a blood clot or embolus, which may proceed to lodge in various organs, including the lungs, heart, or brain, causing ischemia or infarction.

2) In patients suffering from acute inflammatory diseases of the skin or other soft tissues, including joints or surface layers of the bone. Such conditions may be complicated or exacerbated by soft tissue manipulation. Skin with furuncles, ulcerations or open wounds should not be manipulated.

3) Areas of soft tissue calcification, traumatic knee arthritis, or over joints that suffer from an infection.

**References:**

1. Trott A, Mechanisms of surface soft tissue trauma. Ann Emerg Med. 1988 Dec; 17 (12): 1279-83.

2. T VELNAR1, 2, T BAILEY2, et all. The Wound Healing Process: an Overview of the Cellular and Molecular Mechanisms, The Journal of International Medical research 2009; 37: 1528 – 1542 [first published online as 37(5) 12]

3. M. Flanagan, the physiology of wound healing, Journal of wound care. June, vol 9, no 6, http://wenurses.eu/mynurchat/archive/flanaganwoundhealing.pdf

4. Pedro k. Beredjiklian, biologic aspects of flexor tendon laceration and repair, MDJ bone joint surg am, 2003 mar; 85 (3): 539 -550. Http://dx.doi.org/

5. Melissa mcdonagh, foam rollers and myofascial adhesions,

    Http://Journals.Lww.Com/Nsc-Scr/Abstract/2011/03001/The_Effects_Of_Foam_Rolling_On_Myofascial_Release.45.aspx

6. Elaine Atkins, Jill Kerr, Emily Goodlad A Practical Approach to Orthopaedic Medicine: A Practical Approach Elsevier Health Sciences, 12-Apr-2010 - Medical - 480 pages

7. Jonas Vangindertael, Johnathan Fahrner, et al, Deep Transverse friction

8. Theory and science of massage and manual therapy,

    http://www.hendricksonmethod.com/wp-content/uploads/2011/07/HMI_BookExerpts.pdf

9. Thomas Hendrickson, Massage and Manual Therapy for Orthopedic Conditions, 544, 2009

10. Thomas Hendrickson, Massage for Orthopedic Conditions 2002 – p4https://www.google.co.in/search?tbo=p&tbm=bks&q=subject:%22Medical%22&source=gbs_ge_summary_r&cad=0 - 446 pages

11. Sandy Fritz, Mosby's Massage Therapy Review. P 242,552

12. Tahseen Cheema, Complex Injuries of the Hand, p82, JP Medical Ltd, 19-May-2014 - Medical - 272 pages

13. Brian, David R, the Acute Effect Of Self-Myofascial Release On Lower Extremity Plyometric Performance, Spring 2011. Sacred Heart University. http://digitalcommons.sacredheart.edu/cgi/viewcontent.cgi?article=1000&context=masterstheses

14. http://journals.lww.com/nscajscr/Abstract/2011/03001/The_Effects_of_Foam_Rolling_on_Myofascial_Release. 45. Aspx

15. http://www.hendricksonmethod.com/wp-content/uploads/2011/07/HMI_BookExerpts.pdf

16. Soft tissue injuries. A guide to prevention and management, Sports Medicine Australia. www.smartplay.com.au.

17. D. Stasinopoulos, M. I. Johnson; Cyriax physiotherapy for tennis elbow/lateral epicondylitis; Br J Sports Med 2004;38:675-677

18. Michael J. Callaghan; The role of massage in the management of the athlete: a review; Physiotherapy Modalities 1993; 27(1)

19. Joseph MF, et al. Deep friction massage to treat tendinopathy: a systematic review of a classic treatment in the face of a new paradigm of understanding. J Sport Rehabil. 2012 Nov; 21 (4): 343-53. Epub 2011 Dec 30.

20. Warren I. Hammer, Functional Soft-Tissue Examination and Treatment d by Manual Methods; 33105_CH22_Hammer.qxd 1/22/07 9:29 AM Page 1

21. Weerapong P[1], Hume PA et al., The mechanisms of massage and effects on performance, muscle recovery and injury prevention. Sports Med. 2005;35(3):235-56

22. César Fernandez-de-las-Penas, Cristina Alonso-Blanco, Josué Fernandez-Carnero, Juan Carlos Miangolarra-Page; The immediate effect of ischemic compression technique and transverse friction massage on tenderness of active and latent myofascial trigger points: a pilot study; Journal of Bodywork and Movement Therapies (2006) 10, 3–9

23. Amit V. Nagrale, Christopher R. Herd, ShyamGanvir and Gopichand Ramteke; Cyriax Physiotherapy Versus Phonophoresis with Supervised Exercise in Subjects with Lateral Epicondylalgia: A Randomized Clinical Trial; Journal of Manual Manipulative Therapy 2009; 17(3): 171–178.

24. Steve De Coninck. Cyriax transverse friction massage supraspinatus. Available from: http://www.youtube.com/watch?v=8CyF6Bl2J3A [last accessed 03/05/13]

25. Whitney Lowe. Deep friction with the thumb on tendons. Available from: http://www.youtube.com/watch?v=LkPUFOkLMOE [last accessed 03/05/13]

26. J.V. Basmajian, Manipulation, Traction and Massage, Williams & Wilkins, Baltimore, Md., 1985. Pp. 211-280

27. F.B. Moor, S.C. Peterson, E.M. Manwell, M.F. Noble and G. Muech, Manual of Hydrotherapy and Massage, Pacific Press Publishing Association, Mountain View, Ca., 1964. Pp. 129-160

28. B.V. Reed, J.M. Held, "Effects of Sequential Connective Tissue Massage on Autonomic Nervous System of Middle-Aged and Elderly Adults," Physical Therapy, 68:8, August 1988. Pp. 1231-1234

29. S.J. Sullivan, L.R.T. Williams, D.E. Seaborne, M. Morelli, "Effects of Massage on Alpha Motoneuron Excitability," Physical Therapy, 71:8, August 1991. Pp. 555-560

30. F.M. Tappan, Healing Massage Techniques: Holistic, Classic, and Emerging Methods, Appleton & Lange, Norwalk, CT, 1988.

31. J.G. Travell and D.G. Simons, Myofascial Pain and Dysfunction, The Trigger Point Manual, Williams & Wilkins, Baltimore, Md., 1983. Pp. 26, 88-89

32. Diamond MP, Hershlag A: Adhesion formation/reformation. In diZerega GS et al., eds.: Treatment of postsurgical adhesions. New York, 1990, Alan R Liss.

33. Drollette CM, Badaway SZA: Pathophysiology of pelvic adhesions. J Reprod Med 1992; 37: 107-121.

# CHAPTER 6
## Anatomy and Biomechanics of Tibio-Femoral joint

## ANATOMY
The knee joint complex comprises three joints:

1. **Tibio-femoral joint**

2. **Patella-femoral joint**

3. **Proximal tibio-fibular joint**

1. **The tibio-femoral joint** is formed by the distal femur and the proximal tibia. The femur consists of two condyles, medial and lateral. The height of the lateral condyle wall is greater along the trochlear groove, which helps prevent lateral subluxation of the patella. The superior surface of the tibia has two asymmetric plateaus separated in the middle by the medial and lateral eminence. The contact surface of the medial surface is twice as large as the lateral surface.

2. **Patella-femoral joint:** it is the articulation between the patella and the femur. It is a triangular sesamoid bone. Patellar tracking refers to the movement of the patella over the femur during flexion and extension of the knee[12]. Optimal tracking is essential for normal mechanics and is considered normal if the apex of the patella is centred in the femoral trochlear groove through all degrees of flexion. [4]

3. **Proximal tibio-fibular joint:** comprises the articulation of the fibular head to the proximal tibia. These joints play an important part in the optimal function of the tibiofemoral joint. The fibular head glides posteriorly on knee flexion and vice versa for the extension. Hence, a restriction of this motion can affect the mobility and the mechanics of the knee joint complex.

## Biomechanics of tibio-femoral joint

Proximal component - Femur (convex femoral condyle)
Distal component - Tibia (proximal concave surface of the tibial plateau)

**Motion:** possible 3-Planar Movements[15]: figure 1 A&B
• Flexion and Extension are Sagittal Plane movements.
• External and Internal Rotations are Transverse Plane movements.
• Abduction and Adduction are Coronal Plane movements.
• Compression-retraction or proximal-distal movement of the joint

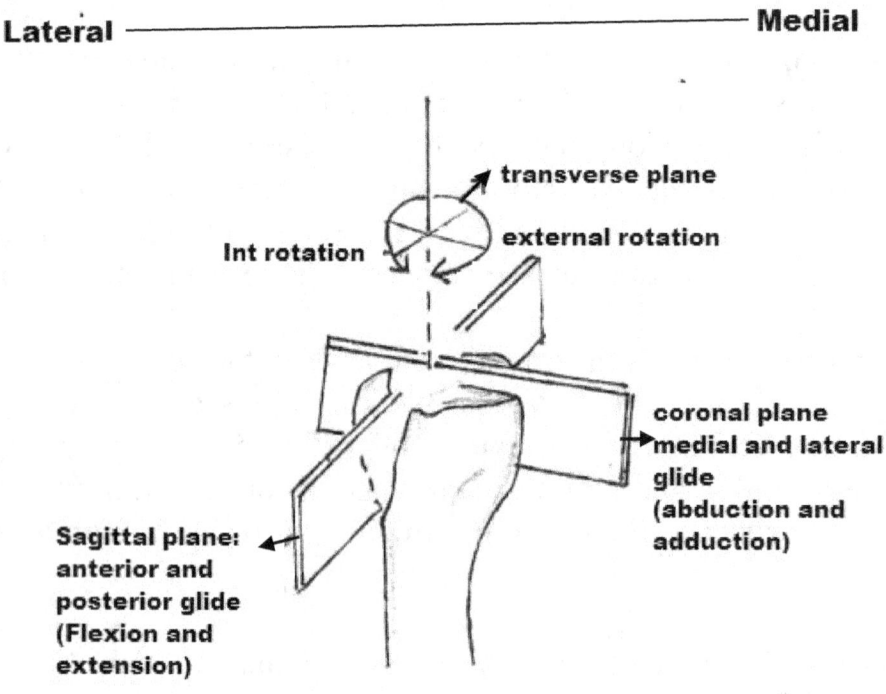

Figure 1 A: Depicts that three dimensional visual clarity on glides of right tibio-femoral joint. Sagittal plane: flexion and extension; coronal plane: medial and lateral glide /abduction and adduction; transverse plane: internal rotation and external rotation.

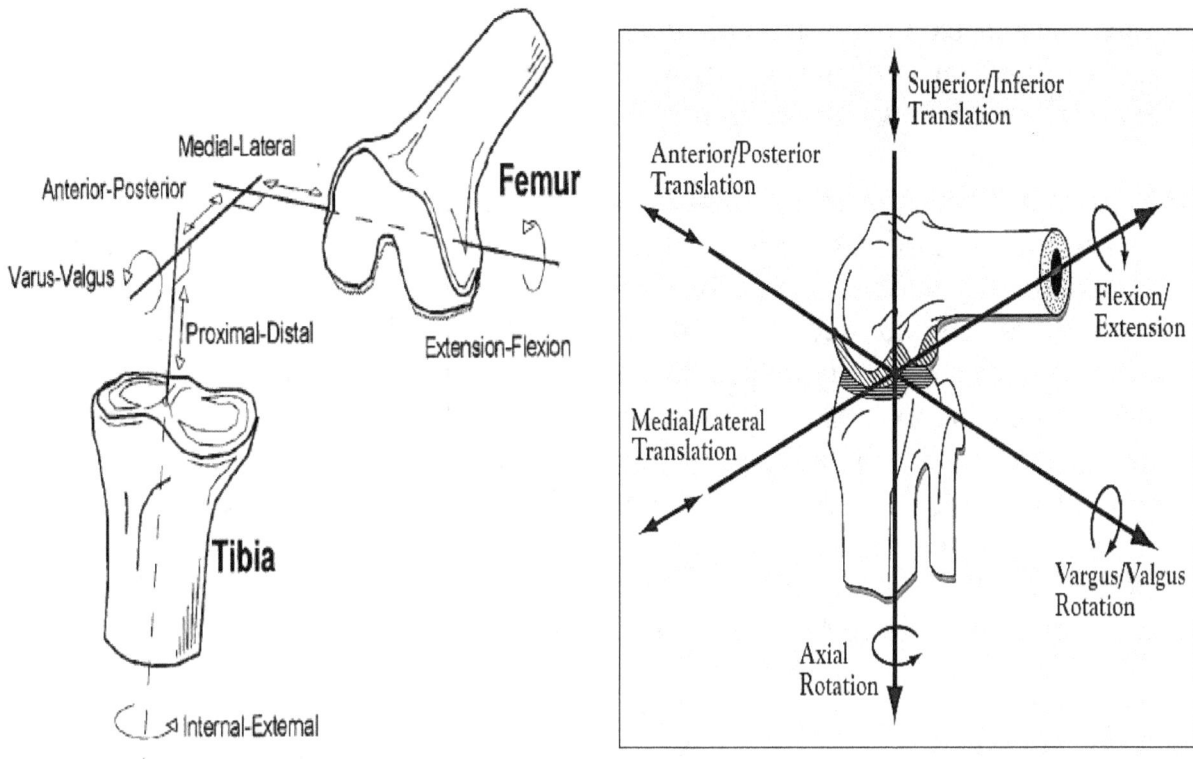

Figure 1B: Schematic diagram illustrating six degrees of motion of the human knee joint; reference from kinematics, in FuFH, Herner CD, Vince KG (edu): knee surgery Baltimore, William & Wilkins, 1994, pp 155-173. In addition to the sagittal, transverse, and coronal planes, this diagram depicts the proximal-distal movement of the knee joint.

## Multiple Degrees of Freedom of knee Joint Motion:

The movement of the knee joint is governed by its ligaments, other supporting soft tissue structures and the geometric constraints of the articular surfaces. The knee can move in six degrees of freedom: three rotations and three translations. The description of knee motion can be accomplished by relating movement to three principal axes: the tibial shaft axis, the epicondylar axis, and the anteroposterior axis, which is perpendicular to the other axes (Fig.1B). Translations along these axes are referred to as proximal-distal, medial-lateral, and anterior-posterior translations, respectively. Rotations about these axes are referred to as internal-external rotation, flexion-extension, and varus-valgus rotation, respectively. [13]

> Flexion and extension are uni-directional sagittal plane movements. Abduction and adduction are uni-directional coronal plane movements. External and internal rotations are uni-directional transverse plane movements.

> Proximal-distal movement/joint compression-retraction: Whenever the Weight-Bearing Axis of the knee joint shifts from the centre, that is, the proximal tibia internally rotates and medially shifts or externally rotates and laterally shifts, then lateral tilt and medial tilt take place respectively along with compression of total joint as total weight shifts to one compartment of the joint. Again, when the weight-bearing axis of the limb comes towards the centre, joint retraction occurs as weight is distributed equally in both compartments. These are evident in weight-bearing close chain movements, for example, the stance phase of the gait cycle. These movements are less important as they are secondary to the position of the weight-bearing axis of the limb and gravity. Once the dysfunction is corrected, the joint retracts to a normal position.

> The glides and rotations of the joint surfaces affect joint mobility. These glides and rotations occur because of the push and pull of soft tissue (muscle, ligaments, and tendons) fibres attached to the bones.

**Note:** the abduction and adduction of the tibia relative to the femur, the concept of abduction of the tibia, go with the medial glide of the proximal tibia. Vice versa, adduction of the tibia goes with the lateral glide of the proximal tibia.

## Laws of Biomechanics[2]:

**Type I** Movement is movement in neutral (neither flexed nor extended). Rotation and side-bending in neutral occur on opposite sides. I.e., the right rotation occurs with the left side bending in neutral.

**Type II** Movement: it is movement in flexion or extension. Rotation and side bending in flexion or extension occurs on the same side. The right rotation occurs with the right side bending in flexion and extension.

Peripheral joints have only Type II movement. There is no Type I movement at the extremity joints.
As we know, the knee is the peripheral joint. Therefore, the movements applicable are type II, whereas both type I and type II movements are applicable in spinal mechanics.

By applying the law on Co-joined Transverse and Coronal Plane Movements of the tibiofemoral joint, it is evident that:

- External Rotation of the proximal tibia always occurs with Adduction (lateral glide).

- Internal Rotation of proximal tibia always occurs with Abduction (medial glide)

- If both internal and external rotation glides are lost, abduction (medial glide) and adduction (lateral glide) will not happen, respectively, as they are a couple of movements.

- The medial and lateral glides are the modified natural coronal plane side bending abduction and adduction motion of the knee.

**Arthrokinematics contrasted with osteokinematics[1, 8]:**

**OSTEOKINEMATIC:** a term, such as abduction or adduction, flexion or extension, observable movements of bones in space. These terms describe the movements that occur around a centre of rotation, namely the joint axis. Joint axis locations are fairly stable, but only because the joint surfaces move in a very specific way; these movements are **gross movements**. They are not in a complete range of motion, as passive movement or terminal glides are excluded.

**ARTHROKINEMATICS:** Unobservable articular accessory motion between adjacent joint surfaces roll, glide, and spin. These accessory motions take place with all active and passive movements. They are necessary for a full, pain-free range of motion[1]. These movements/glides are **more specific** and complete a full range of motion, including passive movements or glides[7].

Arthrokinematic motion cannot occur independently or voluntarily and, if restricted, can limit physiological movement. Movement is necessary to ensure long-term joint integrity. Joint surface movements are sometimes called joint play/glide motions or component motions.

- **Osteokinematics:** i.e. gross movements of bones of tibiofemoral joints[11]
  - Flexion/extension
  - Abduction / adduction
  - Internal rotation / external rotation

> **Arthrokinematics:** specific/Small amplitude motions of the bones at the tibiofemoral joint surface, for example, if we consider it an open kinetic chain.

- Roll and glide: as shown in figure 2(B), posterior roll and glide of the tibia over the femur occur in the same direction when the concave surface tibia moves over the convex surface of the femur during extension to flexion in the sagittal plane.
- The medial glide of the proximal tibia/ abduction of the tibia occurs during extension to flexion in the coronal plane.
- Spin/rotation- internal rotation of proximal tibia occurs during extension to flexion in the transverse plane.

Tibio-femoral Joint surfaces move with respect to one another simultaneously in 3 planar motions. Therefore, the prospective application of arthrokinematics plays an important role in diagnosing and treating dysfunctions over using osteokinematics.

**Arthrokinematics of Tibio-femoral joint:** In flexion and extension of the knee

Extension and flexion of the knee demonstrate a combination of roll-and-glide with spin/rotation according to arthrokinematics.[6, 9]

It is similar to the screw-home" mechanism[3], but in addition, there is lateral glide (adduction) with external rotation and medial glide (abduction) with internal rotation[4].

When viewed in the sagittal plane, the femur's articulating surface is convex while the tibia's in concave[10]. We can predict arthrokinematics glides based on the rules of concavity and convexity. Refer to table 1 and three-dimensional diagrammatic explanations of the mechanics of the tibiofemoral joint in figure 2A and figure 2B

Table 1: Tibio-femoral mechanics in extension and flexion: open chain (sitting on the chair) and close chain kinematics (standing)

| During Knee Extension: in the sagittal plane | | During Knee Flexion: in the sagittal plane | |
|---|---|---|---|
| OPEN CHAIN | CLOSED CHAIN | OPEN CHAIN | CLOSED CHAIN |
| The tibia rolls and glides anteriorly on the stationary femur. (Sagittal plane) | The femur glides posteriorly and rolls anteriorly on the stationary tibia. (Sagittal plane) | The tibia rolls and glides posteriorly on the stationary femur. (Sagittal plane) | The femur glides anteriorly and rolls posteriorly on the stationary tibia. (Sagittal plane) |
| **Knee flexion to full extension: in the transverse and coronal plane** | | **Knee extension to full flexion: in the transverse and coronal plane** | |
| OPEN CHAIN | CLOSED CHAIN | OPEN CHAIN | CLOSED CHAIN |
| The tibia rotates externally (transverse plane) and glides laterally (coronal plane) on the stationary femur. | The femur rotates internally (transverse plane) and glides medially (coronal plane) on the stationary tibia. | The tibia rotates internally (transverse plane) and glides medially (in the coronal plane) on the stationary femur. | The femur rotates externally (transverse plane) and glides laterally (in the coronal plane) on a stationary tibia. |
| **Proximal-distal movement/joint compression-distraction** | | | |
| -in the gait cycle, when the weight-bearing axis of the limb shifts from the centre, that is, when the proximal tibia internally rotates and medially shifts, it leads the WBA of the limb to shift laterally. That, in turn, tilts laterally, along with overall compression of the joint, takes place. Or when the proximal tibia externally rotates and laterally shifts, leading the WBA of the limb to shift medially with medial tilt, along with that overall compression of the joint. Again, joint retraction occurs when the limb's WBA shifts to the centre. These are evident in weight-bearing close chain movements. | | | |

**Note: External/internal rotation during the walking cycle:** [6,14]
A recent study found that screw-home movement occurred as expected during the pre-swing phase and late-swing at a phase angle of about 17°. However, the tibia rotated externally with respect to the femur rather than internally. At the same time, the knee joint started to flex during the loading response (paradoxical screw-home movement[13]), and the angle was 6°.

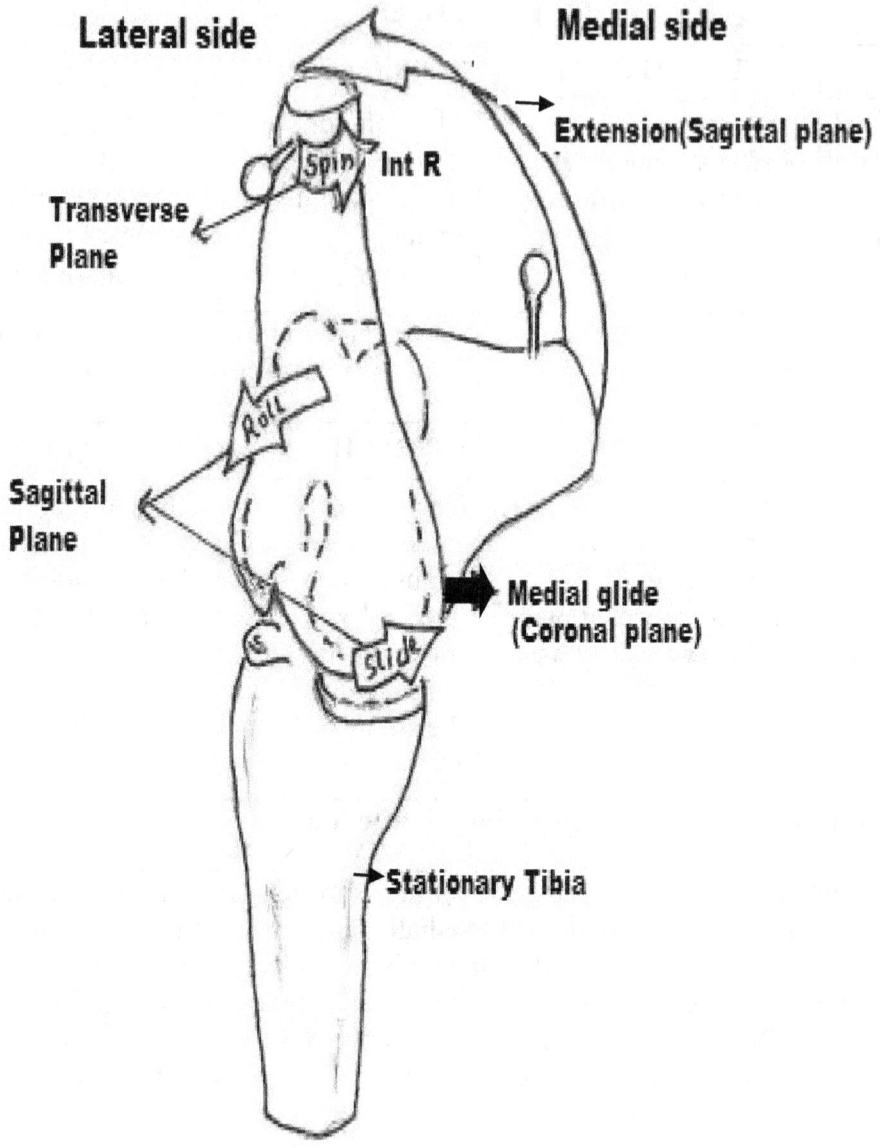

**Figure 2(A) CLOSE CHAIN (sitting to standing) MECHANICS OF KNEE FROM FLEXION TO EXTENSION:** Femoral convex on Tibial concave – rolling occur anteriorly and gliding occurs posteriorly in opposite direction in the sagittal plane. The distal femur internally rotates and medially shifts/glides in transverse and coronal planes respectively.

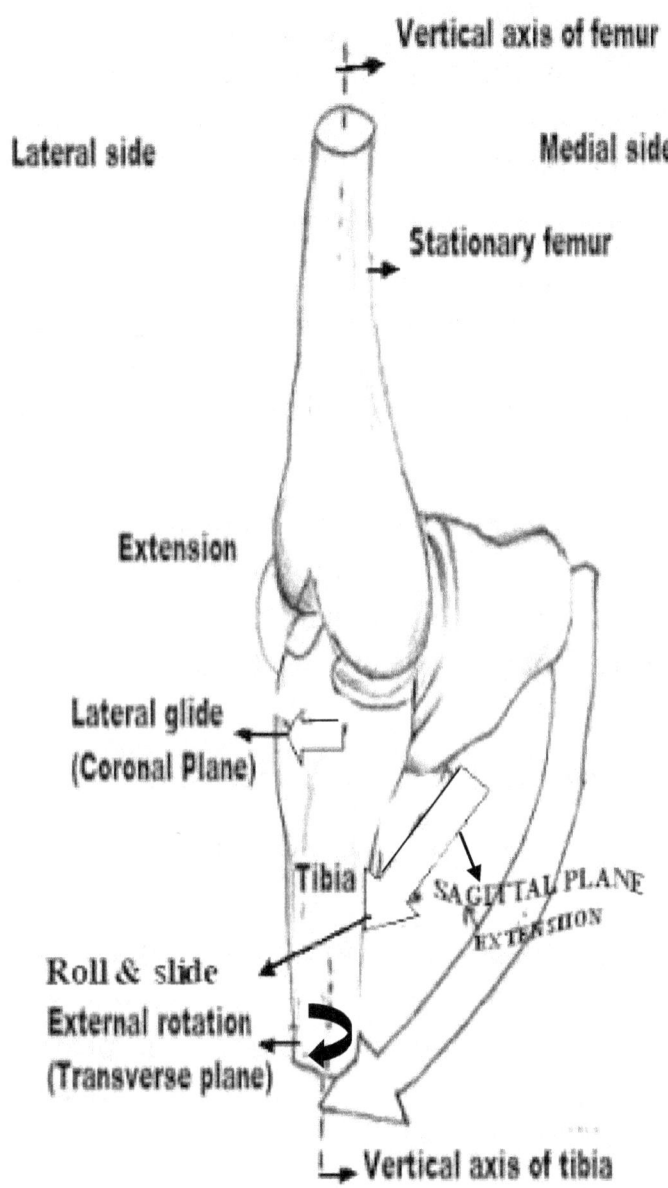

Figure 2(B) OPEN CHAIN MECHANICS OF KNEE FROM FLEXION TO EXTENSION: Tibial concave on femoral convex - roll and glide occur towards anterior that is the same direction in the sagittal plane. The proximal tibia externally rotates and laterally shifts/glides in transverse and coronal planes, respectively.

## Mechanics of tibiofemoral joint in both close-chain and open-chain

### 1. Close chain mechanics (sitting to standing), from knee flexion to extension[5]:

The Tibia (concave surface) is stationary, and the femur (convex surface) is movable. According to the concave and convex rule[10], when the convex surface moves over the concave surface, roll and glide occur in the opposite direction; when the concave surface moves over the convex surface, roll and glide occur in the same direction.

Figure 2(A) shows the close chain mechanics of the tibiofemoral joint from flexion to extension. Femoral (convex) on Tibial (concave)- rolling occurs anteriorly, and gliding occurs posteriorly in opposite directions in the sagittal plane. The distal femur internally rotates and medially shifts/glides in the transverse and coronal planes.

Vice versa, during closed chain mechanics of the tibiofemoral joint from extension to flexion of the knee (standing to sit): the femur (convex) on the tibia (concave)- rolling occurs posteriorly, and gliding occurs anteriorly in the opposite direction in the sagittal plane. The distal femur externally rotates and laterally shifts/glides in the transverse and coronal planes.

### 2. Open chain mechanics, from knee flexion to extension:

The femur (convex surface) is stationary, and the tibia (concave surface) is movable

Figure 2(B), open-chain mechanics of tibio-femoral joint from flexion to extension. Tibia (concave) on the femur (convex) - rolling and gliding occur anteriorly in the same directions in the sagittal plane. The proximal tibia rotates externally and laterally shifts/glides in transverse and coronal planes.

Vice versa during open chain mechanics of the tibiofemoral joint from extension to flexion of the knee, tibia (concave) on the femur (convex): rolling and gliding occur posteriorly in the same directions in the sagittal plane. The proximal tibia internally rotates and medially shifts/glides in the transverse and coronal planes.

## References:

1. Edward P. Mulligan Principles of Joint Mobilization. https://www.physio-pedia.com/images/c/c0/Principles_of_Joint_Mobilization.pdf
2. Sharon, Thomas, et al., Integrative manual therapy for upper and lower extremities, 2008, p 153
3. Screw home echanism, http://www.orthopaedicsone.com/display/Main/Screw-home+mechanism
4. Zappala FG, Taffel CB, Scuderi GR. Rehabilitation of patella-femoral joint disorders. Orth ClinNorth Am. 1992;23 (4): 557.
5. http://blog.nasm.org/uncategorized/knee-biomechanics-screw-home-rotation/
6. https://www.youtube.com/watch?v=YokLbe0v29E
7. Kaltenborn, F.M.(1989).Manual mobilization of the extremity joints (4 Th Ed.). Minneapolis:OPT:http://coph.ouhsc.edu/dthompso/web/namics/arthkin.htm
8. Arthro-kinematic vs osteo-kinematic movements, https://www.youtube.com/watch?v=yPUR4KY6DFc\
9. Arthrokinematics, http://www.physio-pedia.com/Arthrokinematics
10. Jochen schomacher, the convex-concave rule and the lever law, Manual Therapy 14 (2009) 579–582
11. Osteokinematics, arthrokinemaics and kinetics; http://www.mccc.edu/~behrensb/documents/BiomechanicsKineticsCh1.pdf
12. Mandelaum BR, et al. The patella functions to minimize friction and improve the leverage of the quadriceps mechanism, and acts as a protective layer for the femoral condyle cartilage. Articular cartilage lesions of the knee. Am J sports Med. 1998;26;853-61.
13. Savio L-Y. Woo, PhD, Richard E. Debski, PhD, John D. Withrow, and Marsie A. Janaushek. Biomechanics of Knee Ligaments. The American journal of sports medicine, Vol. 27, No. 4 © 1999 American Orthopaedic Society for Sports Medicine.
14. ha yong kim, md, kap Jung Kim, MD, Dae Suk Yang, MD,Sang Wook Jeung, MD, Han Gyeol Choi, MD, Won Sik Choy, MD. Screw-Home Movement of the Tibiofemoral Joint during Normal Gait: Three-Dimensional Analysis. Clinics in Orthopedic Surgery 2015;7:303-309
15. M. A. lafortune,t p. r. cavanagh, j. sommer, a. kalenak. three-dimensional kinematics of the human knee during walking*. j. &mechanics vol. 25, no. 4, pp. 347-357. 1992.

# CHAPTER 7
## Tibio-Femoral Joint: Its Dysfunctions and Pathomechanics

Figure 1: Pathomechanics of KNEE JOINT DYSFUNCTIONS - Gross

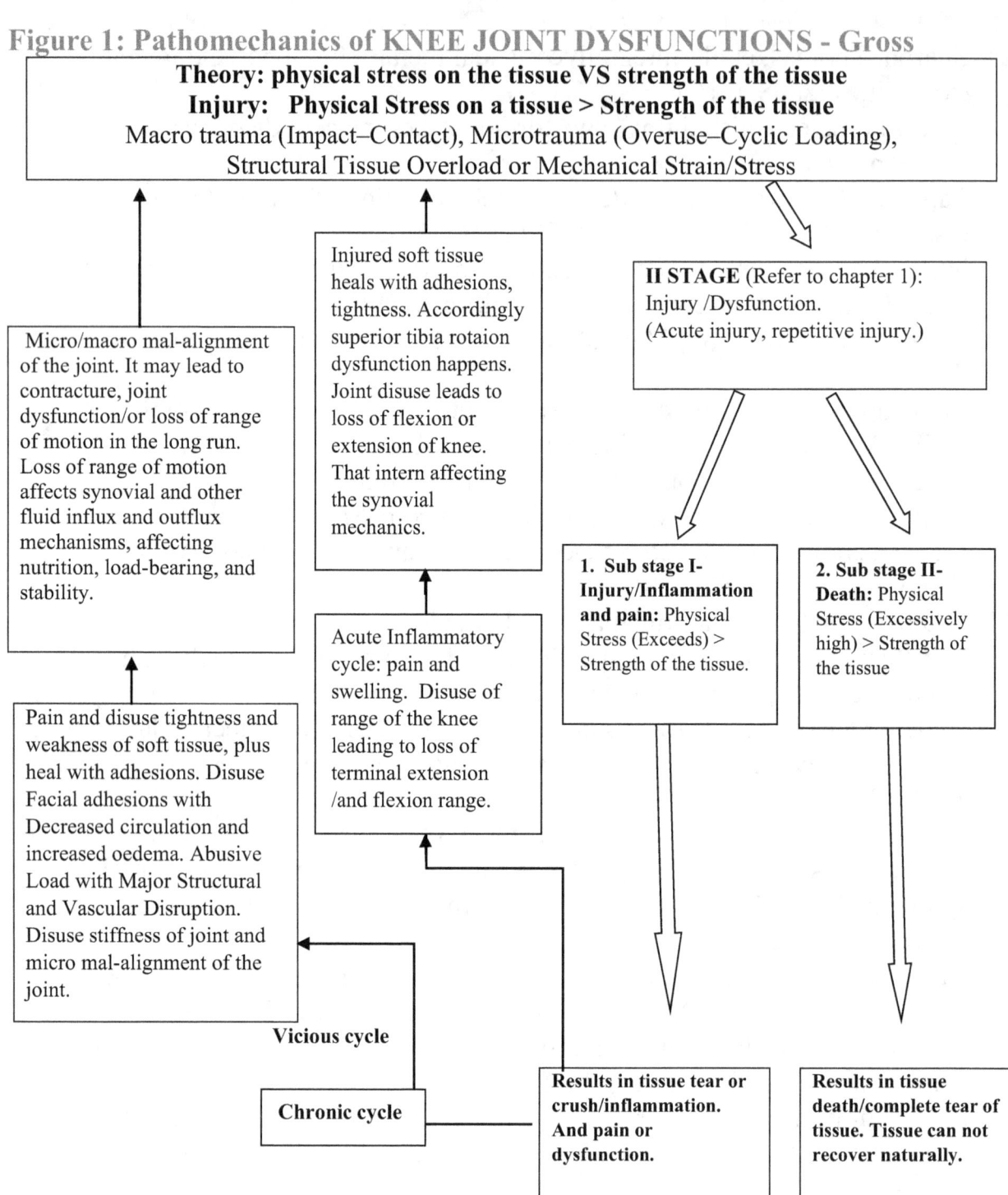

A summary of the above flow chart reveals the **general pathomechanics of Tibio-femoral joint dysfunction**:

According to chapter 1, the II stage is described as the stage of injury/dysfunction of the knee tissue based on the relationship between physical stress acting on the tissue vs strength of the tissue. In this stage, relative physical stress on the tissue is (always greater than) > tissue strength, resulting in tissue injury/dysfunction.

Physical stress could be in the form of micro-trauma, like gradual overuse, or macro-trauma, like sudden excessive load in the form of impact/contact form of sports injuries, which may result in tissue tear or crush, which leads to pain and inflammation. As the pain increases, the patient subconsciously or consciously starts gradually disusing the terminal range, either flexion or extension. That, in turn, leads to disuse of the terminal range of motion; if it is not diagnosed and treated early, it may lead to more loss of joint range. That is why most arthritis patients have knee dysfunction with loss of terminal flexion and extension.

Loss of range of the joint leads to loss of the pressure gradient inside the joint, which affects the fluid exchange, mainly synovial fluid influx and outflux of the joint. If joint range and movements are not restored early, it may lead to arthritic changes.

Disuse of the joint leads to disuse weakness and/or tightness of the soft tissue surrounding the knee joint. After the injury, the affected soft tissue surrounding the joint heals with adhesions. According to the soft tissue, adhesions and tightness, tibial torsion occurs, leading to misalignment.

If post-injury dysfunction is not addressed in a timely manner, it may decrease the strength of the knee joint tissue, i.e., further weakening of the tissue, and may fall into a (chronic dysfunction) viscous cycle.

The above flow chart of pathomechanics of knee dysfunction assists a novice physiotherapist in accurately diagnosing and treating knee joint dysfunction.

## Pathomechanics of tibio-femoral joint dysfunction: arthrokinematic analysis

To accurately diagnose the specific Tibio-femoral joint dysfunction, it is important to predict the associated pathomechanics of dysfunction. The therapist needs to know the important mechanics associated with it.

Tibio-femoral joint surfaces move in three planes in order to achieve the required normal range of motion. If the knee joint surface rolls on its partner without simultaneously sliding and spinning, the surfaces would separate [1](gap or subluxate) and impinge in others (compensate) to complete the range; it may be called a trick movement. Therefore, roll, glide, and spin must occur simultaneously to preserve joint integrity. Therefore, range of motion, diagnosis with spring test, and treatment with manual therapy should be done simultaneously in three planes for accuracy. There are mainly flexed and extended knee joint dysfunctions[2].

Three-dimensional Physiological movements of the Tibio-femoral joint include:
1. Flexion and extension occur in the sagittal plane.
2. Internal and external rotation occurs in the transverse plane.
3. Medial (abduction of the tibia) and lateral glide (adduction of the tibia)/shift occurs in the coronal plane.

Medial and lateral glide/shifts are modified, and the knee's natural coronal plane side bending (abduction and adduction) motions.

Co-joined Transverse and Coronal Plane Movements of Tibio-femoral joint:
• External Rotation of the proximal tibia always occurs with Adduction (lateral glide).
• Internal Rotation of proximal tibia always occurs with Abduction (medial glide)
If there is a loss of internal rotation and external rotation, then abduction (medial glides) and adduction (lateral glides) will not happen, respectively, as they are coupled movements.

If physical stress applied over the tissue is more than the strength of the tissue, it results in injury. Patients start disusing the terminal range because of the pain and inflammation, resulting in extension and flexion lag. Injured soft tissue, which later heals with adhesion/tightness, will lead to proximal tibia rotational dysfunctions. If external rotators of the tibia (TFL, vastus lateralis, lateral gastrocnemius, and Bicep femoris) are involved, they heal with adhesion/tightness. Because of the anatomical position of soft tissue, the proximal tibia is externally rotated and laterally pulled, putting the knee in varus stress (figure 3). In the same way, when internal rotators (pes ansaris, popliteal, semimembranosus) are involved, they will lead to the proximal tibia being internally rotated and medially pulled, putting a knee in valgus stress (figure 2).

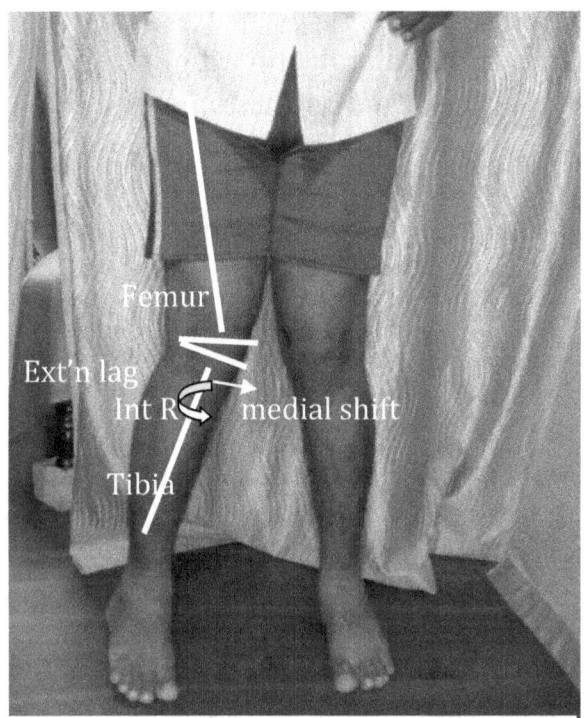

Figure 2: When internal rotators of the tibia heal with adhesions, they will rotate the proximal tibia internally and pull medially, putting the knee in valgus stress.

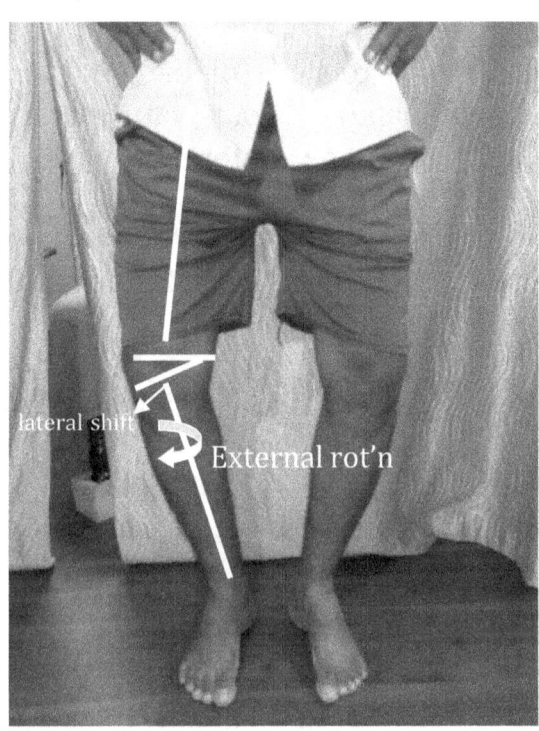

Figure 3: When external rotators of the tibia heal with adhesions they will rotate the proximal tibia externally and pull laterally, putting the knee in varus stress.

## Dysfunctions of Tibio-femoral joint:
Normal biomechanics of the knee joint are altered when there is dysfunction.

## Possible dysfunction of the Tibio-femoral joint will be as follows:
(Refer to figure 4)

1. **Extension lag**: The knee is flexed, i.e., the knee can not extend completely. It also indicates proximal tibia stuck posterior. That is anterior glide loss (in the sagittal plane)
2. **Flexion lag**: The knee is extended, i.e., the knee can not flex completely. It also indicates proximal tibia stuck anterior. That is posterior glide loss (in the sagittal plane)
3. **Flexion and extension lag:** The knee can not completely flex or extend. The proximal tibia can not glide to terminal extension or flexion, Indicating both anterior and posterior glide loss.

**1. Extension lag**: Extension lag occurs because of the dysfunction of one or more components of three planar motions of the tibio-femoral joint. The possible dysfunctions would be as follows:

**Extensions lag with proximal tibia**:

a) Externally rotated (in the transverse plane) and lateral shifted/glide (in the coronal plane). It puts varus pressure on the knee, and in the long run, it may lead to varus knee deformity[3,4]

b) Internally rotated (in the transverse plane) with medial shift/glide (in the coronal plane). It puts valgus pressure on the knee, which may lead to valgus knee in the long run.

c) Both internal, external rotation and medial, lateral glide loss

**2. Flexion lag:** Flexion lag occurs because of the dysfunction of one or more components of the three planar motions of the knee. The possible dysfunction would be as follows:

**Flexion lag with proximal tibia:**

a) Externally rotated (in the transverse plane) with lateral shifted/glide (in the coronal plane).

b) Internally rotated (in the transverse plane) with medial shifted/glide (in the coronal plane).

c) Both internal, external rotation and medial, lateral glide loss.

**3. Both flexion and extension lag:**

The knee can not completely flex or completely extend in these dysfunctions. The proximal tibia can not glide completely in extension and flexion. It is stuck in the mid-range. Therefore, both Extension lag and Flexion lag dysfunctions are included in these dysfunctions.

Figure 4: Flow chart depicting the pathomechanics of possible specific Tibio-femoral joint dysfunctions.

**Pathomechanics: Tibio-femoral joint dysfunctions (specific)**

- **Extension lag**
- **Flexion lag**
- **Flexion and extension lag:** Extension and flexion lag dysfunctions are included. -As an extension lag component will come into play during the weight-bearing cycle of the gait, abnormal forces like varus or valgus will be there, according to proximal tibial rotation.

**The knee is flexed/extension lag.**

**Proximal tibia at the end of the extension lag:** possible dysfunctions
-if soft tissue such as external rotators of the tibia(TFL, bicep femoris, vastus lateralis, lateral gastrocnemius) are involved in the injury, they heal with adhesions and become tight that intern pulls the proximal tibia externally and shifts laterally because of the anatomical position.
Externally rotated with lateral shifted proximal tibia will put varus pressure on the knee and lead to varus knee in the long run.
- If soft tissue such as internal rotators(pes ansaris, semimembranous, popliteus) are involved in the injury, they heal with adhesions and become tight that intern pulls the proximal tibia into internal rotation and shifts medially because of the anatomical position. That puts valgus pressure on the knee, and in the long run, it leads to valgus knee.
If internal and external rotators are involved, both internal and external rotation loss and medial and lateral glide will also be lost. There is no medial or lateral glide of the proximal tibia, so there will not be any varus or valgus force on the knee; therefore, there is no deformity. Only apparent limb length decreases compared to the normal leg as there is severe extension loss.

**The Knee is extended/flexion lag.**

**Proximal tibia at the end of the flexion lag:** possible dysfunctions

-If it is stuck in an externally rotated with lateral shift/glide.
-If it is stuck in Internally rotated with medial shift/glide.
-If there is a loss of both internal and external rotation, then medial and lateral glide also will be lost, respectively.

These dysfunctions do not contribute to varus or vagus knee as they will not occur during the weight bearing cycle of the gait.

**Pathomechanics of knee joint dysfunctions to deformities (Varus and Valgus knee):**

In this section, step-by-step pathomechanics of knee dysfunction to deformities can be analyzed.
The main deformities of the knee are varus, valgus, and knee recurvatum[10]. Each deformity has different step-by-step pathomechanics from knee dysfunctions.

**Dysfunctions** of the knee are **1. Extension lag 2. Flexion lag 3. Both flexion and extension lag**. Moreover, major knee dysfunctions are **varus**[3]**, valgus and knee recurvatum.**

The chapter deals with the in-depth pathomechanics of the varus and valgus knee, as they play an important role in the lower limbs, both above and below the kinetic chain. And in-depth pathomechanics of knee recurvatum is out of the book's scope.

The possible dysfunctions of the tibiofemoral joint are extension lag, flexion lag, or both flexion and extension lag.
The knee has three planar motions, either from extension to flexion or flexion to extension: anterior/posterior roll and glide in the sagittal plane, external/internal rotation in the transverse plane, and lateral/medial glides in the coronal plane. Roll, glide and spin/rotation must occur simultaneously to preserve joint integrity. Suppose roll, glide, and spin/rotation do not occur simultaneously in the required order. In that case, there will be compensatory /trick movement (subluxation of joint: compression in one compartment and gapping in another) to complete terminal flexion or extension[1]. In a gait cycle (figure 10), weight-bearing on the knee occurs in the stance phase. Knee flexion occurs during the swing phase of the gait cycle, which is a non-weight-bearing part. Because of this reason, knee flexion dysfunctions will not contribute to the deformity.
In the above-said dysfunctions of the knee, varus and valgus forces act in the weight-bearing part of the gait cycle, which is the stance phase. When these extension lag dysfunctions fall in the knee extension range, the knee compensates or does the trick movement to complete the terminal extension in the gait cycle. Depending on the dysfunction, varus or valgus forces act on the knee because of the trick movement and soft tissue adhesions, contributing to rotational dysfunction of the tibia. Thus, knee dysfunctions, especially extension lag, must be diagnosed early and treated as early as possible.

# Chapter 7: Tibio-Femoral joint: Its dysfunctions and Pathomechanics

**Analyses of pathomechanics from simple knee extension lag dysfunction to varus and valgus knee:**

For clarity and better understanding, the pathomechanics of knee dysfunction are analysed in an open kinetic chain from flexion to extension.

As the most common knee dysfunction is Extension lag: Analysis of pathomechanics from dysfunction to deformity

**Extension lag:** It can happen because of the dysfunction of one or more components of three planar motions of the knee. Possible dysfunction would be as follows: (Refer to figure 7)

**Extension lag with proximal tibia:**
**a) If stuck in an externally rotated (in the transverse plane) with laterally shifted/glide (in the coronal plane): Refer to figures 6 and 9**
In this dysfunction, the weight-bearing axis of the limb shifts medially. During the weight-bearing stance phase, In order to complete the knee extension, there will be compensatory/trick movement of the knee joint wherein lateral joint space increases and medial joint space decreases, creating a medial tilt (medial sloping of the joint surfaces), which in turn creates varus force on the knee. Therefore, early assessment and timely treatment can prevent chronic deformity of the knee (varum[5] knee arthritis).

**b) If stuck in internally rotated (in the transverse plane) with medially shifted/glide (in the coronal plane). Refer to figures 5 and 8**
In this dysfunction, the weight-bearing axis of the limb shifts laterally. During the weight-bearing stance phase. To complete the terminal knee extension, there will be compensatory/trick movement of the knee joint wherein medial joint space increases and lateral joint space decreases, creating a lateral tilt (lateral sloping of the joint surface), which in turn creates a valgus force on the knee. Therefore, early assessment and timely treatment can prevent chronic deformity of the knee[6, 7] (valgus knee arthritis).

**c)    Internal, external rotation, and medial, lateral glides loss:** There is no option for compensatory/trick movement (compression at one compartment and gapping at one compartment), so there will not be any deformity. However, limb length will get shorter when compared to normal limbs, and there will be more extension lag while walking. Therefore, patients will limp to the short side.

# Chapter 7: Tibio-Femoral joint: Its dysfunctions and Pathomechanics

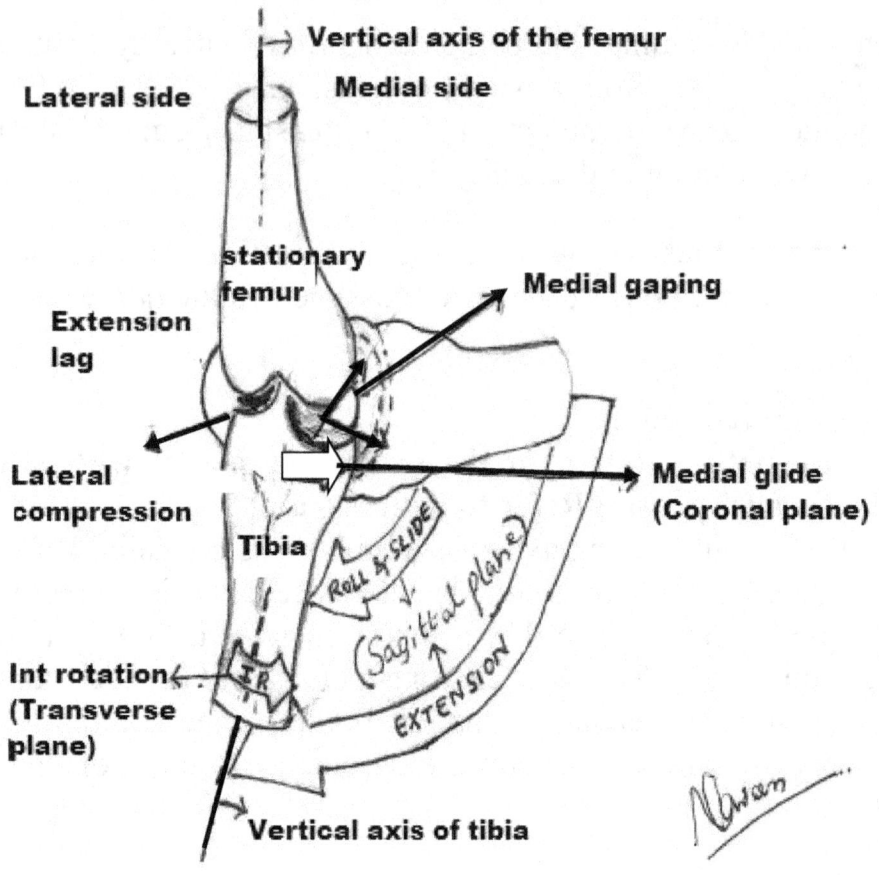

Figure 5: **Right knee extension lag dysfunction (valgus force):** with proximal tibia internally rotated (in the transverse plane) with medially shifted (in the coronal plane). To complete the extension during the gait cycle of the stance phase. There will be compensatory /trick movement of the proximal tibia/lower femur to compress at the lateral compartment and the gap at the medial compartment. Which in turn creates a valgus force at the knee.

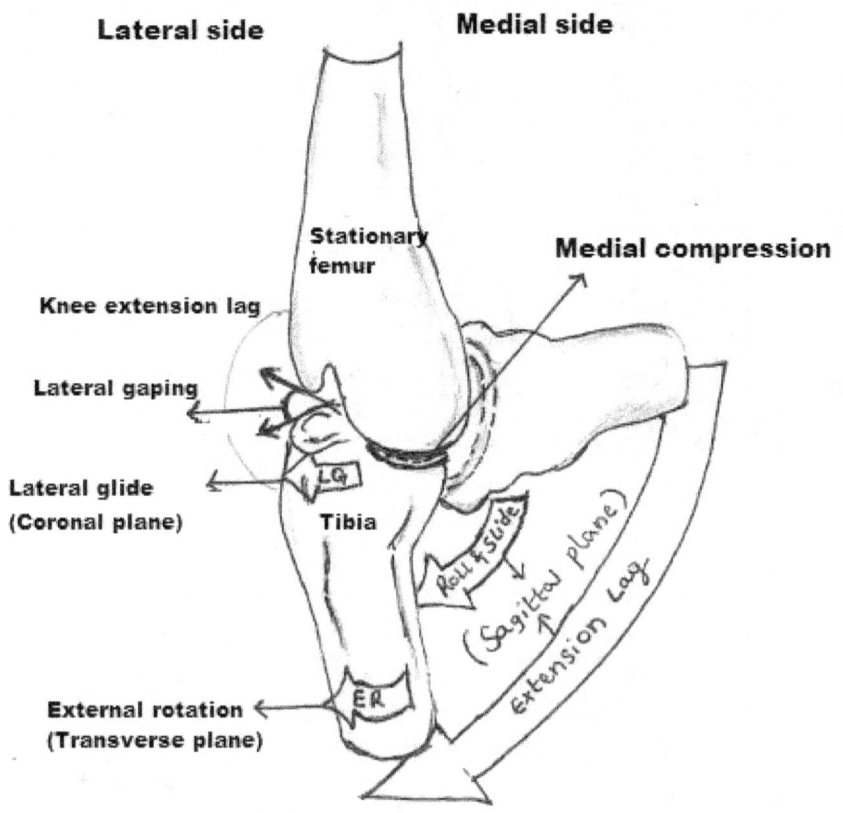

Figure 6: **Right knee extension lag dysfunction (varus force):** with proximal tibia externally rotated (in the transverse plane) and laterally shifted (in the coronal plane) to complete the extension during the gait cycle of the stance phase. There will be compensatory /trick movement of the knee joint, compression at the medial compartment and gapping at the lateral compartment, creating a varus force at the knee.

# Chapter 7: Tibio-Femoral joint: Its dysfunctions and Pathomechanics 150

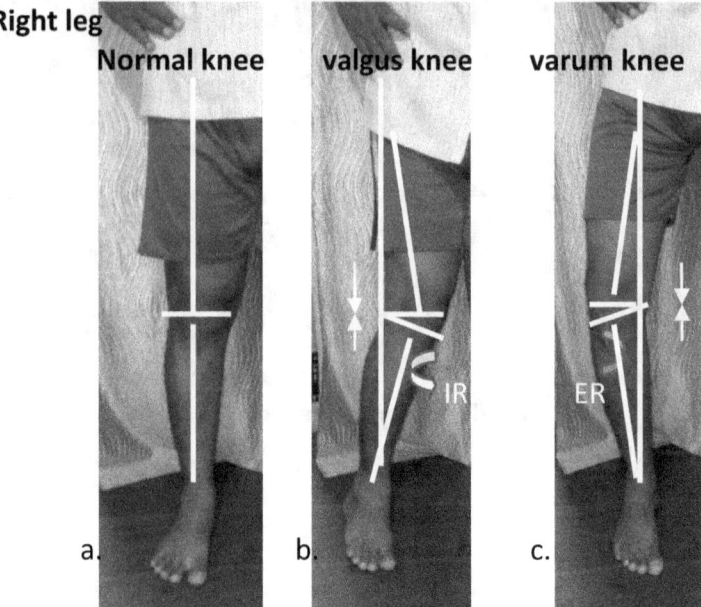

Figure 7: Depicting the a. right normal leg, b. valgus knee and c. varus knee. The vertical line represents the Weight-Bearing Axis of the knee.

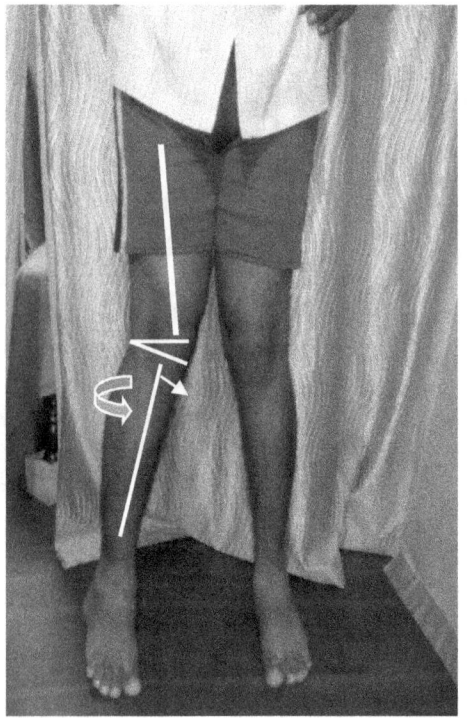

Figure 8: Valgus knee- proximal tibia internally rotated, and medial shifted with medial gapping and lateral compression of the joint.

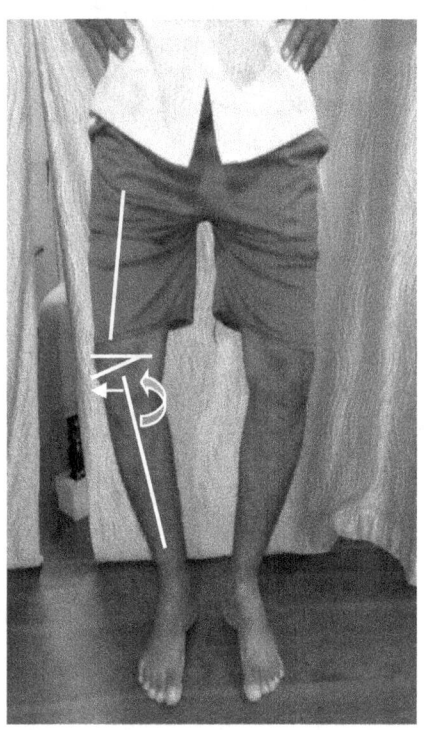

Figure 9: Varus knee- proximal tibia externally rotated and laterally shifted with lateral gapping and medial compression of the joint.

## Pathomechanics of Varus and Valgus knee: from Gait analysis

The author proposes varus and valgus knee pathomechanics from knee extension lag dysfunctions. It can be clearly analyzed by applying knee extension lag dysfunctions in the gait cycle. If we consider the gait cycle[24], the major extension range of the knee happens in the stance phase, from $0^0$ of knee extension to $20^0$ of flexion, the stance phase of the gait cycle where load-bearing takes place (figure 10). This analysis is crucial for analysing the pathomechanics of knee dysfunctions/deformities arising from extension lag. The left leg is depicted in a dark colour, and the gait cycle [11-13] progresses from the left side to the right, as the arrow indicates. The gait cycle starts with the initial contact of the stance phase, where the knee is flexed to $0^0$-$5^0$ and progresses up to the terminal stance phase, at heel off knee extends about $0^0$-$5^0$.[25] During foot flat, the knee is flexed about $15^0$-$20^0$; therefore, the weight-bearing gait cycle uses a total extension range of $0^0$-$20^0$.

Knee extension lag with proximal tibia internally rotated and medially shifted dysfunction, wherein the limb's weight-bearing axis starts shifting towards the joint's lateral compartment (figure 7b). Moreover, medial joint gapping and lateral compression occur to complete the terminal extension during the gait cycle, creating a valgus force on the knee. (as shown in figure 8)

In the same way, knee extension lag with the proximal tibia externally rotated and laterally shifted, wherein the weight-bearing axis of the limb starts shifting towards the medial compartment of the joint( figure 7c). Moreover, lateral joint gapping and medial compression occur to complete the terminal extension during the gait cycle, creating a varus force on the knee. (as shown in figure 9)

In knee extension dysfunction, medial and lateral glides are automatically lost if both internal and external rotation are equally lost. The weight-bearing axis of the limb remains at the centre, and there is no chance of trick movement (compression or gapping) to complete the terminal range; therefore, severe extension lag will happen.

Suppose only knee joint flexion lag dysfunction is present when it is analysed from the gait cycle. In that case, it is evident that only 0° to 60° of the flexion range of motion is utilized in the swing phase of the gait cycle, which is a non-weight-bearing part of the gait cycle, so there is no need for compensatory/trick movement to complete the range. Hence, flexion lag dysfunctions of the knee show that no valgus or varus forces will come into play.

Dysfunction of the knee where there is extension lag with the proximal tibia externally rotating and laterally shifting or internally rotating and medially shifting; in either case, overall joint compression takes place in addition to tilt. Once the dysfunction is corrected, joint retraction takes place.

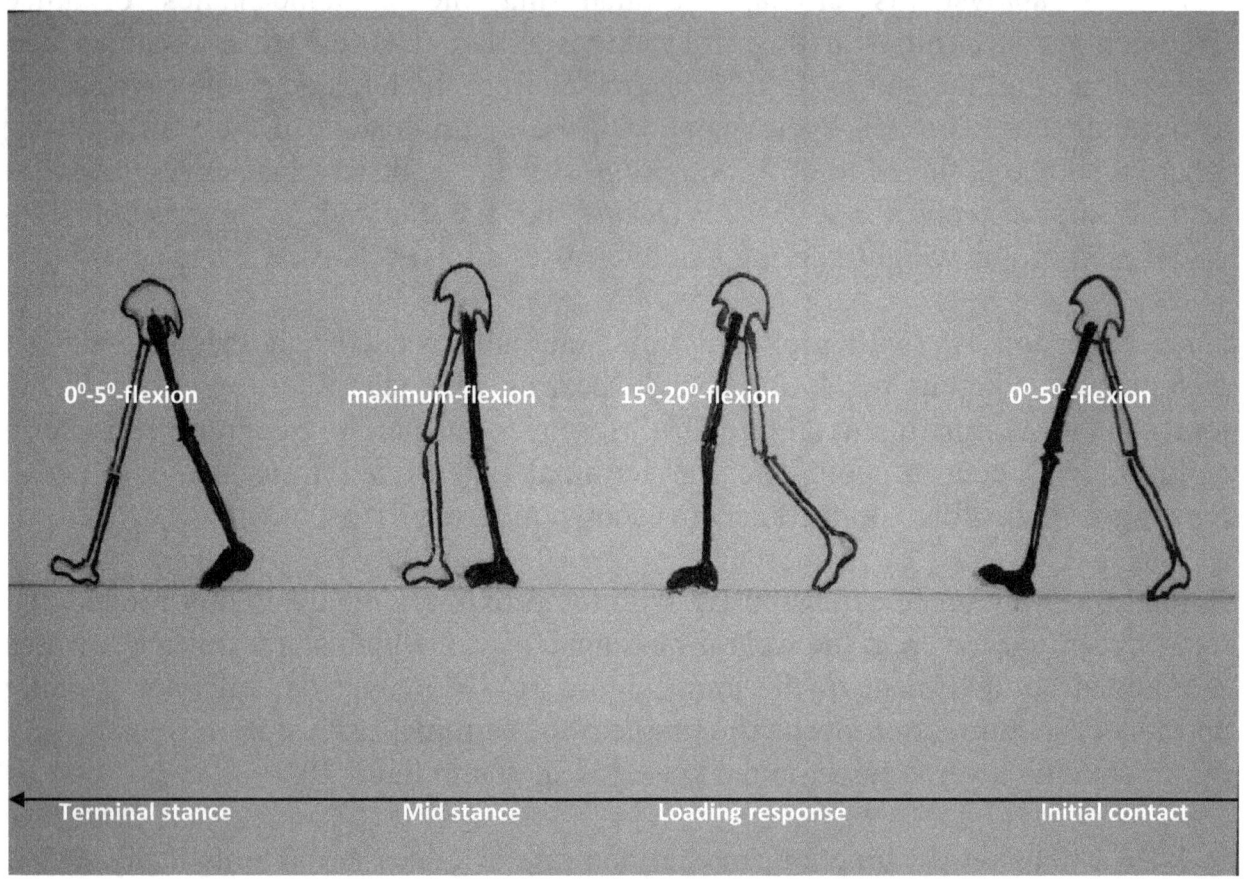

Figure 10: Left knee range (dark colour leg) of motion during the weight-bearing stance phase of the gait cycle.

**Note:** There is compensatory/trick movement in knee extension lag dysfunctions during the weight-bearing phase of the gait cycle and the running, standing and jumping phases of weight-bearing. The impact of trick movement will be more in weight-bearing, running and jumping phases, as the ground reaction force is greater than the gait cycle.

## Analyses of pathomechanics from simple knee /foot/soft tissue dysfunction to knee recurvatum:

In lower-limb deformity patient populations, one of the greatest impediments to energy-efficient ambulation is the development of a genu recurvatum deformity. When this deviation occurs, the thigh and lower limb segments move posteriorly in direct opposition to the anterior advancement of the proximal body mass over the fixed distal base of support. Genu recurvatum is usually an acquired deformity secondary to changes in the distal skeletal joint alignments and compensatory movement patterns. The alignment of the distal base of support determines the load-bearing and functional motion available to the proximal knee joint during ambulation and can either serve to promote or disrupt the required sagittal plane limb advancement[9].

Numerous causes of genu recurvatum are cited in the literature, including plantar flexion contracture, triceps surae spasticity, quadriceps weakness, limb-length discrepancy, and hip extensor weakness[10-13]. Any postural adjustment developed to achieve limb stability and prevent anterior knee collapse may also influence the genesis of this type of deformity.

Unopposed, a posteriorly directed Hyperextension moment may progress into severe deformation. Genu recurvatum deformity refers to a sustained posterior deviation of the knee joint occurring throughout the loading period, from initial contact through forward progression[14]

Some books and research proposed that based on the mechanical loading patterns of the foot and ankle complex, three distinct types of genu recurvatum are identified. The two most common types involve significant transverse plane alignment characterized by excessive external or internal rotation of the talocrural joint axis, with secondary knee joint deviation and axis misalignments. The third type of genu recurvatum is uniplanar and presents with sagittal plane involvement in which compensatory talocrural joint Dorsiflexion loss accompanies the primary knee joint deviation. These three presentations are referred to as external rotatory deformity recurvatum (ERD recurvatum), internal rotatory deformity recurvatum (IRD recurvatum), and non-rotatory deformity recurvatum (NRD recurvatum), respectively[15, 16].

As per clinical experience, case studies, and new pathomechanics proposed in this book, external and internal rotator dysfunction/deformity of the foot with knee extension lag will also contribute to varus and valgus knee.

Knee alignment is influenced by both the alignment of the pelvis and hips above and the ankle and foot below. People who stand with their knees locked out often have an anteriorly tilted pelvis and increased lumbar lordosis. Anterior tilting of the pelvis causes relative flexion of the hip. The flexed position of the hip is countered by extension of the knee, leading to a hyperextended posture. These postural changes can be caused by weak glute and core muscles and tight hip flexors[21].

**Talo-crural joint dysfunction leading to knee recurvatum:**

It is rare that recurvatum deformities present as single-plane involvements. Still, traumatic injuries or unique circumstances can produce a primary sagittal plane deviation of the knee joint with compensatory talo-crural joint dorsiflexion loss or plantar flexed foot[19] (Figure 11A). In this case, the foot and ankle complex is not specifically affected, and the integrity of the anterior-lateral and anterior-medial fore-foot levers remain intact. While the hindfoot remains vertical during loading, the posterior lever decreases as the proximal knee joint deviation progresses posteriorly. Load-bearing stress to the posterior soft tissue structures increases with each degree of continued deformation as the moment arm incrementally increases. The single-plane involvement does not involve excessive transverse plane deviations of the trans- malleolar or knee joint axes and is referred to as the third type of genu recurvatum or non-rotary deformity (NRD) recurvatum.

As shown in Figure 11A, an NRD recurvatum is a uniplanar deformity. Significant sagittal plane recurvatum is noted with no coronal plane deviation. The talo-calcaneal alignment and angle are within normal limits.

Below the knee, the talus shifts to the anterior at the ankle, causing the ankles to remain slightly plantar flexed[20]. Collapsing the arch at the foot level and related weakness of the arch-supporting muscles can also be a factor. As shown in Figure 11A, the foot has increased plantar flexion, which is compensated by hyper knee extension in standing. Meanwhile, in Figure 11B, the foot has normal plantar flexion and normal knee extension.

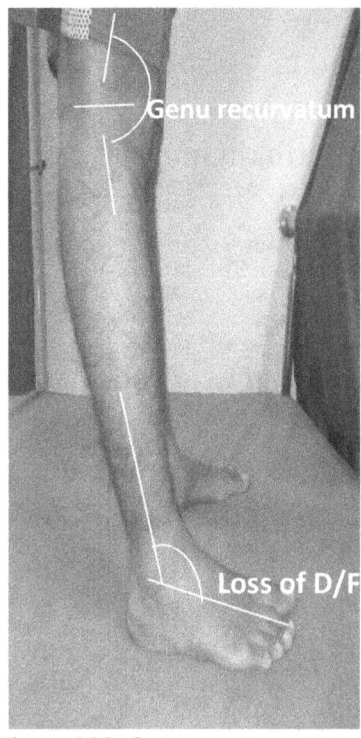

Figure 11A: Compensatory genu recurvatum at the knee secondary to foot dorsiflexion loss.

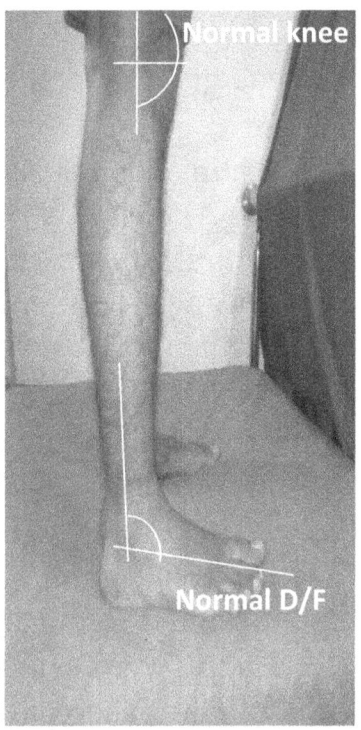

Figure 11B is the normal knee joint.

Loss of dorsiflexion of the foot leads to compensatory knee hyperextension. Usually, when standing, the knee is hyperextended to compensate for the loss of dorsiflexion of the ankle. Therefore, hyperextension force leads to gradual dysfucntion/deformity of **genu recurvatum**.

**Orthotic Design Considerations:** Knee-ankle-foot orthosis[23] is recommended for sagittal plane deformities to assist dorsiflexion. [17, 18, 22]

**Treatment:** the initial stage of dysfunction, talus anterior to posterior glide (Refer to chapter 14), and calf stretching will restore the normal dorsiflexion of the foot and correct the compensatory genu recurvatum.

**Note:** As Genu recurvatum does not come into exact pathomechanics of above and below kinetic chain of the knee dysfunctions, detailed assessment and treatment regarding the genu recurvatum are beyond the book's scope.

**References:**

1. Kaltenborn, F.M. (1989). Manual Mobilization of the Extremity Joints (4th ed.). Minneapolis: OPTP.http://coph.ouhsc.edu/dthompso/web/namics/arthkin.htm
2. Sharon, Thomas, et al., Integrative manual therapy for upper and lower extremities, 2008, p 153
3. AAOS:Bowed legs ,ortho info, http://orthoinfo.aaos.org/topic.cfm?topic=a00230
4. Brooks WC, Gross RH. Genu-Varum in Children: Diagnosis and Treatment. J Am Acad Orthop Surg. 1995 Nov; 3 (6): 326-335.
5. Austin T. Fragomen, MD, Correction of Bilateral Genu Varum for a High Level Athlete, https://www.hss.edu/professional-conditions_Correction-bilateral-Genu-Varum-high-level-athlete.asp
6. Pabitra kumar Sahoo, genu valgum (knock knee):http://www.svnirtar.nic.in/sites/default/files/resourcebook/3._Genuvalgum- Dr_P_K_Sahoo.pdf
7. Genu valgum, https://en.wikipedia.org/wiki/Genu_valgum
8. Knock Knees (Genu Valgum),http://www.nationwidechildrens.org/knock-knees.
9. Deanna J, Cheryl S, Genu Recurvatum: Identification of Three Distinct Mechanical Profiles. Publications>JPO>1998 Vol. 10, Num. 2> pp. 26-32, http://www.oandp.org/jpo/library/1998_02_026.asp
10. Kerrigan C, Deming LC, Molden MK. Knee recurvatum in gait: a study of associated knee biomechanics. Arch Phys Med Rehab 1996;77:645-50.
11. Perry J. Gait analysis-normal and pathological function. Thorofare, N.j.: SLACK In.,1992.
12. Pathological gait analysis :https://www.youtube.com/watch?v=
13. Rose J, Gamble JG. Human walking, 2nd ed. Baltimore: Williams & Wilkins, 1994.
14. Morris ME, Matyas TA, Bach TM, Goldi PA. Electrogoniometric feedback: its effect on genu recurvatum in stroke. Arch Phys Med Rehab 1992;73:1147-54.
15. Kottke FJ, Lehmann JF. Krusen's handbook of physical medicine and rehabilitation, 4th ed. Philadelphia: WB Saunders Co., 1990.
16. Fish, D. Genu recurvatum: mechanical components and clinical presentations of lower-limb pathomechanical deformities. Workshop presented at the New England Chapter AAOP Annual Meeting, 1996.
17. Inman VT, Ralston HJ, Todd F. Human locomotion. In: Rose J, Gamble JG, eds. human walking, 2nd ed. Baltimore: Williams & Wilkins, 1994.

18. Nielsen JP, Fish D. OOS-1 basic seminar in lower extremity pathomechanics and rotational control orthotics. Seminar sponsored by Oregon Orthotic System Inc., 1988-1995.
19. Hennessey WY, Johnson EW. Lower-limb orthosis. In: Braddom RL, ed. Physical medicine and rehabilitation. Philadelphia: WB Saunders Co., 1996.
20. E. Isakov, J. Mizrahi, I. Onna & Z. Susak: The control of genu recurvatum by combining the Swedish knee-cage and an ankle-foot brace, Page 187-191 | Accepted 01 Feb 1992, Published online: 28 Jul 2009
21. James Speck, Fixing Hyperextended Knee Posture:http://www.somastruct.com/genu-recurvatum/
22. Loudon JK, Goist HL, Loudon KL. Genu recurvatum syndrome. J Orthop Sports Phys Ther. 1998 May; 27 (5): 361-7
23. Reduction of genu recurvatum through adjustment of plantarflexion resistance of an articulated ankle-foot orthosis in individuals post-stroke.Clin Biomech (Bristol, Avon). 2016 Jun; 35:81-5. doi:10.1016/j.clinbiomech. 2016.04.011. Epub 2016 Apr 2
24. S.W. Yan-motion analysis; http://rehab.ym.edu.tw/document/motion/3-Normal%20Foot-Ankle-Knee-Hip%20Complex.
25. Loudon J, et al. The clinical orthopedic assessment guide. 2nd ed. Kansas: Human Kinetics, 2008. P.395- 408.

# CHAPTER 8
## Assessment and Treatment methods: Knee joint Complex specific

Joints of knee complex:
1. **Tibio-femoral joint**
2. **Patella-femoral joint**
3. **Proximal tibio-fibular joint.**

The tibio-femoral joint is the main component of the knee, as patella-femoral, tibio-fibular dysfunctions mostly occur secondarily to tibio-femoral dysfunction.[17] The Assessment and treatment methods presented in this book are used for any joints of the body, provided a physiotherapist should have a thorough knowledge of biomechanics and pathomechanics of joints. The chapter deals with assessment and treatment methods applied only to the knee joint to provide more clarity.

**Assessment methods:**
1. Objective methods
2. Subjective methods
3. Palpation of knee joint
4. Spring test

**1. Objective methods[14]:**

The observation component of the injury assessment refers to the visual inspection of the injured body part. Visual observation can be extremely useful in approaching the clinical diagnosis of an injury. When observing a patient, a few rules and regulations are taken into consideration, which aids in the injury assessment procedure.

**When observing:**
Comparison- Be sure to compare BILATERALLY when observing. The bilateral comparison refers to first examining the uninjured limb or body segment to establish a baseline or control for the patient. Comparing an uninjured body segment to an injured one allows the healthcare professional to observe any physical signs of injury and any difference in symmetry.

**Assess for Inflammation:**
Look for any signs of swelling to the injured body segment as compared to the uninjured segment. Look for temperature change within the local area of injury instead of the uninjured segment.

**Assess for Ecchymosis:**
Does the injured body segment show signs of bruising or internal bleeding as a result of an injury?
Are there any signs of pooling blood or discolouration surrounding the local area of injury?

**Assess for Scars:**
Does either the injured or uninjured body segment exhibit any scarring from previous injuries? These observations may be important in determining the cause of injury regarding any laxity, instability, improper healing, or excessive exertion regarding a previous injury.

**Assess for Deformity:**
Does the injured body segment exhibit signs of deformity? The deformity may indicate both the type of the injury and the severity of the injury. Bilateral comparison is essential in visually assessing for deformity and symmetry.

**Assess for postural abnormalities:**
Does the injured body segment affect the overall patient's posture? Again, the bilateral comparison will either rule out or rule in any postural abnormalities.

**Assess for discolouration:**
Does the injured limb exhibit signs of discolouration separate from that of ecchymosis?
Discolouration of the skin or soft tissue surrounding the injury may indicate vascular problems due to injury.

## 2. Subjective methods:

The subjective[13] portion of the injury assessment will contain information addressing the following:

- Past History of Injury
- General Medical Health
- Relevant Illnesses/Potential Labwork
- Recent Medications
- Mechanism of Injury
- Onset/duration of symptoms
- Location/Type/Severity of pain

**Individual components of subjective assessment:**

**History of injury:** This information is a crucial component of the injury evaluation. Addressing any previous injuries to a similar area of the body and any weaknesses due to an injury may lend insight to the clinical diagnosis of an injury and may even impact the type/ duration of the overall treatment.

It is essential to inquire about congenital conditions as certain conditions may predispose an individual to specific injuries.

**General medical health-** The General health portion of the injury assessment covers the present health status of the patient/athlete. Any underlying medical conditions will be assessed and may lend insight to a specific individual's diagnosis/ treatment parameters.

**Present medications-** Questioning and understanding an individual's medications are also essential. Medications, which vary exponentially from each other, affect every individual differently and may contribute to limited or decreased performance in athletics or daily living, but may also predispose an individual to injury.

**Mechanism of injury-** The mechanism of injury (MOI) is an extremely important portion of the medical history, requiring the Health Care Professional to recreate a situation that occurred to another individual. The MOI generally correlates directly with the clinical diagnosis of an injury. The healthcare professional will take the specifics of the injury itself and apply them to the local area of injury. While gathering the MOI, the healthcare professional should also evaluate whether or not the patient heard any abnormal sounds when the injury occurred and evaluate whether or not the patient felt anything abnormal.

**Onset/ Duration of symptoms-** The onset/duration of symptoms is a component of the medical evaluation in which important information regarding the onset of the injury is taken. Whether the condition was acute or not, meaning an immediate occurrence, or chronic, meaning pre-existing or a gradual increase in signs/symptoms?

## 3. Palpation of knee joint complex:

Accurate palpation[12] of knee joint landmarks in standing and sitting can sometimes be difficult due to muscular response to gravity.

In standing, the knee joint posture can be influenced by biomechanical dysfunction above and below the knee. Palpation of the landmarks in supine and prone lying may yield more accurate information about the isolated tibiofemoral and tibiofibular joint structure as the influence of the upper and lower body is reduced. A higher inter and intra-rater agreement has been observed with supine and prone palpation as part of an evaluation protocol (Ellis et al. 1989). An evaluation should include bony palpation and palpation of all soft tissues, especially muscles, tendons and ligaments, and fascia. A distinction needs to be made between positional dysfunction and movement dysfunction. Positional dysfunction describes how it is positioned; movement dysfunction describes how it cannot move. Evaluation and treatment that rely on position alone are, at best speculative. Detailed palpation of the knee is explained in the assessment and treatment chapters.

**Soft tissue:** Superficial to deep palpation is another important method of assessing soft tissue such as ligaments, tendons, muscles, fascia, etc. A detailed explanation can be seen in chapter 13.

**i. Patella:** Begin palpating the patella at its superior patellar pole where the quadriceps muscle group inserts, noting for areas of point tenderness. Then progress centrally down the patella to reach the inferior pole and the origin of the patellar tendon. Return to the starting point of the superior pole by palpating up the medial and lateral patellar borders. With the knee extended and the quadriceps relaxed, palpate the patella to ensure proper alignment in the femoral trochlea and freedom of movement. A dislocated patella can occur with or without the patellar tendon's rupture. A rigid displaced patella accompanied by the inability or unwillingness to extend the knee generally indicates a dislocated patella.

**ii. Tibial Tuberosity:** Palpate the patellar tendon's attachment site on the Tibia. The tibial tuberosity is normally a smooth, rounded protrusion. In adolescent patients, the tuberosity's sensitivity and roughness indicate an inflammation of the tibial tuberosity's growth centre or Osgood-Schlatter's disease.

**iii. Medial femoral condyle and epicondyle:** Flex the knee beyond 90 degrees to better expose the articulating surface of the condyle immediately above the anteromedial joint line. The adductor tubercle, the attachment site for the adductor longus, projects off of the medial femoral condyle. Injuries with rotational or loading type mechanisms may cause a bone bruising or osteochondral fracture, creating pain in the condyles. A contusion or localized inflammation may cause pain.

**iv. Medial tibial plateau:** Locate the medial tibial plateau inferior to the joint line. After palpating along its length, proceed inferiorly to locate the medial tibial flare, a structural necessity to disperse compressive forces at the articulation.

**v. Medial joint line:** Place the knee in at least 45 degrees of flexion to locate the joint lines. Then palpate on either side of the proximal aspect of the patellar tendon until the indentation formed by the femur and tibia is located. Palpate medially and posteriorly along the joint line, noting any crepitus or pain that may indicate possible meniscal, ligamentous or capsular trauma. Externally rotating the tibia makes the border of the medial meniscus more palpable.

**vi. Lateral Joint line:** Position the knee at least 45 degrees of flexion to locate the anterolateral joint line. Begin palpating the joint line lateral to the patellar tendon and progress posteriorly. Internally rotating the tibia makes the lateral meniscus more palpable. Pain along the joint line may indicate meniscal pathology.

**vii. Fibular head:** Locate the fibular head below and slightly posterior to the lateral joint line. Two ropes-like structures may be felt arising from the fibular head. The Lateral Collateral Ligament projects off its superior portion; the insertion of the biceps femoris tendon is slightly posterior to this structure.

**viii. Anterior tibial border:** The sharp subcutaneous ridge of the tibia extends from the tuberosity to the anterior part of the medial malleolus.

**ix. Anterio-medial surface:** The area medial to the anterior border of the tibia.

**x. Anterio-tibial lateral surface:** The area between the anterior border of the tibia and the interosseous border of the tibia.

**4. Spring test:** A spring test is essential in assessing joint dysfunction. This book shows the detailed application of spring test assessment to lower limb joints: knee joint complex, ankle, foot, and hip joint.

"**Spring Tests**," a fundamental concept of Manual Therapy[10], have been improved by Dr. Jerry Hesch. The method of spring testing applied is an enhancement referred to as "Springing with Awareness." Specifically, this approach allows the clinician to experience and interpret the visco-elastic joint structure's recoil instead of simply letting go of the spring. This advanced testing is fundamental to experiencing hypomobility and hypermobility with confidence empirically. In this way, the therapist will find that the application of techniques will enhance clinical palpatory literacy. "Springing with Awareness" has application throughout the body in joints and dense connective tissue. The spring test allows the Therapist to evaluate the true motion loss in each plane instead of perceived loss. There is more precision in assessment and ultimately greater success in restoring normative joint function through precisely targeted treatment. Clinicians consistently report confidence in the clinical application of this evaluation and treatment paradigm. For several reasons, specific joint mobility tests (also called spring tests) may yield information about the perceived movement that may be greater than the actual movement which occurs. The bony landmarks used are at a distance to the joint and may thus amplify perceived motion. The spring test may be applied in one plane and yet may produce triplane motion in the joint, and the kinesthetic information may seem to be amplified.

It is nearly impossible to perform a joint spring test in a close kinetic chain, i.e., in standing/sitting foot touching the ground. It is much easier to perform isolated joint spring tests with the client in an open kinetic chain, i.e., supine and prone. The term 'spring' seems very appropriate when testing the quality of knee joint play as there is a very discernable elastic feel in loading the knee joints, imparting the actual spring test, and in the quality of recoil.

Force transducers can measure spring tests, for example, the MicroFET muscle testing device (Hoggan Health Industries, Draper, UT, USA). It is a handheld instrument that measures the amount of force applied by the clinician. After taking up the slack in the joint, the clinician can then apply an additional force and determine how much force is applied when joint play is perceived. Both sides are compared. The clinician can measure pre-and post-treatment force. Most force transducers used in the clinic describe force in pounds or kilograms, although the force described in Newtons' (N) accounts for the influence of gravity. All three measures will be presented to benefit the interdisciplinary audience. The spring tests average 59 N (13 1b, 6 kg) for taking up the slack and up to 118 N (26 lb, 12 kg) to apply the spring test. The force needed may vary from person to person. The above averages serve as a guideline with which to develop the skill of applying the spring tests. The appropriate amount of force is the least amount that yields valuable information without increasing pain. The initial load takes 2-3 seconds, and performing the spring test takes 1-2 seconds to assess the recoil.

Knee joint dysfunction, more than any other joint dysfunction, has been inadequately defined in the traditional method on the basis of gross motion testing and limited bony landmark palpation. While modern research has provided insight into the anatomy and dysfunction in this area, the evolution of treatment methods has lagged behind. This is the author's proposal for a new approach to evaluating and treating knee dysfunctions. This complex body area is finally addressed through advanced palpatory skills, accessory motion tests, and a practical treatment approach. This approach recognizes that at times the specific joints of the knee may be involved, and at other times, the entire knee structure has movement dysfunction, which influences the kinetic chain, both above and below. Also addressed are the concepts that soft tissue (muscles, tendons, and ligaments) function can affect and be affected by joint dysfunction. Treatment is based on soft tissue factors as well as the viscoelastic nature of the joints.

## Assessment of knee joint dysfunction: Dynamic VS Static

**Static diagnosis:** x-ray and M.R.I fall under static diagnosis, giving information on one plane at a time. They are instrumental in diagnosing fractures, dislocations, inter-vertebral prolapse, etc. A dynamic structure for any joint anatomy may be suspected of varying conformation depending on its flexion, extension, rotation, and lateral bending orientation. However, accepted diagnostic imaging, especially magnetic resonance imaging (MRI), has been mostly static and limited to neutral positioning. Such convention ultimately may prove deceptive and fraught with bias[19, 20].

Orthopaedic manual physiotherapy is an important assessment tool such as comparing the symmetry and three planar spring tests, which include skilled passive movements of the joints and palpation of related soft tissues. A manual therapist applies these movements at varying speeds and amplitudes to gain a dynamic structural assessment of the musculoskeletal system. A manual therapist also gains more accurate information on three planes of movement and the total range of joints which X-rays, MRI, or stationary testing cannot obtain. The findings from dynamic assessment help us prioritize a patient's sources of pain in order of clinical importance, which is critical in the management of all pain syndromes[18]. Determining primary, secondary, and tertiary sources of pain is essential for designing and implementing treatment programs that help us prevent or minimize future pain episodes.

**Dynamic postural evaluation:** When evaluating the movement, it is necessary to slowly and gently move the extremities passively or through assisted activities, through the range of motion, maintaining a neutral position throughout (without deviation from the median, pure unidirectional, uniplanar movement). This process is called dynamic postural evaluation[21]. It is essential to maintain articular balance throughout the movement. If the limb is not allowed to deviate from mid-line during movement, the limitations of the motions will be obvious. With static postural dysfunction on any one plane, it is impossible to have full accessory and physiological ranges of motion of the joint(s) involved.

If the patient quickly and grossly moves the body part through an apparent full range of motion without maintaining articular balance, compensatory (trick) movements will not be noted. For example, knee flexion to complete knee extension on a sagittal plane is done (unidirectional /uniplanar). If any dysfunction exists, i.e., loss of anterior glides of the tibia over the femur with proximal tibia externally rotated, lateral shifted or proximal tibial internally rotated and medially shifted or both internal-external rotation loss with a medial, lateral glide loss. The limitation of the extension loss/pain at the limited range will be obvious.

**Postural dysfunction and articular balance:**

Whenever there is postural dysfunction on a sagittal, coronal or transverse plane, there will be a compromise of the articular balance of the joints in that region. Articular balance is the normal neutral relationship of two articular surfaces at rest and throughout the complete physiologic range of motion.

Example: on observing a patient with varus knee, walks with supination of the foot or weight falls on the lateral border of the foot (one of the postural dysfunction of the knee). The articular balance of the knee joint will be affected by the proximal tibia, which is externally rotated and laterally shifted.

**Accessory joint movement and physiological range of motion:** Whenever there is hypomobility of accessory movements and joint play in the joint, there must be correlated loss of joint physiological range of motion. There may be facial dysfunction and adhesions surrounding the joint's connective tissue. The soft tissue surrounding the joint may also have hypertonicity (protective muscle spasm). However, suppose the body receives a command from the brain cortex to move the joint despite the hypomobility. In that case, it will involuntarily compromise the accessory joint, and the trick movement occurs to complete the range.

If the moving joint surface rolls on its partner without simultaneously gliding and spinning, the surfaces would separate (gap or subluxate) in some places and impinge in others, called trick movement/compensatory movement. Roll, glide, and spin must occur simultaneously to preserve joint integrity.

We can predict and understand the relationship between bony shapes at a joint surface and the surface movements by applying the rules of concavity and convexity (Kaltenborn 1989, p. 27).

**Essential Treatment techniques used in musculoskeletal dysfunctions: Manual therapy prospective**

1. Joint mobilization and sustained glide
2. Muscle energy technique
3. Taping
4. Progressive strengthening
5. Deep transverse friction
6. Corrective Orthotics

**1. Joint mobilization[6,7] and sustained glide** (Enhancing the Traditional 5 Point Joint Mobilization Scale)

**Traditional 5-point Scale of joint mobilization[8]:**

**Grade I Oscillation**
It is a small amplitude movement conducted from the beginning of the available range of motion.

**Grade II Oscillation**
It is a large-amplitude movement conducted within the range. It does not reach either end of the range.

**Grade III Oscillation**
It is a large-amplitude movement that does reach the end of the range of motion.

**Grade IV Oscillation**
It is a small amplitude movement conducted at the very end of the range of motion.

**Grade V Oscillation**
It is a high velocity, low-amplitude thrust at the end of the available range and within its anatomical range. This grade of mobilization is also called "joint popping", also called a "manipulation".

**I** to **v** point scale, joint mobilization[9] make a lot of sense for acute conditions, but for chronic conditions, much more comfortable and efficient joint mobilization are **Grade vi**, and **Grade vii**.

Key concepts: one MUST keep the slack taken up at all times! Always oscillate forward from the position of taking up the slack, and maintain the tightened position throughout the treatment. It would help if we mobilized a joint many times to maximize the gain, e.g. 30 reps.

**Sustained glide**[11]: It is divided into two parts, **grade vi** and **grade vii**
**Grade vi:** Sustained Creep without Oscillation
**Grade vii:** Sustained Creep with forwarding Thrusts Avoiding Recoil

**Grade vi: Sustained Creep without oscillation or sustained glide**
Take up the slack in a joint and maintain the position with constant force, typically for 2 to 5 minutes. In some joints, the duration can be increased up to 5 to 10 minutes. Creep is a fundamental property of joints, defined as deformation over time. The element of a specific length of time makes this a distinct departure. This is usually done passively by a therapist or can be done passively by an external device like a knee log which will be addressed in the treatment part of the knee dysfunctions.

**Grade vii: Sustained Creep with forwarding Thrusts Avoiding Recoil**
This differs from lesser grades; the slack is taken up, though there is a subtle difference. In essence, there is no recoil with this technique; whenever the barrier is increased with a forward spring, recoil is avoided by actively preventing it. In contrast, with the lesser grades, such as grade 3, recoil is allowed after each forward portion of oscillation such that the new barrier is encountered again with the next forward part of the oscillation.

The procedure for this technique is to take up the slack in a joint and perform repeat mobilizations, to be gentle, but applying repeated moderate velocity, low amplitude forces. Always keep the slack taken up; as motion is gained, it is followed, such that there is a new position of the slack being taken up. This assures that the energy in the next mobilization will be applied directly against the barrier. Each thrust has the potential to move the joint past the barrier into a new range of motion. A typical number of repetitions: 30.

## 2. Muscle Energy Technique

Muscle energy technique[1,4,5] (or MET) is based on the principle of reciprocal inhibition; a theory explains that muscles on one side of a joint will always relax to accommodate the contraction of muscles on the other side of the joint when direct/indirect pressure is applied. In this book, the direct technique is applied.

The muscle energy technique is applied to a patient to lengthen shortened or spastic muscles, improve weakened ligament and muscle strength, and improve range of motion. This procedure is performed when a patient is asked to contract a muscle for approximately 5-seconds against an anti-force applied by the therapist. The muscle contraction is performed by the client 2 or 3 times in a row in the hope of stretching the muscle further each time.

### 3. Taping technique:

Taping techniques are used to correct the alignment and stabilise the given dysfunction by restoring normal alignment and reducing the inflammation, which assists in healing in acute conditions[2,3].

The taping technique helps in 3-dimensional correction, assists during mobilisation, and gives the desired direction of sustained glide in subacute and chronic conditions.

Taping aims to:

Prevent injury, reduce the severity of the injury, provide support, limit pain, limit specific movement of the joint, allow desired movements of the joints, and provide proprioception.

Some of the good tapes available in the market are K-tape/transpore Tape etc.

### 4. Progressive strengthening: a detailed insight into progressive strengthening is already covered in chapter 2

### 5. Soft tissue deep transverse friction[23, 24]: a detailed insight into soft tissue adhesions and treatment using deep transverse friction (knee joint complex) is covered in chapter 13.

### 6. Orthotics:

**Orthotics** (Greek: *Ορθός, ortho*, "to straighten" or "align")[16,22] is
a speciality within the medical field concerned with the design, manufacture and application of orthosis. An orthosis (plural: orthosis) is "an externally applied device used to modify the structural and functional characteristics of the neuromuscular and skeletal system".[15]

Orthotics combines knowledge of anatomy and physiology, pathophysiology, biomechanics, and engineering. Patients who benefit from an orthosis may have a condition such as spina bifida or cerebral palsy or have experienced a spinal cord injury or stroke. Equally, an orthosis is sometimes used prophylactically or to optimize performance in sports.

An orthotist is the primary medical clinician responsible for prescribing, manufacturing, and managing orthosis. An orthosis may be used to:

- Control, guide, limit and/or immobilize an extremity, joint or body segment for a particular reason.
- To restrict movement in a given direction.
- To assist movement generally.
- To reduce weight-bearing forces for a particular purpose.
- To aid rehabilitation from fractures after the removal of a cast.
- To otherwise correct the body's shape and/or function, to provide easier movement capability or reduce pain.

**References:**

1. Masters, Yashvant, The effect of combining muscle energy technique with soft tissue massage on hamstring extensibility a research project submitted in partial fulfilment of the requirements for the degree of Master of Osteopathy Unitec Institute of Technology, 2014. http://unitec.researchbank.ac.nz/handle/10652/2527
2. http://www.physioadvisor.com.au/health/taping-techniques-lower-body/
3. https://www.physiotherapyalberta.ca/public_and_patients/the_you_movement_blog/what_is_taping_and_does_it_work
4. https://en.wikipedia.org/wiki/Muscle_energy_technique
5. http://c.ymcdn.com/sites/www.opso.org/resource/resmgr/OMT_Binder/14_-_BASIC_PRINCIPLES_OF_MUS.pdf
6. Mulligan, Principles of Joint Mobilization, https://www.physio-pedia.com/images/c/c0/Principles_of_Joint_Mobilization.pdf
7. Farzin Halabchi, Joint Mobilization and Traction Techniques in Rehabilitation, http://medicine.tums.ac.ir:803/Users/farzin_halabchi/Lectures/Sports%20Rehabilitation/8)%20Joint%20Mobilization%20&%20Traction.pdf
8. http://www.physio-pedia.com/Maitland's_Mobilisations
9. http://www.physio-pedia.com/Manual_Therapy
10. Jerry Hesch, Hesch Method of Manual Therapy Basic Information, http://www.heschinstitute.com/hesch-method-basics.html
11. Jerry Hesch, Enhancing the Traditional 5 Point Joint Mobilization Scale, http://www.heschinstitute.com/enhanced-mobilization-scale.html
12. Calmbach et al., Evaluation of Patients Presenting with Knee Pain: Part I. History, Physical Examination, Radiographs, and Laboratory Tests, http://www.aafp.org/afp/2003/0901/p907.pdf
13. Subjective Examination in Physiotherapy, http://www.strengthphysio.com/subjective-assessment-physiotherapy/
14. http://www.physio-pedia.com/Template:Clinical_Examination
15. Jump up^ Redford, John B.; Basmajian, John V.; Trautman, Paul (1995). Orthotics: clinical practice and rehabilitation technology. New York: Churchill Livingstone Inc. pp. 11–12.
16. https://en.wikipedia.org/wiki/Orthotics.
17. Thay Q. Lee, The Influence of Tibial and Femoral Rotation on Patellofemoral Contact Area and Pressure; J Orthop Sports Phys Ther • Volume 33 • Number 11 • November 2003
18. http://www.practicalpainmanagement.com/resources/diagnostic-tests/using-dynamic-mri-diagnose-neck-pain-importance-positional-cervical-cord

19. J Orthop Sports Phys Ther. 2009 Aug; 39(8):628-34. doi: 10.2519/jospt.2009.2968.
20. Differences in static and dynamic measures in the evaluation of talonavicular mobility in gait.Dicharry JM[1], Franz JR, Della Croce U, Wilder RP, Riley PO, Kerrigan DC.
21. Dynamic structural assessment
http://www.neilkingpt.com/index.php?option=com_content&view=article&id=33&Itemid=155
22. Isabel A. C. Baert & Jo Nijs & Mira Meeus & Enrique Lluch & Filip Struyf. The effect of lateral wedge insoles in patients with medial compartment knee osteoarthritis: balancing biomechanics with pain neuroscience. Clin Rheumatol (2014) 33:1529–1538.
23. Janet McMurray, Scott Landis, Kris Lininger, Russell T. Baker, Alan Nasypany, Jeff Seegmiller. A Comparison and Review of Indirect. Myofascial Release Therapy, Instrument-Assisted Soft Tissue Mobilization, and Active Release Techniques to Inform Clinical Decision Making.30, September 2015 international journal of Athletic Therapy & training
24. Salvi Shah, Akta Bhalara. Myofascial Release. International Journal of Health Sciences & Research (www.ijhsr.org) 69 Vol.2; Issue: 2; May 2012.

# CHAPTER 9
## Assessment and Treatment of Tibio-Femoral Joint Dysfunctions of Knee

**Surface Anatomy and important palpatory landmarks of the Knee:**

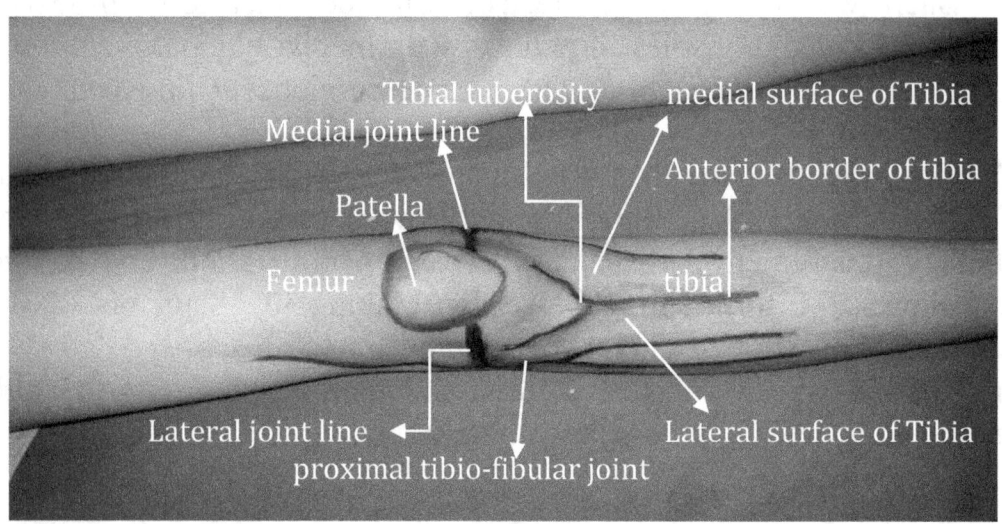

Figure 1a: Surface anatomy of the knee: Showing important landmarks that assist in assessing and treating knee dysfunctions.

As shown in Figure 1a, the knee is easy to find right between the leg and the thigh. You can visualize the popliteal fossa on the posterior aspect of the knee - it is a diamond-shaped area right over the part where the knee bends[3].

The popliteal artery can be palpated for a pulse, but it is not always easy to find unless the patient is lying prone with the knee bent. Press your fingers deep into the popliteal fossa to feel the pulse. [12]

# Chapter 9: Assessment and Treatment of Tibio-Femoral joint of Knee

The bones are easy to find using the following clues, [10, 11]:

a) The condyles of the femur and tibia give the knee its shape and are easy to palpate on either side of the knee. They are the largest bony prominences on either side of the knee above the articulation.

b) The head of the fibula is located just inferior to the lateral condyles. The bony prominence on the lateral side is inferior to the knee articulation.

c) The patella is anterior to the knee joint and may be located by sight or palpation. It is the bony knee cap located anterior to the knee joint.

d) The **anterior crest or border**, the most prominent of the three, commences above the tuberosity and ends below the anterior margin of the medial malleolus. It is sinuous and prominent in the upper two-thirds of its extent but smooth and rounded below. It gives attachment to the deep fascia of the leg.

e) The **medial surface** is smooth, convex, and broader above than below. Its upper third, directed forward and medial ward, is covered by the aponeurosis derived from the tendon of the sartorius and by the tendons of the Gracilis and Semitendinosus, all of which are inserted nearly as far forward as the anterior crest; in the rest of its extent, it is subcutaneous.

f) The **lateral surface** is narrower than the medial. Its upper two-thirds present a shallow groove for the origin of the Tibialis anterior. Its lower third is smooth and convex, curves gradually forward to the anterior aspect of the bone, and is covered by the tendons of the Tibialis anterior, Extensor hallucis longus, and Extensor digitorum longus, arranged in this order from the medial side.

g) Medial and lateral joint line: The medial joint line is the palpatory space on the medial surface of the knee between the femur and tibia. The lateral joint line is the palpatory space on the lateral surface of the knee between the femur and the tibia.

The leg is shaped primarily from the superficial posterior muscles that form the calf. They may be visible under the skin, along with superficial veins.

**Assessment and treatment of tibio-femoral joint dysfunction[4]:**
1. Flexion lag
2. Extesion lag
3. Extension and Flexion lag

## 1. Knee flexion lag: extended knee
Flexion ROM: If it is full - Normal
If there is Lag - indicating dysfunction (knee is extended)
Possible dysfunctions are as follows:

- A. Flexion lag: with proximal tibia externally rotated with lateral shift/glide.
- B. Flexion lag: with proximal tibia internally rotated with medial shift/glide.
- C. Flexion lag: with proximal tibia internal rotation, medial glide and external rotation, lateral glide loss.

## Spring test:
**Osteo-kinematic (gross) spring test:** For flexion lag (when knee can not flex completely).
- The knee is stuck in the extension.
- The extended knee joint dysfunction.

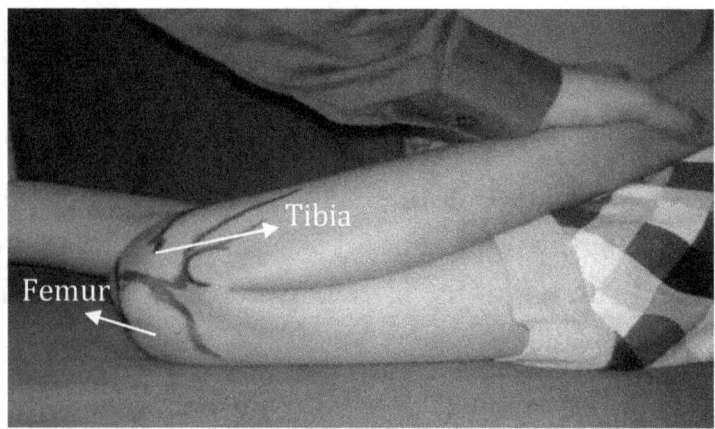

Figure 1b: Osteo-kinematic assessments of knee flexion lag dysfunction: open-chain flexion of the knee in the prone, concave surface of proximal tibia rolls and glides posteriorly on the convex surface of the stationary femur.

**Osteo-kinematic assessment of right knee flexion in an open kinetic chain:** first, as shown in Figure 1b, the patient is prone, and the therapist approaches the patient from the right side[1, 2]. The therapist's left-hand grasps the lower anterior surface of the tibia, and the patient is asked to actively flex the terminal range of the knee in the first method. Secondly, passive assessment of the spring test is done in only one plane, the sagittal plane; the therapist takes up the slack passively in flexion (sagittal plane), not in the transverse nor coronal plane. After reaching the terminal flexion, the therapist applies additional force to test the spring. In the first (active movement) and second (passive movement with spring test) methods, there is a chance of compensatory/trick movement, that is, either gapping at one compartment or compression at the other takes place, according to knee dysfunction to complete the terminal flexion. In the second method, it **may be** normal; if it does not spring, it indicates flexion lag (knee dysfunction). This method of spring test is a gross assessment compared to the Arthro-kinematic three-planar spring test, which is more specific and three-planar.

**Three planar Arthro-kinematic (Specific) spring test:** Three planar Arthrokinematic assessment is more efficient than osteokinematic assessment, as slack is taken in three planes simultaneously, so there is no chance of compensatory/trick movement. A possible 3-planar (sagittal, transverse, and coronal planes) assessment, i.e., a combination of 3-planar Arthrokinematic spring test assessment, is a better choice to screen out accurate possible dysfunction. Therefore, all dysfunctions are assessed in three planar Arthrokinematic[1] spring tests.

**A. Flexion lag: with proximal tibia externally rotated and lateral shifted/glide.**

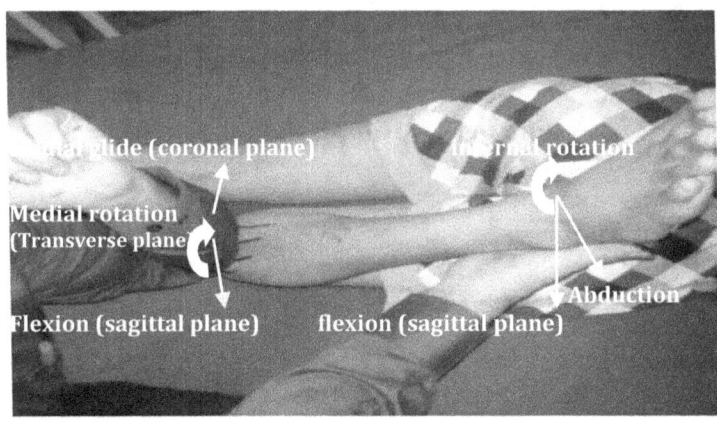

Figure 2: depicts arthrokinematic assessment and treatment of knee flexion lag dysfunction with the proximal tibia externally rotated and laterally shifted.

**Three planaarArthro-kinematic spring tests**: Shown in Figure 2,
**Position of the patient:** The patient is prone, and the right knee is to be assessed.
**Position of the therapist and procedure:** The therapist approaches the patient's right side. The Left Pisiform/olecranon is placed on the proximal lateral surface close to the tibial tuberosity. Then, an internal rotation (transverse plane), medial glide (coronal plane), flexion/ posterior glide of the proximal tibia (sagittal plane), and three planar movement barriers are reached. Simultaneously, the therapist's right wrist slightly extended, fingers flexed as shown in Figure 2, grasp the posterior distal, tibia and further internal rotation, abduction, flexion, three planar movement barriers are reached, which reinforces three planar movement barriers at the proximal tibia. After reaching the movement barrier at the proximal tibia, flexion slack is taken with 12 kg force. Additionally, 8kg force is applied in terminal flexion to test the spring/end feel. If it does not spring, the test will be positive - indicating dysfunction.

**Note:** For the spring tests, the knee averaged 118 N (26lb, 12 kg) for taking up the slack and up to 235 N (53 lb, 24 kg) to apply the spring test. The force needed may vary from person to person, and the condition of dysfunction. The above averages serve as a guideline to develop the skill of applying the spring tests[14]. The appropriate amount of force is the least amount that yields useful information without increasing pain. The initial load takes 2-3 seconds, and performing the spring test to assess the recoil takes 1-2 seconds.

**Treatment:**
**-Mobilization:** Shown in Figure 2
**Position of the patient:** is prone.
**Position of therapist and procedure:** this is the same as the assessment position explained above. After reaching the movement barrier in three planes, tibial posterior glide/flexion slack is taken with 12 kg force, and further posterior glide/flexion is done according to the grades of mobilization. Five glides are given three times in one session. Each time, a 5-second rest is given.

**-Muscle energy technique**[7]: Shown in figure 2
**Position of the patient:** is the same as above
**Position of therapist and procedure:** The position is the same as the assessment position as explained above; after reaching the movement barrier in three planes, flexion slack is taken with 12 kg force. After that, the patient is asked to extend, and simultaneously, the therapist resists producing an isometric contraction. After 5 seconds of relaxation, three new planar movement barriers are reached (internal

rotation, medial glide, and flexion/posterior glide). Again, repeat the same three times per session.

**-Taping[8]:** Shown in Figure 3

**Position of the patient:** The patient is in the supine and right knee to be treated.

**Position of the therapist and procedure:** The therapist approaches the patient from the right side. One end of the tape is pasted on the proximal lateral surface of the tibia; the ulnar border of the therapist's left-hand needs to stabilize the medial lower surface of the femur. Then, the right hand of the therapist's thumb/olecranon is placed on the proximal lateral surface of the tibia, and internal rotation and medial glide slack are taken at the proximal tibia with 12 kg force. Simultaneously stabilizing the medial distal femur with left thenar eminence, the other end of the tape is pasted at the medial lower thigh (femur). To some extent, it will assist in correcting internal rotation (transverse plane) and medial glide (coronal plane), Thereby assisting in restoring normal alignment, stabilization, and reduction in pain.

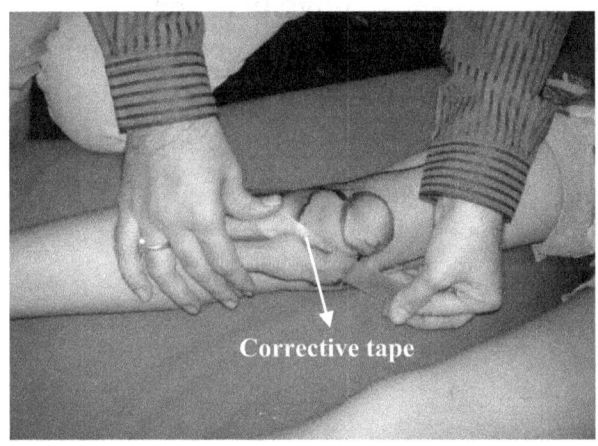

Figure 3: Taping technique to correct proximal tibia, which is externally rotated and laterally shifted in the knee dysfunction.

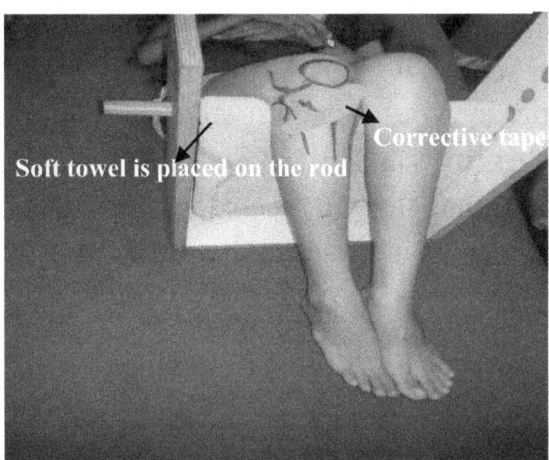

Figure 4: External device (stand) to correct knee flexion dysfunctions with tape. A soft towel is placed on the rod to give a cushioning effect.

**-Sustained glide[5, 6]:** It is a technique in which a slow and sustained glide for 2-5 minutes is given manually by the therapist or an external device, which glides the proximal tibia posteriorly. The author has designed the external device, as shown in Figure 4, which depicts the stand with a rod placed in between the hole of the frame to adjust the height; once the height is adjusted, the therapist places the patient's knee with corrective tape on in a flexed position. The corrective tape will assist the proximal tibia glide medially and rotate internally. The proximal tibia's posterior glide occurs with the leg's weight on the rod. The advantage is that the glide is gradual and less painful for the patient, and the therapist's time and energy will be saved. According to the patient's condition and tolerance, weight can be added to the dorsal ankle to increase flexion at the knee.

**-Deep transverse friction**[9]: DTF is given to affected knee soft tissue, as shown in chapter 13.
**-Progressive/progressive strengthening** is advised according to the patient's condition and tolerance. A detailed explanation is covered in Chapter 2.

**B. Flexion lag: with proximal tibia internally rotated with medial shift/glide.**

**Spring test:** Shown in figure 5
**Position of the patient:** is in the prone and right knee to be assessed.
**Position of therapist and procedure:** The therapist approaches the patient's right side. The therapist places his left Pisiform/olecranon on the proximal medial surface of the tibia closest to the Tibial tuberosity. Then, an external rotation (transverse plane), lateral glide (coronal plane), posterior glide/flexion (sagittal plane) of the proximal tibia, and three planar movement barriers are reached. Simultaneously, the therapist extends his right wrist and slightly flexes his fingers to grasp the posterior distal tibia. Then an, external rotation (transverse plane), adduction (coronal plane), and flexion (sagittal plane) movement barriers are reached, which in turn reinforce three planar movement barriers at the proximal tibia. After reaching the three planar movement barriers at the proximal tibia, flexion slack is taken with 12 kg force, and additionally, 8kg force is applied in terminal flexion to test the spring/end feel; if it doesn't spring, then the test will be positive - indicating dysfunction.

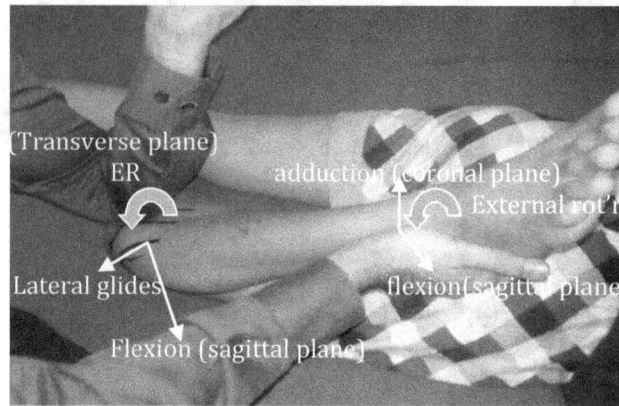

Figure 5: Depicts both arthrokinematic spring test and treatment of knee flexion lag dysfunction with the proximal tibia internally rotated and medially shifted.

**Treatment:**

**-Mobilization:** Shown in Figure 5
**Position of the patient:** the patient is prone, and the right knee is to be treated.
**Position of therapist and procedure:** as explained above, after reaching the movement barrier in three planes - external rotation (transverse plane), lateral glide (coronal plane), and flexion (sagittal plane) then knee flexion slack is taken with 12 kg force, and further posterior glide is done according to the grades of mobilisation. Five glides are given three times in one session. Each time, a 5-second rest is given.

**-Muscle energy technique:** Shown in Figure 5
**Position of the patient:** the patient is prone, and the right knee is to be treated.
**Position of the therapist and procedure:** as explained above, knee flexion/tibial posterior glide slack is taken with 12 kg force after reaching the movement barrier in three planes. After that, the patient is asked to extend the knee, and simultaneously, the therapist resists producing an isometric contraction. After 5 sec rest, three new planar movement barriers, external rotation, lateral glide, and flexion, are reached. Again, repeat the same three times per session.

**-Taping:** Shown in figure 6
**Position of the patient:** The patient is in the supine and right knee to be treated.
**Position of therapist and procedure:** The therapist approaches the patient's right side. One end of the tape is pasted on the proximal medial surface of the tibia; the left hand of the therapist needs to stabilise the femur's lateral lower surface—the right hand of the therapist placed on the superior medial surface of the tibia, then an external rotation and lateral glide slack are taken at proximal tibia with 12 kg force. Then, the other end of the tape is pasted at the distal lateral thigh (femur). To some extent, it will assist in correcting external rotation (transverse plane) and lateral glide (coronal plane), Thereby assisting in restoring normal alignment, stabilization, and reduction in pain.

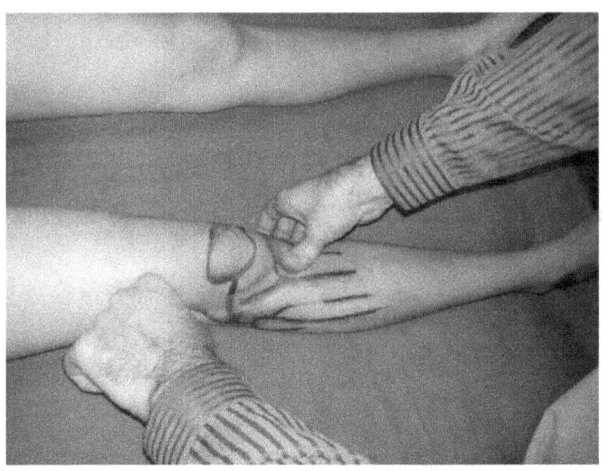

**Figure 6:** Taping technique to correct knee dysfunction with proximal tibia internally rotated and medially shifted.

**-Sustained glide:** Shown in Figure 7

**Position of the patient:** is supine with hip and knee flexed as shown.

**Position of the therapist and procedure:** As explained above, with the correction tape on to glide the proximal tibia into external rotation (transverse plane) and lateral glide (coronal plane). The sustained glide is also employed to correct the flexion/posterior glide of the proximal tibia in the sagittal plane. The therapist places the patient's knee flexed on the external device stand to correct the knee flexion dysfunction. The horizontal rod will assist the proximal tibia glide posteriorly with the own weight of the leg; additionally, if required, according to the patient's condition and tolerance, to increase flexion, additional weight can be placed on the dorsal surface of the ankle.

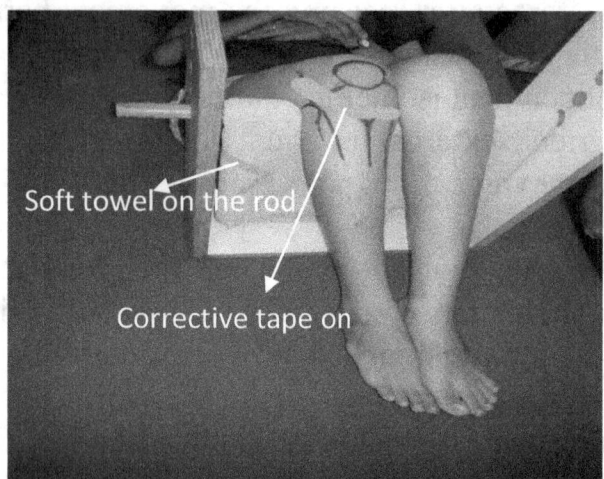

Figure 7: Sustained posterior glide of proximal tibia: stand for correction of knee flexion dysfunctions with corrective tape. A soft towel is placed on the rod to give cushioning.

**-Deep transverse friction**: DTF is given to affected knee soft tissue, covered in chapter 13.

**-Progressive strengthening** is advised according to the patient's condition and tolerance. A detailed explanation is covered in Chapter 2.

## C. Flexion lag: with the proximal tibia, both internal, external rotation and medial, lateral glide loss:

As it is known that internal rotation occurs with medial glide, and external rotation occurs with lateral glide. If rotational glides are lost, medial and lateral glides also will be lost.

For the assessment and treatment of this dysfunction, previous dysfunctions A and B assessment and treatment sections should be included. Moreover, the proximal tibia medial and lateral glide spring test and treatment at the flexion barrier can be included.

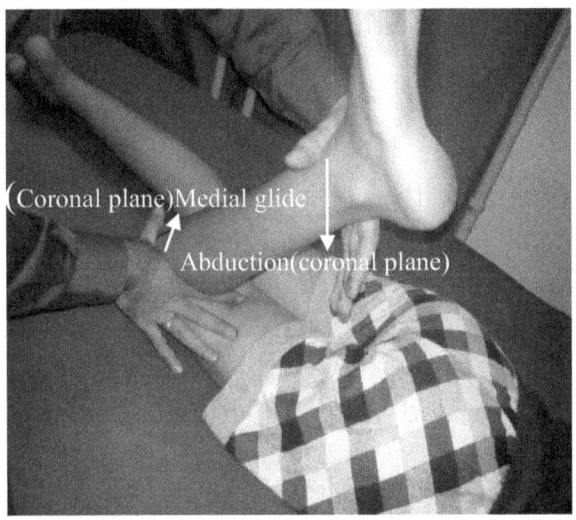

Figure 8: Spring test of the right proximal tibia- medial glide loss at flexion barrier.

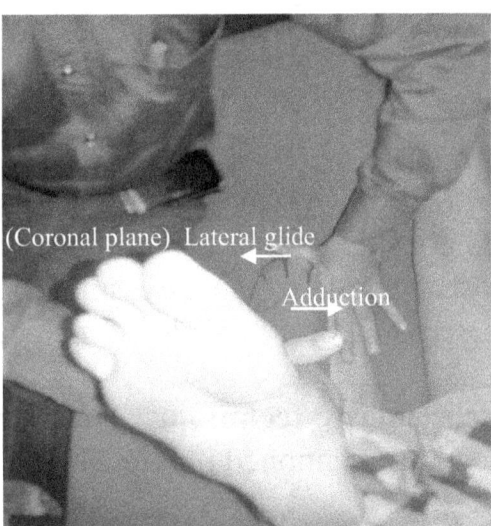

Figure 9: Spring test of the proximal tibia- lateral glide loss at flexion barrier.

**Spring test: Proximal tibia- lateral to medial glide:** Shown in Figure 8
**Position of the patient:** is prone, right knee to be assessed.
**Position of the therapist and procedure:** The therapist approaches the patient's right side. Then, the right knee is taken into the possible extent of flexion (flexion barrier). The therapist's right hand's webspace of thumb and forefinger is placed on the proximal-lateral surface close to the tibial tuberosity. The medial glide movement barrier is reached. Simultaneously, the therapist's left-hand web space of the thumb and forefinger grasps the medial surface of the distal tibia to impart abduction, which in turn reinforces the medial glide movement barrier at the proximal tibia. Then, the medial glide slack is taken with 12 kg force, and 8kg

force is applied to test the spring/end feel. If it does not spring, the test will be positive – It indicates dysfunction.

**Spring test: Proximal tibia - medial to lateral glide:** Shown in Figure 9
**Position of the patient:** is prone, right knee to be assessed.
**Position of the therapist and procedure:** The therapist approaches the patient's right side, and the right knee is taken into the possible extent of flexion (flexion barrier). The therapist's left hand's webspace of thumb and forefinger is placed on the proximal-medial surface close to the tibial tuberosity, and then the lateral glide movement barrier is reached. Simultaneously, the therapist's right-hand web space of the thumb and forefinger grasps the lateral surface of the distal tibia to impart adduction, which in turn reinforces lateral glide movement at the proximal tibia. Then, the lateral glide slack is taken with 12 kg force, and 8kg force is applied to test the spring/end feel. If it does not spring, the test will be positive–it indicates dysfunction.

**Treatment:**
**-Mobilization:** As known, internal rotation occurs with medial glide, and external rotation occurs with lateral glide. If rotations are lost, the medial and lateral glides are lost. Therefore, the assessment and treatment of both A and B dysfunctions discussed previously should be included, as mentioned previously.

**-Muscle energy technique**: Treatment of both A and B dysfunctions should be included, as mentioned previously.

**-Taping**: Treatment of both A and B dysfunctions should be included, as mentioned previously.

**-Sustained glide:** Treatment of both A and B dysfunctions should be included, as mentioned previously.

**-Deep transverse friction**: DTF is given to affected knee soft tissue, as shown in chapter 13.

**-Progressive strengthening** is advised according to the patient's condition and tolerance. A detailed explanation is covered in Chapter 2.

## 2. Knee extension lag/flexed knee:

Possible dysfunctions are:

A. Extension lag: with proximal tibia externally rotated and laterally shifted/glide
B. Extension lag: with proximal tibia internally rotated and medially shifted/glide
C. Extension lag: with the proximal tibia, both internal, external rotation, and medial, lateral glide loss

**i) Osteokinematic (gross) spring test**: shown in figure 10.

**Position of the patient:** is supine, right knee to be examined.

**Position of the therapist and procedure:** The therapist approaches the patient's right side. The therapist's left hand web space of the thumb and forefingers is placed on the tibia's proximal anterior surface, and then the extension/anterior glide movement barrier is reached. Moreover, the therapist's right hand's fingers and wrist are flexed to grasp the patient's distal posterior tibia surface, giving upward-directed movement to reinforce the extension barrier at the proximal tibia. The proximal tibia anterior glide slack is taken with 12kg force, and additionally, 8kg force is applied in extension to test the spring/end feel. If it does not, spring indicates dysfunction. In osteokinematic assessment, even though there is dysfunction, it may spring, as there is a chance of trick movement to complete the terminal extension by compressing at one compartment and gapping at another. Therefore, it is not accurate.

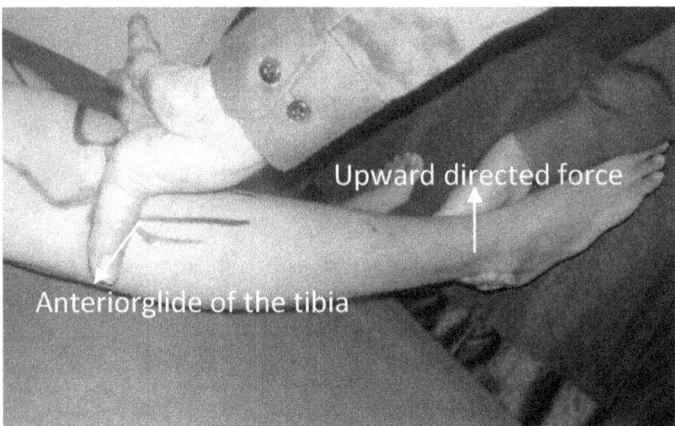

Figure 10: Osteo-kinematic/gross assessment of knee extension lag.

**ii) Arthrokinematic (Specific) spring test:** Arthrokinematic assessment is more efficient than the osteokinematic assessment, as osteokinematic assessment involves gross movement, and there is a chance of compensatory or trick movement while completing the full terminal range. Therefore, the better choice to screen out accurate dysfunction is to include possible joint glides in three-dimensional planes- sagittal, transverse, and coronal simultaneously in the spring test assessment. Therefore, all dysfunctions are assessed in three planar arthrokinematic spring tests.

## A. Extension lag: with proximal tibia externally rotated with lateral shift/glide

**Spring test:** shown in Figures 11A &11B

**Position of the patient:** is supine, right knee to be assessed.

**Position of the therapist and procedure:** The therapist approaches the patient's right side. The therapist's left-hand pisiform, as shown in figure 11A (or) with thumb/ olecranon of the elbow, as shown in figure 11B, is placed on the proximal-lateral surface close to the tibial tuberosity. Then, with internal rotation (transverse plane) glide, medial glide (coronal plane), and anterior glide (sagittal plane) of the proximal tibia, three planar movement barriers are reached. Simultaneously, the Therapist's right wrist is slightly extended with fingers flexed, grasping the lower posterior tibia, and internal rotation, abduction, and upward force are applied to reinforce the three planar movement barriers at the proximal tibia. After reaching the three planar movement barriers, extension slack is taken with 12kg force. Additionally, 8kg force is applied in extension to feel the spring. If it does not spring, it indicates dysfunction.

Figure 11A (with pisiform bone) and 11B (with thumb): depict the arthro-kinematic spring test, and treatment of knee dysfunction - extension lag with superior tibia externally rotated with lateral shift/glide.

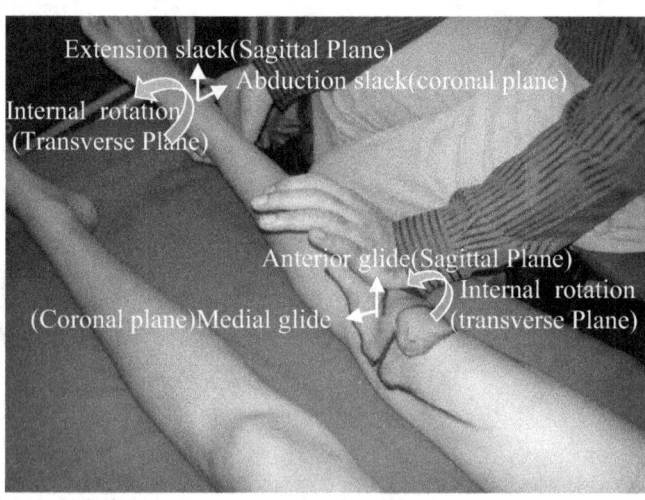

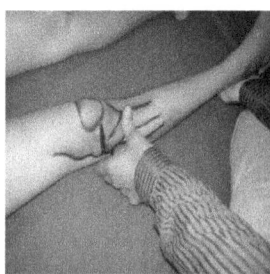

## Treatment:
**-Mobilization:** shown in figure 11a

# Chapter 9: Assessment and Treatment of Tibio-Femoral joint of Knee

**Position of the patient:** is supine, lying

**Position of the therapist and procedure:** the therapist approaches the patient's right side. As explained above, after reaching the movement barrier in three planes at the proximal tibia, the extension slack is taken with 12kg of force. Further mobilization is done according to the grades of mobilization. Three glides are given three times in one session. Each time, 5 seconds of rest is given.

-**Muscle energy technique**: shown in Figure 11a

**Position of the patient:** is in supine lying.

**Position of therapist and procedure:** The therapist approaches the right side of the patient, and as explained above, after reaching the movement barrier in three planes, extension slack is taken with 12 kg force. Then, the patient is asked to flex, and simultaneously, the therapist resists producing an isometric contraction. After 5 sec relaxations, a further new movement barrier in three planes is reached: internal rotation, medial glide, and anterior glide. Again, repeat the same three times. Each time, 5 seconds of rest is given.

-**Taping**: Shown in figure 12

**Position of the patient:** is supine

**Position of the therapist and procedure:** The therapist approaches the patient from the right side, and as explained above, One end of the tape is pasted on the proximal lateral surface of the tibia; the therapist's left-hand ulnar part of the lower forearm should stabilize the medial lower surface of the femur. Then, the therapist's right thumb/pisiform is placed on the proximal lateral surface of the tibia and rotated internally by taking the slack of 12kg force. The other end of the tape is pasted over the lower medial thigh (femur). To some extent, it will assist in achieving internal rotation (transverse plane) and medial glide (coronal plane) as they are coupled movements.

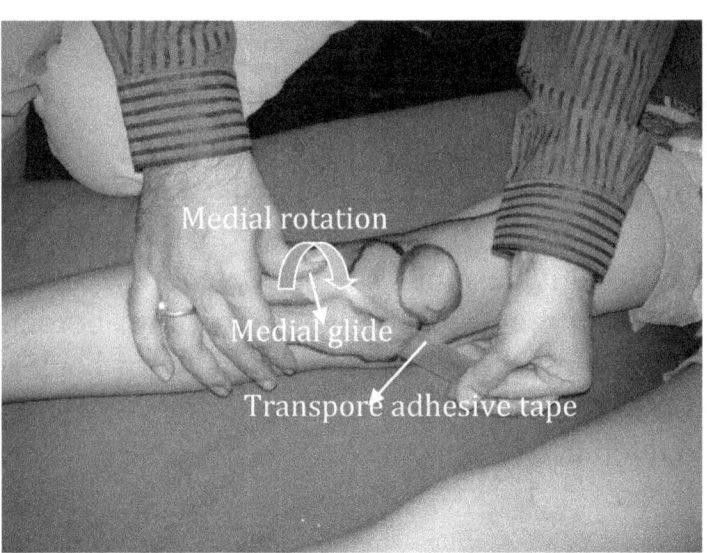

Figure 12: taping technique for dysfunction - Extension lag with proximal tibia externally rotated and laterally shifted.

**-Sustained lateral to medial glide of the proximal tibia at extension barrier:** Shown in Figure 13

**Position of the patient:** is on right side lysing.

**Position of the therapist and procedure:** along with the tape mentioned above, a sustained glide is employed to correct the right proximal tibia lateral to medial glide at the extension barrier with a specially designed stand. The stand consists of a rectangular base [1/2 inch of thickness, 15 inches of length, 5.5 inches of breadth], and at the centre, there is a projection [2 inches of height, 10 inches of length, ½ inch of thickness].

The right proximal-lateral tibia is placed on the projected part of the stand. With the help of body weight, the proximal tibia will glide medially on the femur. It can be kept for 2-5 minutes, depending on the condition and tolerance of the patient. As medial glide and internal rotation are couple movements, if medial glide increases, internal rotation also increases.

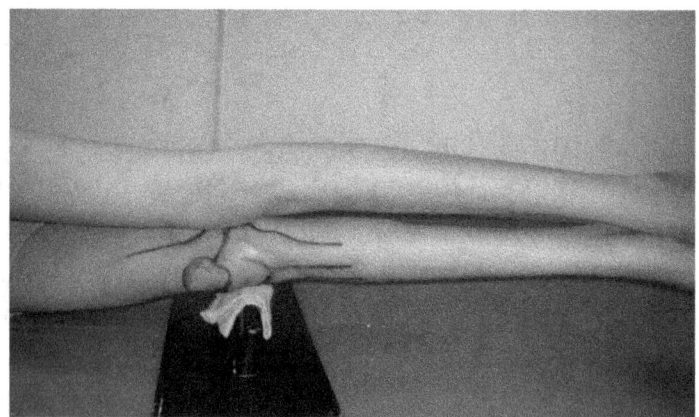

Figure 13: Sustained lateral to medial glide of the proximal tibia at extension movement barrier is given withstand. Soft cushioning is kept between the stand and the knee.

**The sustained anterior glide of the proximal tibia:** Shown in Figure 14

**Position of the patient:** the patient is prone, and the right knee is to be treated.

**Position of the therapist and procedure:** along with the tape on, a further sustained glide is employed to correct the right proximal tibia anterior glide in extension (sagittal plane) with a specially designed stand, as mentioned above.

The distal anterior surface of the right femur/just above the superior border of the patella is placed on the projected part of the stand. With the help of body weight, the proximal tibia glides anteriorly on the femur. It can be kept for 2-5 minutes, depending on the condition and tolerance of the patient.

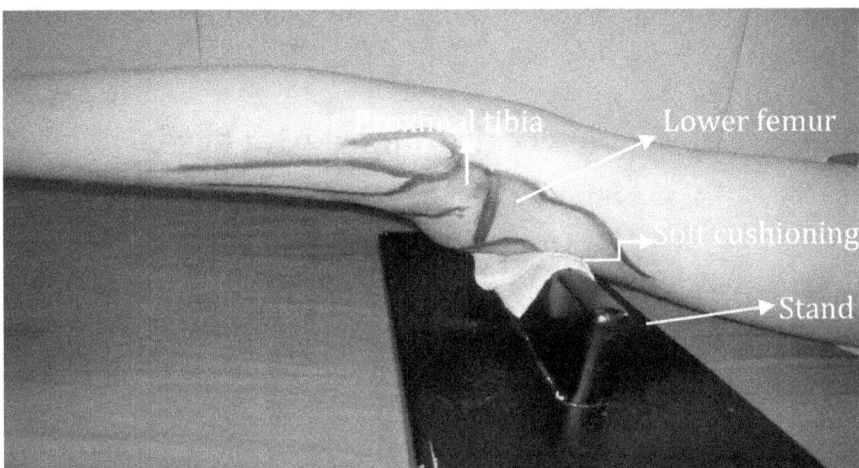

Figure 14: Shows the sustained anterior glide of the proximal tibia into an extension on the specially designed stand. Soft cushioning is kept between the projected part of the stand and the knee.

**-Deep transverse friction**: follow the assessment and treatment of knee soft tissue with Deep Transverse Friction, covered in chapter 13 of this book.

**-Orthosis:**
Note: If dysfunction is not diagnosed early and treated, the above dysfunction may end up as the varus knee. If the varus knee is severe, then along with manual therapy techniques, a therapist can advise suitable orthotics for gradual correction[13]. Varus knee below kinetic chain pathomechanics will lead to an adducted and inverted (supinated) foot, where the patient walks with bowed legs with the weight falling on the lateral border of the foot. For the varus knee, footwear correction would be a lateral raise, as shown in Figures 15a and 15b. Lateral wedge can range from $2^0$-$6^0$. With this correction, valgus force is applied to the affected knee, assisting in the gradual correction of the varus knee.

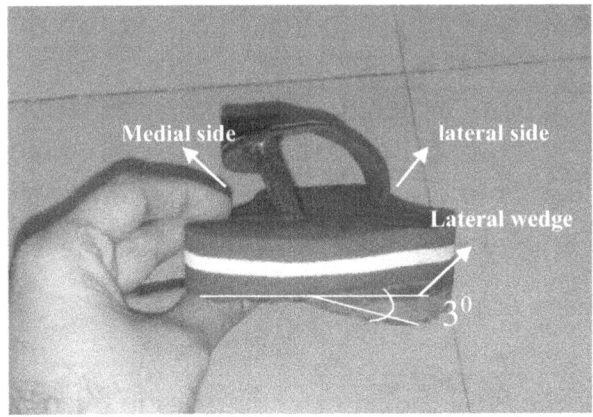

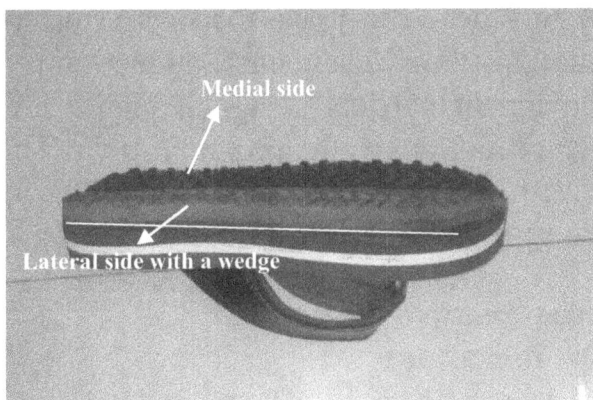

Figure 15a: Lateral raise of left footwear with $3^0$ lateral wedge. (Frontal view)

Figure 15b: Plantar view.

**-Progressive strengthening:** is advised according to the patient's condition and tolerance. A detailed explanation is covered in Chapter 2.

## B. Extension lag: with proximal tibia internally rotated with medial shift/glide:

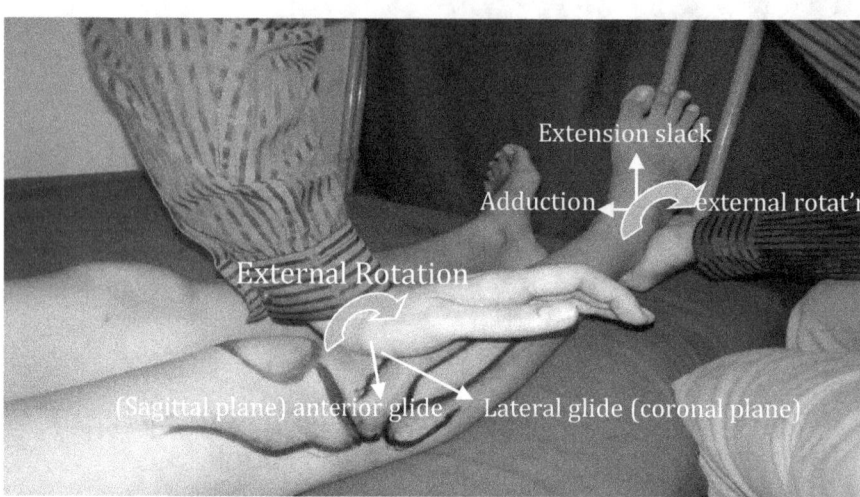

Figure 16: Shows both spring test and treatment of knee dysfunction: Extension lag with proximal tibia internally rotated with medial shift/glide.

**Spring test:** shown in figure 16
**Position of the patient:** is supine, right knee to be examined.
**Position of the therapist and procedure:** The therapist approaches the patient's right side. The knee is taken into the possible range of extension. The therapist left Pisiform/olecranon placed on the proximal-medial surface close to the tibial tuberosity. Three planar movement barriers of the proximal tibia - external rotation (transverse plane), lateral glide (coronal plane), and anterior glide (sagittal plane) are reached. Simultaneously, the therapist's right wrist is slightly extended with fingers flexed to grasp the lower posterior surface of the tibia. Then, an external rotation (transverse plane), adduction (coronal plane), and anterior glide/extension movement barriers (sagittal plane) are reached, which in turn reinforces three planar motions at the proximal tibia. Then, proximal tibia extension slack is taken with 12kg force, and additionally, 8kg force is applied in terminal extension to test the spring/end feel. If it does not spring - it indicates dysfunction.

**Treatment:**
**-Mobilization:**
**Position of Patient:** The patient is lying supine, and the right knee is to be treated.

**Position of the therapist and procedure:** The therapist approaches the patient's right side as explained in the assessment above; three planar movement barriers are reached at the proximal tibia. Then, the extension slack is taken with 12kg force, and further, the anterior glide of the proximal tibia/extension is done according to the grades of mobilization. Three glides are given three times. Each time, a 5-second rest is given.

**-Muscle energy technique:** Shown in figure 16
**Position of the patient:** is in supine lying, and the right knee is to be treated.
**Position of the therapist and procedure:** The therapist approaches the patient's right side; as mentioned above, three planar movement barriers are reached at the proximal tibia, and three planar slacks are taken with 12kg force. Then, the patient is asked to flex the knee, and simultaneously, the therapist resists producing an isometric contraction. After 5 seconds of relaxation, a new movement barrier is reached in three planes (i.e., external rotation, lateral glide, and anterior glides/extension). Again, repeat the same three times per session.

**-Taping:** Shown in figure 17
**Position of the patient:** is in supine lying, and the right knee is to be treated.
**Position of the therapist and procedure:** The therapist approaches the patient's right side. One end of the tape is pasted on the proximal medial surface of the tibia, and the therapist's left hand stabilize the lateral lower surface of the femur. The therapist's right-hand thumb/pisiform/olecranon of the elbow is placed on the proximal-medial surface of the tibia, close to the tibial tuberosity, and rotated externally with a slack of 12kg force. Then, the other end of the tape is pasted at the distal lateral thigh (femur) to achieve external rotation (transverse plane) and lateral glide (coronal plane).

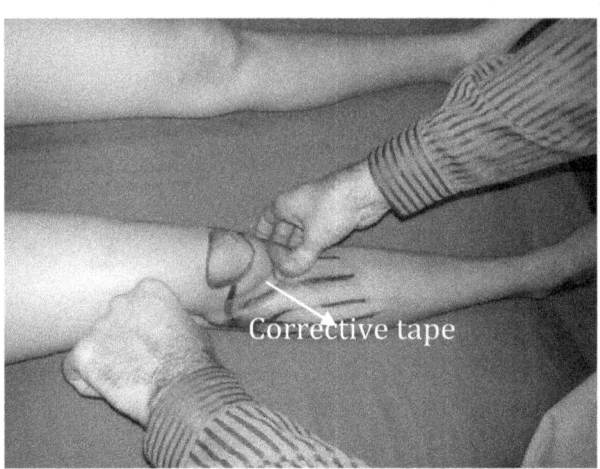

Figure 17: External rotation and lateral glide taping of the proximal tibia in knee dysfunction- Extension lag with superior tibia internally rotated and medial shifted.

**-Sustained medial to lateral glide of the tibia:** Shown in Figure 18
**Position of the patient and procedure:** The patient is on the left side, and the right knee is to be treated. Along with the correction tape (figure 17), further sustained glide is employed to give medial to lateral glide with a specially designed stand (dimension of stand previously mentioned). The left leg is slightly extended at the hip, flexed at the knee; the right leg's hip is flexed, the knee is extended, and the pillow is kept under the right leg, below the stand, to increase the height. The medial surface of the right proximal tibia is placed on the projected part of the stand, and then the weight of the leg glides the proximal tibia laterally. It can be kept for a duration of 2-5 min, depending on the condition and tolerance of the patient. If required, additional weight can be placed over the lateral surface of the distal tibia according to patient tolerance and condition.

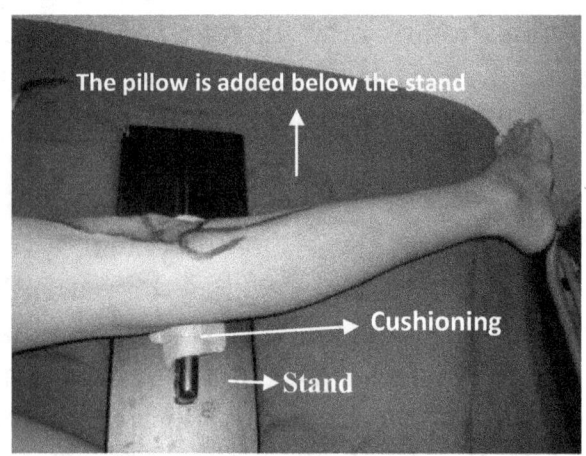

Figure 18: Shows the sustained lateral glide (coronal plane) of the proximal tibia at the extension barrier on a specially designed stand with corrective tape on. Cushioning is added between the medial side of the knee and a stand.

**The sustained anterior glide of the tibia:** Shown in figure19
**Position of the patient and procedure:** is prone lying, and the right knee is to be treated. Along with the correction tape, further sustained glide is employed to increase the anterior glide/extension (sagittal plane) of the proximal tibia with a specially designed stand (dimensions of the stand are previously mentioned).

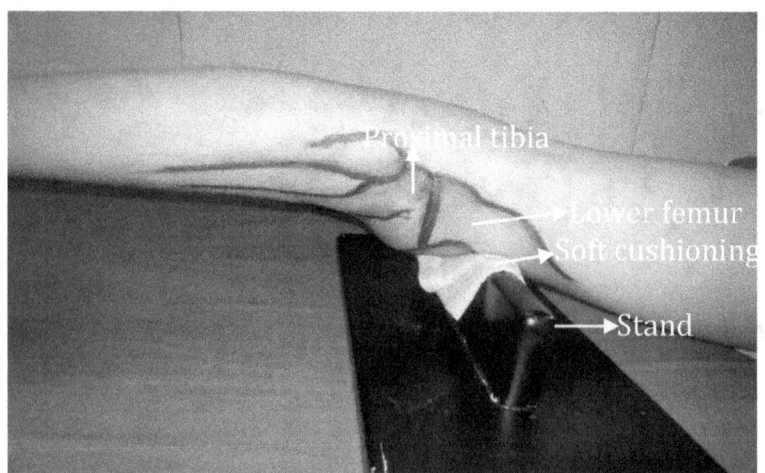

Figure 19: Shows the sustained extension glide of the proximal tibia, with corrective tape on, with the help of a specially designed stand. Cushioning is kept between the stand and the knee.

The position of the patient is prone; the distal anterior surface of the femur or just above the superior border of the patella is placed on the projected part of the stand, and then leg weight makes the proximal tibia glide anteriorly on the femur. Duration can be kept for 2-5 minutes, depending on the condition and tolerance of the patient.

**-Orthotics:**
Note: As already discussed, if the initial dysfunction is not diagnosed early and treated, the above dysfunction may end up in the valgus knee. If the valgus knee is severe, suitable orthotics and manual therapy can be advised for gradual correction. As we know from below the knee kinetic chain, the pathomechanics of the valgus knee will lead to abduction and eversion of the foot (pronated foot). That is, the patient walks on the medial border of the foot[13]. Therefore, footwear correction would be a medial raise for the valgus knee, as shown in Figures 20a and 20b. The medial wedge should be added; it may range from $2^0$-$6^0$. This correction of the footwear will lead to varus force on the knee, which will gradually assist in the correction of the dysfunction/deformity.

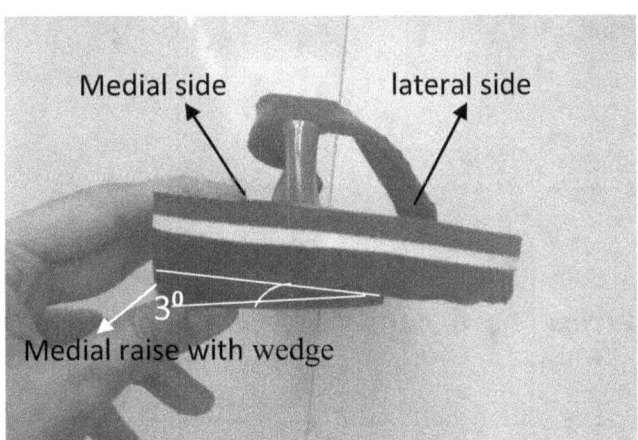

Figure 20a: Medial raise of left footwear with $3^0$ wedge. Frontal view. If needed medial arch can be added.

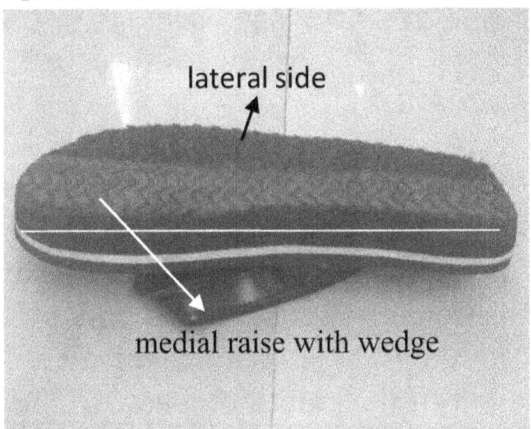

Figure 20b: Plantar view

**-Progressive strengthening** is advised according to the patient's condition and tolerance. A detailed explanation is covered in Chapter 2.

## C. Extension lag: with the proximal tibia, both internal, external rotation and medial, lateral glide loss:

As we know, internal rotation occurs with the medial glide, and external rotation occurs with the lateral glide. Therefore, medial and lateral glides will also be lost once rotations glides are lost, as they are coupled movements.

The above A and B sections of knee extension lag dysfunctions, which are already covered above, are included in the assessment and treatment. Moreover, the proximal tibia medial and lateral glide spring test and treatment at the extension barrier can be included.

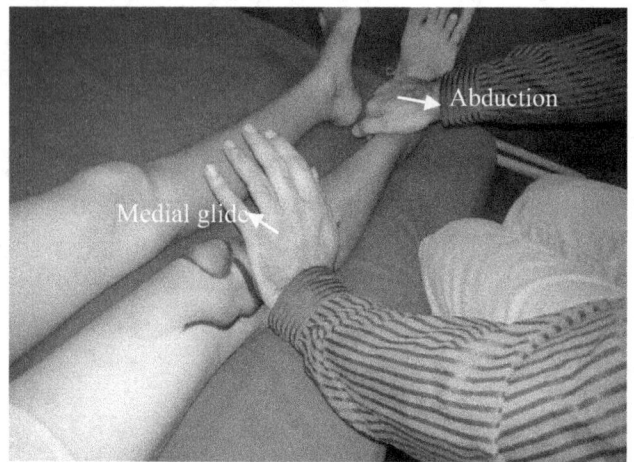

Figure 21: Right knee: spring test of proximal tibia medial glide loss, at extension barrier.

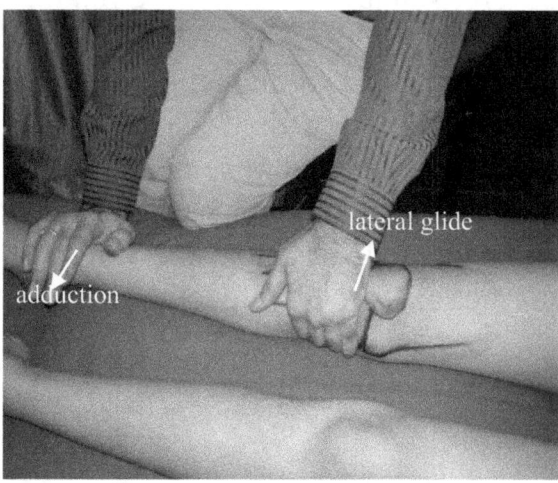

Figure 22: Right knee: Spring test of proximal tibia lateral glide loss at extension barrier.

### Proximal tibia- lateral at extension barrier

**Spring test:** Shown in Figure 21

**Position of the patient:** is supine; affected knee to be treated is right.

**Position of the therapist and procedure:** The therapist approaches the patient from the right side of the patient, and then the right knee is taken into the possible extent of the extension barrier. The therapist's right hand's pisiform/ webspace of thumb and forefinger is placed on the proximal-lateral surface of the tibia; simultaneously, the therapist's right wrist and finger are flexed to grasp the medial surface of the distal tibia, and then abduction is done, which intern reinforces medial glide at the proximal tibia. After reaching the movement barrier in extension and medial glide, proximal tibia medial glide slack is taken with 12 kg force, and additionally, 8 kg force is applied to test the spring/end feel. If it does not spring, then the test is positive, indicating dysfunction. If it springs, then the test is negative, i.e., the knee's proximal tibia medial glide (coronal plane) is normal.

**Proximal tibia- medial to lateral glide: at extension barrier**
**Spring test:** Shown in Figure 22,
**Position of the patient:** is supine; affected knee to be treated is right.
**Position of the therapist and procedure:** The therapist approaches the patient from the right side, and then the right knee is taken into the possible extent of the extension (extension barrier). The therapist's left wrist and finger flexed to grasp the proximal-medial surface of the tibia to reach the lateral glide barrier. Simultaneously, the therapist's right wrist extended, and fingers flexed to grasp the distal lateral surface of the tibia to reach the tibia adduction barrier. Which, in turn, reinforces lateral glide at the proximal tibia. Then, lateral glide slack at the proximal tibia is taken with 12 kg force, and 8 kg force is applied to test the spring/end feel. If it does not spring, then the test is positive–it indicates dysfunction. If it springs, it indicates the test is negative, i.e., the knee's proximal tibia lateral glide (coronal plane) is normal.

**3. Knee flexion and extension lag:**
If there is extension and flexion lag of the knee, that indicates dysfunction.
That is, both flexion and extension of the knee are not complete.
Therefore, apply the assessment and treatment procedures for both 1 and 2 of the knee dysfunctions mentioned above.

**References:**

1. https://www.youtube.com/watch?v=yPUR4KY6DFc
2. http://www.mccc.edu/~behrensb/documents/OsteoArthrokinematics.pdf
3. Lippert, L.S. (2011). Clinical Kinesiology and Anatomy, 5th ed. Philadelphia, PA: F.A. Davis.
4. Sharon, Thomas, et al., Integrative manual therapy for upper and lower extremities, 2008, p 153
5. Lopez-Lopez A, Mobilization versus manipulations versus sustained apophyseal natural glide techniques and interaction with psychological factors for patients with chronic neck pain: a randomized controlled trial.Eur J Phys Rehabil Med. 2015 Apr;51(2):121-32. Epub 2014 Oct 9
6. Maria Moutzouri, The effects of the Mulligan Sustained Natural Apophyseal Glide (SNAG) mobilisation in the lumbar flexion range of asymptomatic subjects as measured by the Zebris CMS20 3-D motion analysis system, *BMC Musculoskeletal* Disorders20089:131.
7. Martin Meyer, Muscle Energy Techniques, http://www.apemedical.com.au/useruploads/files/muscle_energy_techniques_pt1.pdf
8. https://www.youtube.com/watch?v=TEjKhf-qDJU
9. https://www.youtube.com/watch?v=W_IrZOtWqpg
10. https://www.youtube.com/watch?v=RzydPGGyPw0
11. Gwilym G. Davis; Region Of The Knee. Surface Anatomy, "Applied Anatomy: The Construction Of The Human Body".
12. http://www.orthopaedicmedicineonline.com/downloads/pdf/B9780702031458000879_web.pdf
13. Paul Frowen, et al., Neale's Disorders of the Foot; Elsevier Health Sciences, 12-Apr-2010 - Medical - 716 pages
14. Jerry Hesch Hesch Method of Manual Therapy Basic Information, http://www.heschinstitute.com/hesch-method-basics.html

# CHAPTER 10
## Anatomy, Biomechanics, and Pathomechanics of patellofemoral joint

### Anatomy[31]: The patella mainly articulates with the femur
### Femur

- Trochlear groove consists of medial and lateral femoral condyles with intervening shallow depression (5-6 mm)
- The lateral wall of the trochlear groove is more prominent and projects further anteriorly.
- Structural abnormalities of the trochlear groove predisposing an individual to lateral tracking of the patella: flattening or hypoplasia of the trochlear groove (normal groove angle is 130 degrees)

### Patella

- The articular surface is divided by a medial ridge into 2 large facets: medial & lateral.
- The less distinct ridge divides the medial facet into 2 facets in most: medial & lateral.
- Indistinct transverse ridges divide the medial & lateral facets into superior, middle, and inferior facets.
- The lateral facet is usually larger than the medial.

Figure 1: Depicts the patella-femoral joint of the knee and associated soft tissue around the patella.

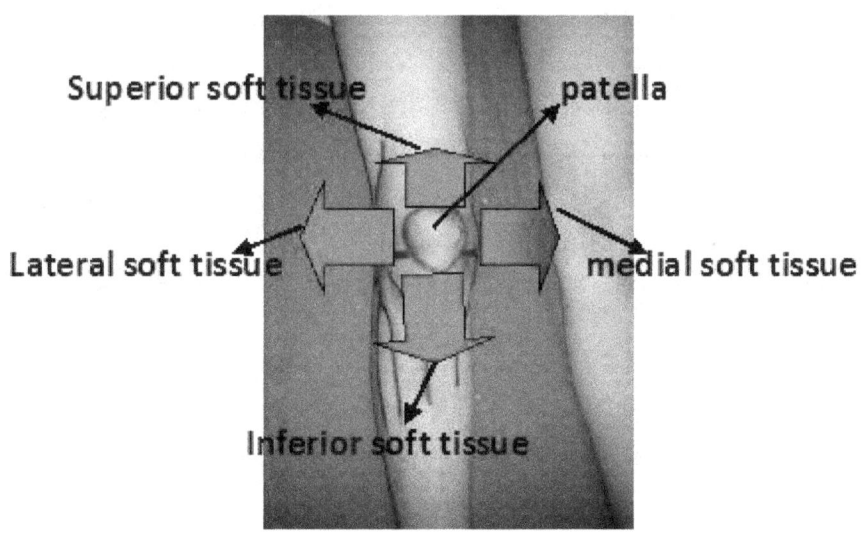

**Quadriceps and other soft tissues which influence patellar mechanics[37]:** Shown in Figure 1

**Rectus femoris tendon:** 8-10 cm in length, triangular in shape with insertion 3-5 cm in width at the superior pole of the patella

**VMO tendon[30,32,33]:** inserts obliquely at the superomedial border of the patella, oriented 55-70 degrees in relation to the sagittal plane, tendon only a few mm in length; primary stabilizer of patella medially against Vastus lateralis

**Vastus lateralis:** inserts obliquely at the superolateral aspect of the patella, oriented 22-45 degrees in relation to the sagittal plane, 2.8 cm in length

Lateral expansion of the vastus lateralis with a superficial and deep layer forms the lateral retinaculum; the deep layer is the lateral patella-femoral lig: this is a static guide for the patella; this may decrease medial excursion and increase lateral tracking[35, 38]

**Ober:** fascial band extending from ITB to the lateral and inferior margin of the patella (importance of ITB flexibility)

The medial side also has a Patello-Femoral lig, but it is much weaker than the lateral side.
Dysplasia of the extensor mechanism may be responsible for Patello-femoral symptoms, with even small variations being liable to affect the delicate muscle complex that controls Patello-femoral kinematics.
Increased tension of the lateral retinaculum increases stress on the lateral patellar facet and predisposes to mal-alignment and instability[9]. Similarly, excessive tension of the iliotibial band, through its expansion on the quadriceps and patellar tendon, causes a lateral patellar shift predisposing to lateral dislocation[10]. A similar effect is determined by true VMO hypoplasia[11,12]. It has been demonstrated that the VMO[34] is oriented at $47° ± 5°$ with respect to the medial femoral axis, while the orientation of the vastus lateralis is $35° ± 4°$ [13]. Furthermore, relaxation of the VMO at 20° of knee flexion determines a 30% reduction of lateral stability[14]. Despite normal development of the medial structures, an imbalance of neuro-muscular activation and coordination also determines an alteration of patellar behaviour during flexion-extension [15].

The passive stabilizers of the PF joint include the MPFL (medial patella-femoral ligament), the medial patella-tibial ligament (MPTL) and the retinaculum. It has been shown that MPFL and MPTL contribute 60% and 22% of the force that opposes lateral displacement of the patella[16] and that the force needed to determine a lateral patellar displacement is less at 20° of knee flexion [17]. Furthermore, MPFL injury has been proven to reduce by almost 50% the force needed to dislocate the patella laterally with the knee extended [18]. For this reason, the scientific community has shown a growing interest in studying this important anatomical structure in recent years.

Medial patella-femoral ligament damage is one of the leading causes of lateral dislocation of the patella [19-21]. Although reconstruction of an injured MPFL gives better results today than in the past, a recent systematic review of the literature suggested that there is a need for a better understanding of the capacity of the reconstructed MPFL to prevent alterations in PF kinematics and cartilage degeneration [22].

Kinematic *ex vivo* studies can provide extremely realistic models of knees with intact MPFL. However, analyzing the mechanical behaviour of the patella in cases of MPFL injury or reconstruction is less straightforward[23-27]. There are also conflicting results regarding MPFL tension at rest with the knee extended [19, 20]. These differences are likely attributable to the use of different reference systems, to difficulties defining the points of MPFL insertion on the femur and the patella[19,27-29], and to differences in specimen preparations due to the complexity of MPFL dissection and resection.

**Articulation**

No contact between the femur and patella in full extension[1]; the patella lies over an area of thin, smooth synovial tissue on the anterior shaft of the femur, proximal to the trochlear surface (superio-trochlear tubercle) from extension to flexion, the patella: begins laterally and moves medially as the patella enters the trochlear groove and the tibia derotates; it follows the groove until the knee is flexed to 90 degrees when the patella again moves laterally until it covers the condyle at 135 degrees with flexion, patella enters the trochlear groove from the lateral side seats in the trochlea at 20 degrees; at this point, the congruence and compressive forces provide stability from 0-20 degrees, stability comes from soft tissues Q angle = 10-12° males and 15-18° for females; several studies have found increased Q angles in those with patellar dislocations[36].

## Biomechanics:

Proximal component - the femur (convex femoral condyles)

Distal component - patella (3 concave facets of the patella)

Joint type - saddle joint

Motion - superior, inferior glide, and medial/lateral shift, as well as medial and lateral tilt associated with knee extension and flexion

### *Functions of the patella:*

The primary function[8] is to increase the force production of the quadriceps; it acts like a pulley to increase the mechanical action of the quadriceps, centralising the quadriceps' divergent muscles.

Patellar compression force: to pull the patella against the anterior surface of the femur, and it increases with flexion

Quadriceps angle: the angle formed by the angle of the pull of the quadriceps and the line representing the patellar tendon. Male-12 degrees, female- 15 degrees

### *Patellofemoral contact areas:*

**0 degrees**: Patella completely above the femoral articular surface

**30 degrees**: The inferior aspect of the patella contacts the uppermost portion of the femoral condyles; contact begins between the LFC and the lateral facet of the patella, but by 30 degrees is evenly distributed on both sides

**60 degrees**: Contact between the superior half of the patellar surface and part of the femoral groove slightly inferior to the contact area at 30 degrees; contact area larger than at 30 degrees.

**90 degrees**: Contact between the superior half of the patella and an area of the femoral groove just above the notch; contact area larger than at 60 degrees

**120 degrees**: Contact between the superior aspect of the patella and the areas on the femoral groove immediately surrounding the notch in a kidney shape; quadriceps tendon contact with the trochlea also helps to share the compressive load.

# Chapter 10: Anatomy, Biomechanics and Pthomechanics of the Patello-Femoral joint

**Dynamic biomechanics: Patellofemoral joint reaction forces:**
Directly related to the quadriceps force generation, it increases as the angle of flexion increases. PFJR (patella-femoral joint reaction) force reaches 3.3xBW (bodyweight) when ascending and descending stairs, knee bend to 130 degrees and increases force to 7.8x BW. Open chain: PFJR force zeroes at 90 degrees flexion at rest; force increases rapidly to a maximum of 1.4x BW at 36 degrees flexion and decreases rapidly to 0.5 BW at the full extension, force increase faster when contact area increases, so stress/unit area increases rapidly to 90 degrees. Abnormal tracking results in even higher forces/unit area owing to smaller contact areas. Hungerford showed that a minor lateral shift of the patella could decrease the contact area by 60% and increase stress by 2.5xBw; surgical procedures attempt to re-centre the patella to redistribute the loads; Macquet (Macquet procedure) showed that a 2 cm elevation of the tibial tubercle increased the quadriceps moment and decreased the PF joint reaction force by 50% at 45 degrees flexion. One study showed a 50% decrease in patellar stress when the Q-angle was reduced from 15 to 5 degrees at 30 degrees of flexion.

**Dynamic stabilizers**: ITB, lateral retinaculum, VL, VMO[34], adductor Magnus. PFJR forces during isokinetic exercise at 60 and 180 degrees were lower (< 1.0 BW) at angles less than 20 degrees and were highest at 70-75 degrees of knee flexion (5.1x BW at 60 degrees/Sec and 4.9x BW at 180 deg/Sec) following ACL reconstruction using central 1/3 patellar tendon; PF contact pressures were not different from controlled knees. VMO is active throughout the ROM, maximum at 70 degrees. SAQ (short arc quadriceps) trains both the VMO and VL. EMG demonstrates increased activity in the VMO with concurrent hip adduction[40]

**Patello-femoral evaluation**
**Factors related to patellar dysfunction:**

**Staticfactors[9, 3]:**
Femoral anteversion

External tibial torsion

PatellaAlta[4] (patellar tendon length >120% patella)

PatellaBaja (Patellar tendon<80% patellar length)

Increased Q angle[2]

**Subjective:**
Diffuse anterior knee pain.
Pain is often exacerbated while using stairs.
Crepitus, giving way (buckling), and swelling can be noticeable.

**Pathomechanics of patella-femoral joint dysfunction:**
Patello-femoral main dysfunctions are:

- **Patella superior or inferior**
- **Patella medial or lateral**
- **Patella medially tilted or laterally tilted[39].**

Patellar dysfunctions occur secondarily to tibiofemoral and soft tissue (which attaches to the patella) dysfunction[5, 6]. Adhesions or tightness of soft tissue around the patella will lead to misalignment of the patella, thereby influencing the patellar mechanics.

Screening of the hip and foot mechanics should also be considered[7], as abnormal mechanics of these may affect the normal mechanics of the tibiofemoral joint and soft tissue related to the patella, thereby secondarily influencing normal patellar mechanics.

Patellar mobility may be affected secondary to tibiofemoral dysfunction, soft tissue (which attaches the patella), and adhesions/tightness. Treatment's main objective should be correcting the primary problem, i.e., restoring normal tibiofemoral mechanics and soft tissue attached to the patella[6]. Once it is done, normal patellar mechanics will be restored.

**References:**

1. Amis AA, Senavongse W, Bull AM. Patellofemoral kinematics during knee flexion-extension: an in vitro study.J Orthop Res. 2006;24:2201–2211.
2. Insall J, Goldberg V, Salvati E. Recurrent dislocation and the high-riding patella.Clin Orthop Relat Res. 1972;88:67–69.
3. Blackburn JS, Peel TE. A new method of measuring patellar height. J Bone Joint Surg. 1977;59:241–242.
4. Luyckx T, Didden K, Vandenneucker H, et al. Is there a biomechanical explanation for anterior knee pain in patients with patella alta?: influence of the patellar height of patellofemoral contact force, contact area, and contact pressure. J Bone Joint Surg Br. 2009;91:344–350.
5. Smillie, IS. The biomechanical basis of osteoarthritis of the knee in total knee replacement. Paper presented at Total knee replacement organised by the Institution of Mechanical Engineering; London. 1974.
6. Takai S, Sakakida K, Yamashita F, et al. Rotational alignment of the lower limb in osteoarthritis of the knee.Int Orthop. 1985;9:209–215.
7. http://www.mikereinold.com/influence-hip-foot-patellofemoral-pain/
8. http://www.healthline.com/human-body-maps/patella-bone
9. Ficat, P.; Hungerford, DS. Disorders of the Patellofemoral Joint. Williams & Wilkins; Baltimore: 1977.
10. Terry GC, Hughston JC, Norwood LA. The anatomy of the iliopatellar band and iliotibial tract.Am J Sports Med. 1986;14:39–45.
11. Insall J. Current Concepts Review: patellar pain. J Bone Joint Surg Am. 1982;64:147–152.
12. Fox TA. Dysplasia of the quadriceps mechanism: hypoplasia of the vastus medialis muscle as related to the hypermobile patella syndrome. Surg Clin North Am. 1975;55:199–226.
13. Farahmand F, Senavongse W, Amis AA. Quantitative study of the quadriceps muscles and trochlear groove geometry related to instability of the patellofemoral joint. J Orthop Res. 1998;16:36–143.
14. Goh JC, Lee PY, Bose K. A cadaver study of the function of the oblique part of vastus medialis.J Bone Joint Surg Br. 1995;77:225–231.
15. Voight ML, Wieder DL. Comparative reflex response times of vastus medialis obliquus and vastus lateralis in normal subjects and subjects with extensor

mechanism dysfunction. An electromyographic study. Am J Sports Med. 1991;19:131–137.
16. Desio SM, Burks RT, Bachus KN. Soft tissue restraints to lateral patellar translation in the human knee. Am J Sports Med. 1998;26:59–65.
17. Senavongse W, Farahmand F, Jones J, et al. Quantitative measurement of patellofemoral joint stability: force-displacement behavior of the human patella in vitro. J Orthop Res. 2003;21:780–786.
18. Senavongse W, Amis AA. The effects of articular, retinacular, or muscular deficiencies on patellofemoral joint stability: a biomechanical study in vitro. J Bone Joint Surg Br. 2005;87:577–582.
19. Amis AA, Firer P, Mountney J, et al. Anatomy and biomechanics of the medial patellofemoral ligament. Knee. 2003;10:215–220.
20. Nomura E, Horiuchi Y, Kihara M. Medial patellofemoral ligament restraint in lateral patellar translation and reconstruction. Knee. 2000;7:121–127.
21. Philippot R, Chouteau J, Wegrzyn J, et al. Medial patellofemoral ligament anatomy: implications for its surgical reconstruction. Knee Surg Sports Traumatol Arthrosc. 2009;17:475–479.
22. Buckens CF, Saris DB. Reconstruction of the medial patellofemoral ligament for treatment of patellofemoral instability: a systematic review. Am J Sports Med. 2010;38:181–188.
23. Parker DA, Alexander JW, Conditt MA, et al. Comparison of isometric and anatomic reconstruction of the medial patellofemoral ligament: a cadaveric study. Orthopedics. 2008;31:339–343.
24. Ostermeier S, Stukenborg-Colsman C, Hurschler C, et al. In vitro investigation of the effect of medial patellofemoral ligament reconstruction and medial tibial tuberosity transfer on lateral patellar stability. Arthroscopy. 2006;22:308–319.
25. Ostermeier S, Holst M, Bohnsack M, et al. In vitro measurement of patellar kinematics following reconstruction of the medial patellofemoral ligament. Knee Surg Sports Traumatol Arthrosc. 2007;15:276–285.
26. Sandmeier RH, Burks RT, Bachus KN, et al. The effect of reconstruction of the medial patellofemoral ligament on patellar tracking. Am J Sports Med. 2000;28:345–349.
27. Bedi H, Marzo J. The biomechanics of medial patellofemoral ligament repair followed by lateral retinacular release. Am J Sports Med. 2010;38:1462–1467.

28. Baldwin JL. The anatomy of the medial patellofemoral ligament. Am J Sports Med. 2009;37:2355–2361.
29. Nomura E, Inoue M, Osada N. Anatomical analysis of the medial patellofemoral ligament of the knee, especially the femoral attachment. Knee Surg Sports Traumatol Arthrosc. 2005;13:510–515.
30. Zaffagnini S, Colle F, Lopomo N, et al. The influence of medial patellofemoral ligament on patellofemoral joint kinematics and patellar stability. Knee Surg Sports Traumatol Arthrosc Nov. 2012;24 doi:10.1007/s00167-012-2307-9..
31. Smirk C, Morris H. The anatomy and reconstruction of the medial patellofemoral ligament. Knee. 2003;10:221–227.
32. Conlan T, Garth WP Jr, Lemons JE. Evaluation of the medial soft-tissue restraints of the extensor mechanism of the knee. J Bone Joint Surg Am. 1993;75:682–693.
33. Hautamaa PV, Fithian DC, Kaufman KR, et al. Medial soft tissue restraints in lateral patellar instability and repair.Clin Orthop Relat Res. 1998;(349):174–182.
34. Panagiotopoulos E, Strzelczyk P, Herrmann M, et al. Cadaveric study on static medial patellar stabilizers: the dynamizing role of the vastus medialis obliquus on medial patellofemoral ligament.Knee Surg Sports Traumatol Arthrosc. 2006;14:7–12.
35. Nha KW, Papannagari R, Gill TJ, et al. In vivo patellar tracking: clinical motions and patellofemoral indices.J Orthop Res. 2008;26:1067–1074.
36. Yamada Y, Toritsuka Y, Horibe S, et al. In vivo movement analysis of the patella using a three-dimensional computer model. J Bone Joint Surg Br. 2007;89:752–760.
37. Amis AA. Current concepts on anatomy and biomechanics of patellar stability. Sports Med Arthrosc. 2007;15:48–5
38. Asano T, Akagi M, Koike K, et al. In vivo three-dimensional patellar tracking on the femur.Clin Orthop Relat Res. 2003;413:222–232.
39. http://www.patellofemoral.org/pfoe/PDFs/Patellofemoral_Pain_ICRS.pdf

# CHAPTER 11
## Assessment and Treatment of Patellar Dysfunctions

**Assessment of patella-femoral joint**

Patello-femoral joint dysfunctions are secondary to tibiofemoral and/or soft tissue dysfunction[10,11]. The assessment and treatment of the tibiofemoral joint and soft tissue surrounding the patella are of primary importance over patellar mobilization. Patellar dysfunctions can be assessed by palpating surrounding tissue with Cyriax deep friction and comparing the position of the patella symmetry with the normal side.

**Acute Phase treatment:**

The goal is to control pain and inflammation and prevention of quadriceps atrophy.

**Rest**: Controlled activity through an assistive device( like a walker or stick) depending upon evaluation

**Ice**: 2-3 times daily for 5-10 min

**Knee braces**: For stabilization of the knee on weight-bearing activities of daily life.

**Taping:** This can be used for the correction of the alignment and to provide stabilization.

**NSAIDs**: NSAIDs (non-steroidal anti-inflammatory drugs) can be used to decrease inflammation and pain. And isometrics to quadriceps can be introduced to maintain strength.

**Stiffness/chronic phase treatment:**

In the stiffness phase of patellar dysfunction, graded mobilization of the patella and soft tissue release around the patella need to be done. Suppose patellar dysfunctions occur because of the primary dysfunction of the above and below kinetic chain, i.e., tibiofemoral, foot, and hip dysfunction. In that case, it needs to be addressed first and gradually; progressive strengthening can be added according to patient conditions and tolerance.

**Note**: Detailed soft tissue assessment and treatment of knee joint complex is covered in chapters 5 and 13 of this book.

## Patellar dysfunctions and assessment:

Patellar dysfunctions are always secondary to soft tissue adhesions, tightness and tibiofemoral dysfunctions[3,4] (refer to Chapter 13). The main dysfunctions of the patella are:

**Superior, inferior, medial,** and **lateral** or a combination of one or more may give rise to **patellar tilt**[2]

## Patellar superior, inferior and medial, lateral symmetry testing:

As shown in Figure 1, a horizontal line divides the patella into superior and inferior halves, which will enable us to compare the symmetry with the normal side[5]. When soft tissue attached to the inferior border of the patella, like ligamentum patella, becomes tight/has adhesions, the patella shifts inferior from the horizontal line. Similarly, when soft tissue attached to the superior border of the patellar-like quadriceps tendon becomes tight/has adhesion, it is seen that the patella shifts **superior** from the horizontal line, as shown in Figure 1. Likewise, when soft tissue attached to the medial border of the patellar becomes tight/has adhesions, it is seen that the patella shifts **medially** from the vertical line, as shown in Figure 2. Similarly, when soft tissue attached to the lateral border of the patellar becomes tight/has adhesions, it is seen that the patella shifts **laterally** to the vertical line, which divides the patella into medial and lateral halves shown in Figure 2. A combination of more than one of the above may lead to **patellar tilt**.

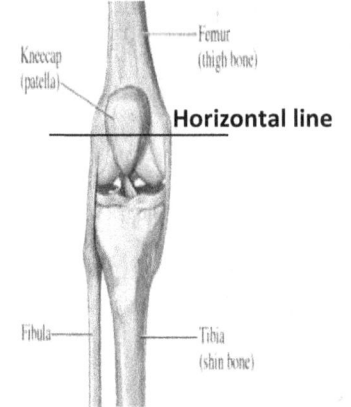

Figure 1: horizontal line dividing the patella into superior and inferior halves.

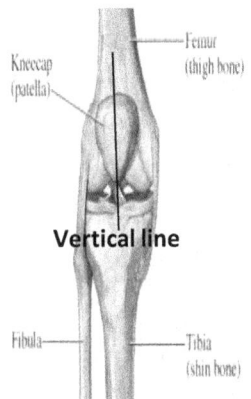

Figure 2: vertical line dividing the patella into medial and lateral halfs.

## Patellar inferior and superior mobility testing:

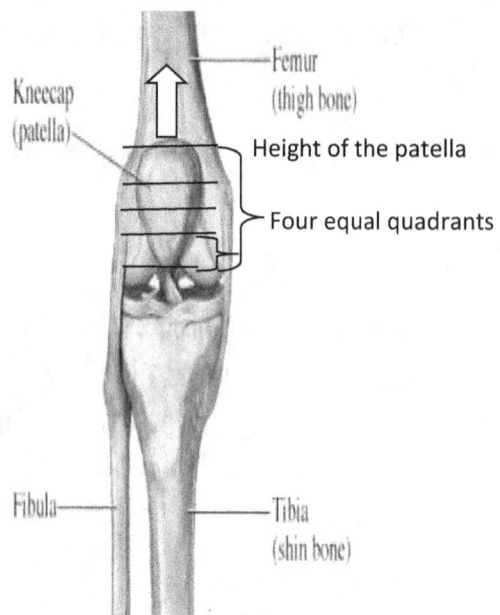

Figure 3: Height of patella divided into four equal compartments, shown as horizontal lines for testing superior and inferior patellar mobility.

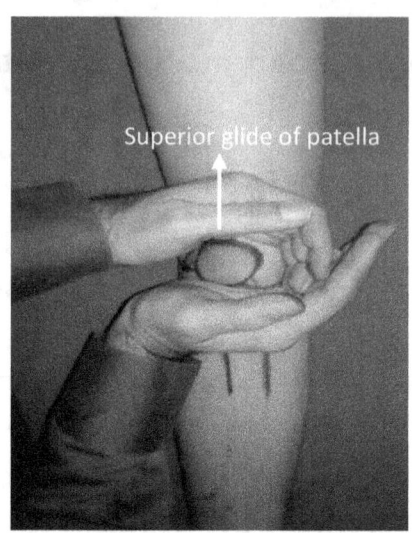

Figure 4: Superior glide of the patella.

**Patellar superior mobility testing[6]**: Shown in Figures 3 and 4.
Position of the patient: Superior glide testing was performed on the right knee in a supine and resting position.
Position of the therapist and procedure: The therapist approaches the patient from the right side. The therapist's right hand's Palmar surface of the 5th metacarpal wrapped around the inferior border of the patella, and simultaneously therapist's left hand's Palmar surface of the 5th metacarpal wrapped around the superior border of the patella, as shown in figure 4. By grabbing the patella firmly and gliding it superiorly, the extent of displacement is described in relation to the height of the patella and measured in 4 equal quadrants as horizontal lines depicted in Figure 3. Patellar displacement less than one quadrant superiorly is considered tightness/adhesions of inferior structure, i.e. ligamentum patella. Displacement of more than three quadrants is considered hypermobile.

**Patellar inferior mobility testing:** The testing position of the patient and therapist is the same as mentioned above. Patellar displacement of less than one quadrant inferiorly is considered tightness/adhesions of superior soft tissue attachments of the patella and quadriceps tendon. Patellar inferior displacement of more than three quadrants is considered hypermobile.

**Patellar medial and lateral mobility testing[7]:**
**Patellar medial mobility testing:** Shown in Figures 5 and 6.
Position of the patient: Medial glide testing was performed on the right knee in the supine.
Position of the therapist: The therapist approaches the patient from the right side. The therapist's right hand's Palmar surface of the 5th Metacarpal wrapped around the inferior border of the patella, and simultaneously, the therapist's left hand's Palmar surface of the 5th metacarpal wrapped around the superior border of the patella as shown in Figure 6. By grabbing firmly, glide the patella medially. Assess the amount of excursion of the patella. The extent of displacement is described in relation to the width of the patella and measured in 4 equal quadrants, vertical lines depicted in Figure 5. Patellar displacement of less than one quadrant medially is considered tightness/adhesions of lateral soft tissue attachments of the patella. Displacement of more than three quadrants is considered hypermobile.

**Patellar lateral mobility testing:** The testing position of the patient and therapist is the same as mentioned above. Patellar displacement of less than one quadrant laterally is considered tightness/adhesions of medial soft tissue attachments of the patella. Patellar lateral displacement of more than three quadrants is considered hypermobile.

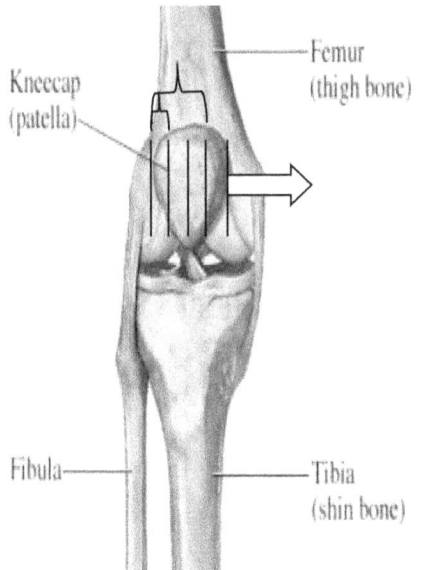

Figure 5: The width of the patella is divided into 4 equal compartments by vertical lines for testing medial and lateral patellar mobility.

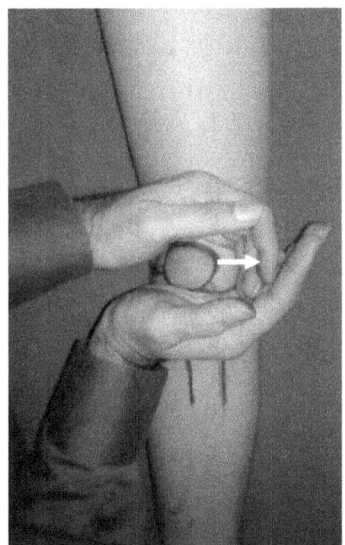

Figure 6: Right knee-medial glide of the patella.

**Note:** Similarly, patellar inferior and superior mobility testing can be done. Sometimes, combined mobility testing also gives very useful information about patellar dysfunction.

**Treatment of patellar dysfunctions**: It includes restoring normal mobility and alignment of the patella, and associated soft tissue adhesions release as well as stretching. Detailed associated knee soft tissue tightness/adhesion treatment is covered in chapter 13 of the book.

**Patellar mobilization**[8,9]: The author suggests two grades of mobilization of the patella. According to the assessment of patellar positional dysfunctions, specific mobilization can be implemented.

**1. Grade I**: patellar mobilization in four directions, i.e., a) Superior glide, b) Inferior glide, c) Medial glide, d). Lateral glide.

The patella can be mobilized in **a single glide or combined glide**. The single glide of the patella would be superior glide, inferior glide, medial glide, or lateral glide. A combined glide can be given with superior to inferior, inferior to superior, medial to lateral glide, and lateral to medial glide.

While mobilizing, the patella's opposite side of the soft tissue will be stretched. That is, if the right knee patella is mobilized.
- a) When mobilized superiorly, the inferior part of the patellar soft tissue is automatically stretched. As shown in Figure 7
- b) When mobilized inferiorly, soft tissue that attaches to the patella's superior border will be stretched. As shown in Figure 8
- c) When mobilized medially, soft tissue that attaches to the patella's lateral border will be stretched. As shown in Figure 9
- d) When mobilized laterally, the soft tissue which attaches to the medial border will be stretched. As shown in Figure 10

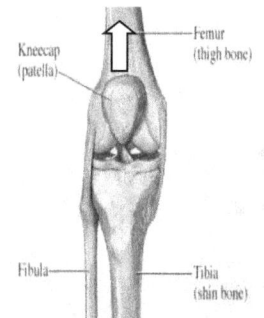

Figure 7: superior glide and inferior soft tissue stretch.

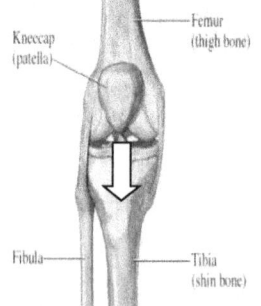

Figure 8: inferior glide and superior soft tissue stretch.

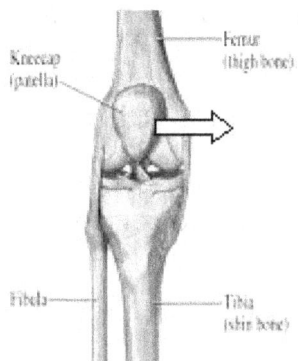 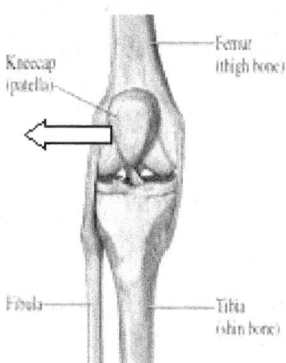

Figure 9: Medial glide and lateral soft tissue stretch.

Figure 10: Lateral glide and medial soft tissue stretch.

**Combined glides of the patella**:

The basic principles of patellar mobilization remain the same as mentioned above. Additionally, a combination of the mobilizations can be introduced. These are as follows.

a) Lateral to medial glide and /or medial to lateral glide. Figure 11
b) Superior to inferior glide and/or inferior to superior glide. Figure 12

As shown above, mobilization of the patella and simultaneous stretch of opposite side soft tissue can be done.

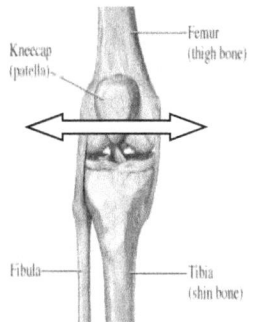 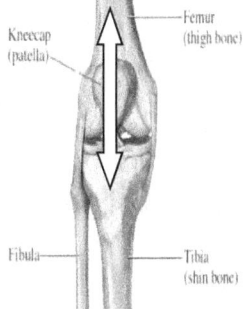

Figure 11: Medial to lateral and lateral to medial glide of the right patella.

Figure 12: Superior to inferior and inferior to superior glide of the right patella.

**2. Grade II:** Maintaining uni-directional patellar glide and stretch; another opposite directional glide and stretch can be added. That is, maintaining one horizontal glide; additionally, vertical superior to inferior glide and inferior to superior glide can be added. In the same way, maintaining one-directional vertical glide; additionally, horizontal medial to lateral and lateral to medial glide of the patella can be done. These are explained in detail below:

i) Maintaining superior glide, medial to lateral, and lateral to medial glide is given. As shown in Figure 13
ii) Maintaining inferior glide, medial to lateral, and lateral to medial glide is given. As shown in Figure 14
iii) Maintaining medial glide, superior to inferior and inferior to superior glide, is given. As shown in Figure 15
iv) Maintaining lateral glide, superior to inferior and inferior to superior glide, is given. As shown in Figure 16

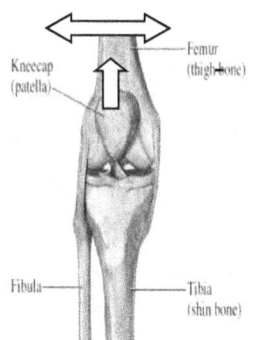

Figure 13: Superior glide with medial to lateral and lateral to medial glide is given.

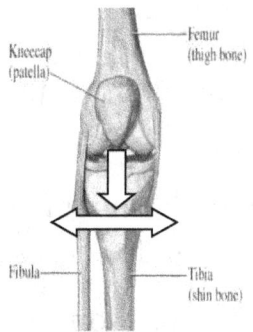

Figure 14: Inferior glide with medial to lateral and lateral to medial glide is given.

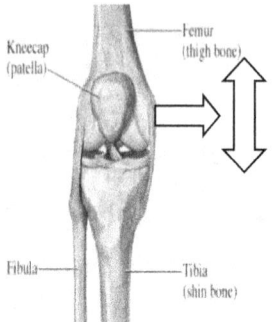

Figure 15: Medial glide with superior to inferior and inferior to superior glide is given.

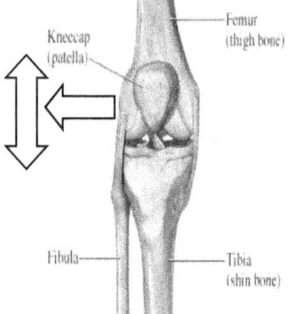

Figure 16: Lateral glide with superior to inferior and inferior to superior glide is given.

**The number of glides per session:** 5 glides with 1 to 3 times in one session, according to the patient's condition and tolerance, each time 5 Sec rest is given.

**References:**

1. Stefano zaffagnini, David et al., Patellofemoral anatomy and biomechanics: current concepts, Published online 2013 October 24, 2013 April; 1(2): 15–20. ISSN: 2282-4234
2. E. G. McNally, at al, Assessment of patellar maltracking using combined static and dynamic MRI; European Radiology, June 2000, Volume 10, Issue 7, pp 1051–1055
3. Boden BP, Pearsall AW, Garrett WE, Feagin JA: Patellofemoral instability: evaluation and management. J Am Acad Orthop Surg. 1997;5:47-57.
4. Fulkerson, JP: Patellofemoral disorders: evaluation and management. J Am Acad Orthop Surg. 1994;2:124-132.
5. Heidi Dawson, Patellofemoral pain syndrome: Assessment and treatment;http://www.multibriefs.com/briefs/exclusive/pfps_what_why_how.html#.WN3QLvmGPIU
6. John miller, Patellofemoral Pain Syndrome.http://physioworks.com.au/injuries-conditions-1/patellofemoral-kneecap-pain-syndrome
7. Measuring the position and mobility of the patella; https://mikereinold.com/measuring-position-and-mobility-of/
8. https://www.youtube.com/watch?v=VZfoIUIpT40
9. Patellar Mobilisation (Part 2 of a set of tutorials by Dirk Kokmeyer on Arthrofibrosis Rehab) http://www.kneeguru.co.uk/KNEEnotes/courses/arthrofibrosis-rehab-tutorials-dirk-kokmeyer-pt-scs-comt/patellar-mobilisation-part-2-set
10. http://www.axelsonchiropractic.com/uploads/8/7/3/1/8731168/art-kneepain.pdf
11. Joe jphson et al.; the use of augmented soft tissue mobilization as a conservative treatment for patella femoral pain syndrome. http://rapidrehabilitation.com/wp-content/uploads/2014/09/ATYM-PFPS.pdf

# CHAPTER 12
## Proximal Tibio-fibular joint: Biomechanics, Pathomechanics, and Treatment

**Proximal tibiofibular joint**: [Shown in figure 1]
The postero-lateral surface of the tibia and the head of the fibula form an arthrodial articulation known as the proximal tibiofibular (PTF) joint. The capsule surrounding the PTF joint, although reinforced by anterior and posterior ligaments, is thicker anteriorly. The popliteus tendon helps reinforce the capsule's posterior aspect as it crosses the joint. At the insertion of the biceps femoris, the proximal fibula provides lateral stability to the knee. Three distinct movements occur between the proximal tibia and the fibular head
1) Antero-posterior glide
2) Supero-inferior motion and
3) Rotation.

The ability of the PTF joint to withstand longitudinal or axial stresses is a direct function of its anatomy. The proximal aspect of the fibula seems best able to undergo tensile and torsional stresses. Compressive forces appear best managed distally, where the interosseous membrane ensures lower leg function by actively involving the fibula in load transference. The fibula has been shown to bear one-sixth of axial loading on the leg, with a key role in dissipating torsional stresses produced by ankle motion[2].

The PTF joint primarily reduces torsional stress at the ankle, minimises lateral bending of the tibia, and decreases weight-bearing torsion.[1,2] Abnormal force accumulation and altered biomechanics or trauma frequently affect a joint that, when injured, can contribute to chronic pain and considerable disability[3,4,5].

Figure 1: proximal tibio-fibular joint.

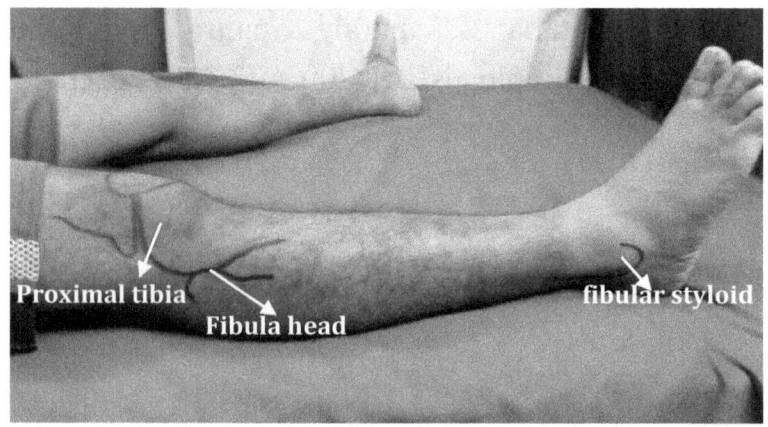

## Mechanics of PTF joint:

### Mechanics: related to foot dysfunction (when the knee is not involved)

The fibular head goes anterio-lateral with dorsiflexion; the fibular head goes posterior-medial with plantar-flexion.[8]

The fibular head goes into superior with eversion of the foot; the fibular head goes inferior with inversion of the foot.

Plantar flexion goes with the inversion of the foot, and dorsiflexion goes with the eversion of the foot.

### Mechanics: related to knee dysfunction (when the foot is not involved)

As we know, with regard to dysfunctions of the knee, the proximal tibia externally rotates with lateral shifts or internally rotates with medial shifts. When the proximal tibia externally rotates, the normally fibular head goes posterior. Even though the tibia rotates internally, the fibular head becomes posterior as the bicep femoris will not let the fibula head go anterior.

### proximal tibio-fibular joint dysfunction[9]:

**PTF dysfunctions** are mainly involved secondary to either knee or foot dysfunctions.

Dysfunctions[6,7,8] of this joint occur mainly secondary to either tibia-femoral dysfunction or ankle inversion/and dorsiflexion, eversion/and plantar flexion dysfunction.

**PTF dysfunctions secondary to knee dysfunction:** The fibular head is always posterior in most knee dysfunctions. As we know, in knee dysfunctions, the proximal tibia can externally rotate and laterally shift or internally rotate and medially shift. If it is externally rotated, the fibular head goes into the posterior along with the tibia's external rotation. Even though it is internally rotated, it will be posterior because the bicep femoris pulls the fibular head posterior opposite to the internal rotation of the tibia.

**PTF dysfunctions secondary to foot dysfunctions:**
The fibular head is anterior-lateral when the foot is dorsiflexed, and the fibular head is posterior-medial when the foot is plantar-flexed

The fibular head is superior when the foot is everted, and the fibular head is inferior when the foot is inverted.

The **dysfunctions of tibio-fibular joint** are as follows: they can be one or more combinations of the following. [11-13]
1. Fibular head posteriormedial
2. Fibular head anterior lateral
3. Fibular head, both anterior and posterior glide loss
4. Fibular head superior
5. Fibular head inferior
6. Fibular head inferior and superior glide loss

**Assessment and treatment of proximal tibio-fibular joint dysfunction:**
**1. Fibular head anterior-lateral**
**Spring test:** [As shown in figure 2]
Position of the patient: lying Supine, affected right knee is in extension.
Position of Therapist: The therapist approaches the patient from the right side of the patient.
Procedure: The clinician ensures symmetry of both limbs by confirming that the knee and feet are close together and exactly adjacent. The bilateral foot is plantar-flexed to reach the posterior glide of the fibular head barrier. The clinician then palpates the affected fibular head anterior border with the thumb and compares it with another limb for symmetry. The left therapist's thumb is placed at the anterior border of the fibular head; the posterior slack is taken with (3-5)kg force. Additionally, 5kg force is applied to feel the spring/end feel. If it does not spring, it indicates the fibular head is anterior.

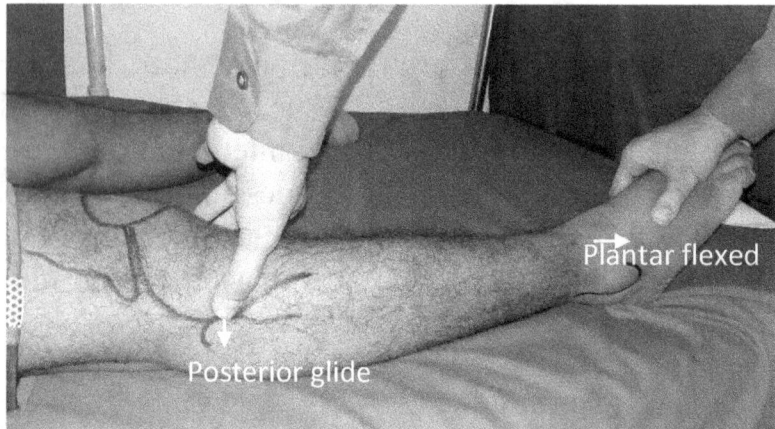

Figure 2: Spring test for fibular head anterior. At the fibular head, the arrow line indicates posterior directed slack and glide. At the ankle, the arrow line indicates plantar flexion of the foot.

**Treatment:**

**i). Mobilization:** [As shown in figure 2]
Position of the patient: same as assessment position as explained above
Procedure: The fibular head slack is taken into the posterior with (3-5)kg force; the posterior glides are given further according to the grades of mobilization. Five glides are given three times, and 5 Seconds rest is given each time.

**ii). Muscle energy technique:** [As shown in figure 2]
Position of the patient: same as assessment position as explained above
Procedure: posterior slack is taken at the fibular head with (3-5)kg force with a plantar flexion barrier at the ankle. The patient is asked to dorsiflex, and the therapist resists simultaneously, producing an isometric contraction. After 5 Sec relaxations, further slack of ankle plantar flexion and fibular head posterior glide slack is taken. Again, repeat the same three times, and each time, 5 Sec rest is given.

**iii). Taping[8]:** [As shown in figure 3]
Position of the patient: The patient is side-lying.
Procedure: A pillow is placed between the legs, the knee is slightly flexed ($30^0$-$40^0$), and the foot is plantar-flexed to assist the fibular head in gliding posteriorly. One end of the tape is pasted at the anterior border of the fibular head, then the therapist's thumb is placed at the anterior border of the fibular head, and posterior slack is taken with (3-5)kg force. Then, additionally, the posterior glide is done with 5kg force, and the other end of the tape is pasted over the calf.

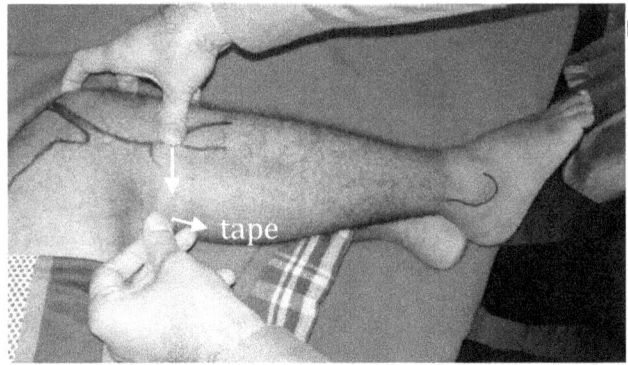

Figure 3: fibular head anterior to posterior taping.

**iv) Sustained glide:** [As shown in figures 2 and 3]
Procedure: along with the correction tape, the fibular head posterior glide barrier is reached by plantar flexing of the foot. Then, the therapist's right thumb is placed on the anterior border of the fibular head, and posterior slack is taken with (3-5)kg

force. Fibular head posterior glide is maintained with an additional 5kg force for the duration of 2-5 min, depending on the condition and tolerance of the patient.

## 2. Fibular head posterior-medial
**Spring test:**
<u>Position of the patient:</u> The patient should be prone-lying, with the affected right knee in extension and the foot outside of the bed [as shown in Figure 4].
<u>Position of Therapist:</u> The clinician approaches from the right side of the patient.
<u>Procedure:</u> Ankle is dorsi-flexed to assist fibular head anterior glide. The clinician ensures symmetry by confirming that the knee and feet are close together and exactly adjacent. The therapist palpates the bilateral posterior border of fibular heads with the thumb for symmetry. Followed by fibular head anterior slack is taken with (3-5)kg force, and additionally, 5kg force is applied to feel the spring/end feel. If it does not spring, the fibular head is posterior. The fibular head posterior is very commonly seen in knee dysfunctions.
Dysfunction of the fibular head can predispose to irritability of the peroneus-longus and, subsequently, the peroneus nerve. It can also predispose to dysfunctions of the lateral collateral ligaments and the ilio-tibial band.

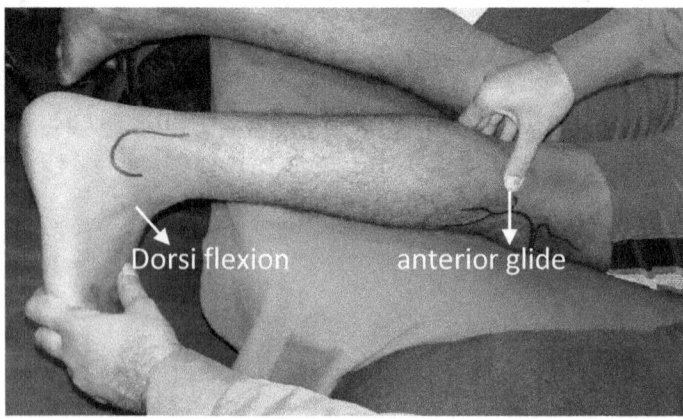

Figure 4: Spring test for fibular head posterior. The Arrow line indicates anterior directed slack and glide, and the ankle is dorsi flexed.

**Treatment:**
**i) Mobilization[8]:** [As shown in figure 4]
<u>Position of the patient:</u> is the same as the assessment position as explained above.
<u>Procedure:</u> The dorsiflexion barrier is reached at the ankle, and the fibular head anterior slack is taken with (3-5)kg force. Then, further posterior to anterior glides are given according to the grades of mobilization. Five glides are given three times, and 5 second rest is given each time.
**ii) Muscle energy technique:** [As shown in figure 4]

Position of the patient: is the same as the assessment position as explained above
Procedure: The dorsiflexion barrier is reached at the ankle, and anterior glide slack is taken at the fibular head with 5kg force. Then, the patient is asked to plantar-flex, and simultaneously, the therapist resists producing an isometric contraction. After 5-second relaxations, the further dorsiflexion barrier is reached, and fibular head anterior slack is taken. Again, repeat the same three times. Each time, 5 seconds of rest is given.

### iii) Taping: [As shown in figures 5 and 6]
The patient is lying on the side, and the pillow is placed between the legs [as shown in Figure 5.]
Procedure: Once the ankle dorsiflexion barrier is reached, one end of the tape is pasted at the posterior border of the fibular head. Then, the therapist's thumb is placed on the posterior border of the fibular head, and the anterior slack is taken with (3-5)kg force. Additionally, the anterior glide is done with 5kg force. The other end of the tape is pasted over the superior medial surface of the tibia[10] [as shown in Figure 6.]

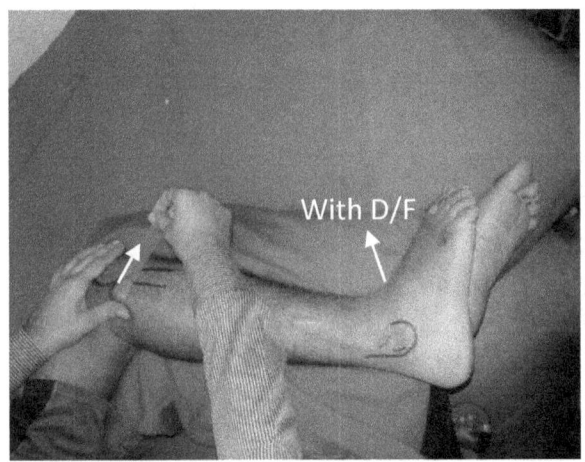
Figure 5: Lateral side view: taping of fibular head posterior to anterior with ankle dorsi flexion to reinforce further anterior glide.

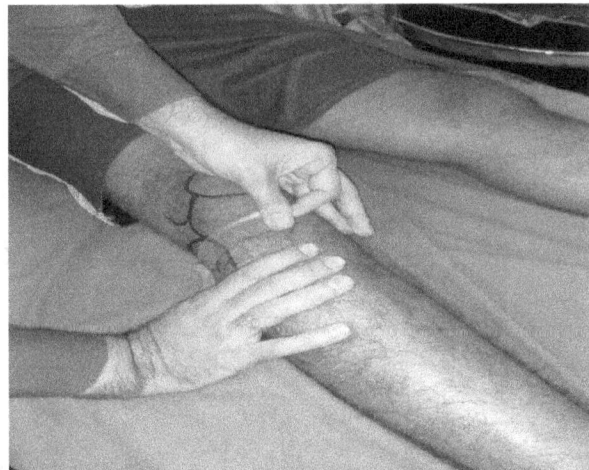
Figure 6: Anterior view of taping.

### iv) Sustained glide: [As shown in figure 4]
Position of the patient: same as assessment position as explained in the spring test.
Procedure: along with the corrective tape, further anterior glide slack is taken with 3-5kg force, and additionally, 5kg force is applied to maintain further anterior glide for the duration of 2-5 min, depending on the condition and tolerance of the patient.

**3. Fibular head, both anterior and posterior glide loss**

**Spring test and treatment:** Both spring tests, which are explained in 1 and 2 dysfunctions, are included, as they are needed to test the anterior and posterior glide of the fibular head. If the spring test is positive, the treatment follows both 1 and 2 dysfunctions.

### 4. proximal/Superior Fibula:
**Spring test:** [As shown in figure 7]
<u>Position of the patient:</u> The patient should be lying on the left side, and the pillow should be placed between the two legs; the affected right PTF joint is to be examined, and the knee should be flexed around $10^0$-$30^0$.
<u>Position of the therapist and procedure:</u> The therapist approaches the patient from the right side and ensures symmetry of both limbs by confirming that the knee and feet are close together and exactly adjacent. The therapist then palpates the affected proximal/superior border of the fibular head with the left thumb and compares it with others for symmetry. The therapist's left thumb is placed at the superior border of the fibular head, and the right hand assists in an inversion of the foot, which assists the fibula's inferior glide. The inferior directed slack of the fibula is taken with (3-5)kg force, and 5kg force is applied to test the spring/end feel. If it does not spring, then the fibular is superior.

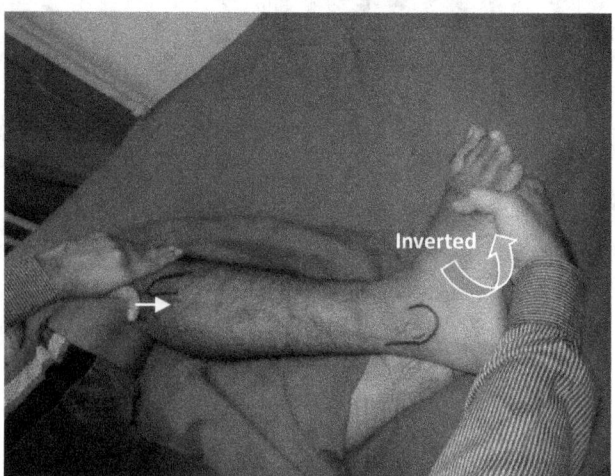

Figure 7: Spring test for fibular proximal/superior. The Arrow line indicates inferior directed slack and glide. The ankle is inverted further to assist the inferior slack and glide of the fibula.

### Treatment:
**i) Mobilization**: [As shown in figure 7]
patient and therapist position for treatment is the same as the assessment position, as explained above. Additionally, the patient's foot is inverted, which will further assist in reaching the inferior glide of the fibula. The fibula's inferior slack is taken with (3-5)kg force. Then, proximal/superior to distal/inferior glides are given

according to the grades of mobilization. Five glides are given three times. Each time, a 5-second rest is given.

**ii) Muscle energy technique:** As shown in Figure 7, the patient and therapist's position for treatment is the same as the assessment position as explained above; additionally, the patient's foot is inverted and adducted, which further assists the inferior glide of the fibula. Inferior slack at the fibular head is taken with (3-5)kg force, and additionally, 5kg force is applied. Following this, the patient is asked to Evert the foot, and the therapist resists simultaneously, producing an isometric contraction. After 5 Sec relaxation, further fibular head inferior slack is taken. Again, repeat the same three times, and a 5-second rest is given each time.

**iii) Taping:** It has three parts: one on foot, one at the proximal fibula, and the other at the distal/inferior fibula.

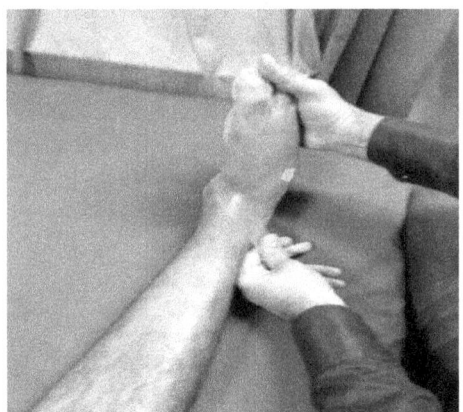

Figure 8: (a) Tapping the foot into inversion and adduction to assist inferior fibular glide.

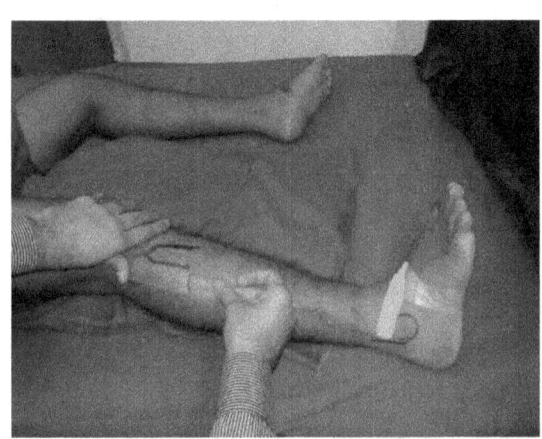

Figure 9: (b) Taping at proximal fibula to glide fibula inferiorly.

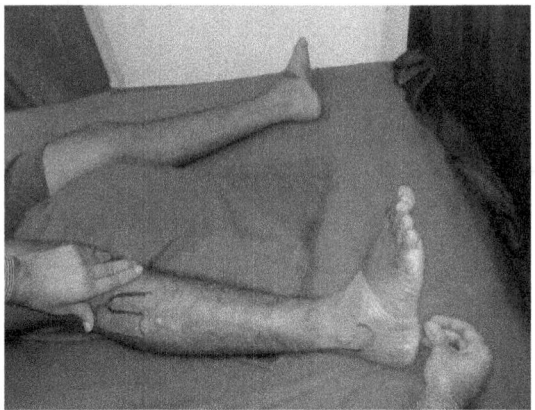

Figure 10: (c) Taping at distal fibula to glide fibula inferiorly.

(a) Inversion and adduction taping of the right foot: [As shown in Figures 8, 11, and 12]

Position of the patient: the patient is supine; the right fibula is to be treated.
Position of the therapist: The therapist approaches from the right side of the patient.
Procedure: One end of the tape is pasted at the dorsal 4th and 5th metatarso-tarsal joint junction and wrapped around the plantar side of the foot; the other end of the tape is pulled and pasted over the lateral malleolus to maintain inversion and adduction of the foot.

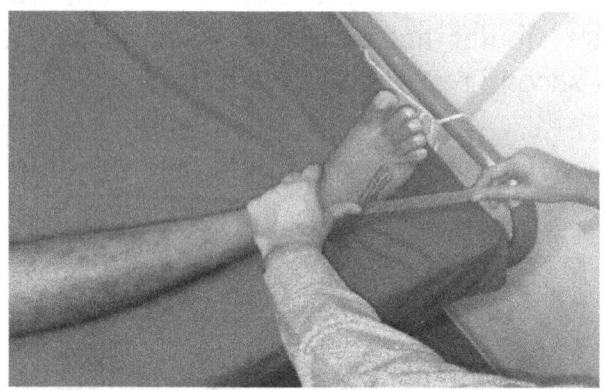

Figure 11: Taping for inversion and adduction of the foot. The initial end of the tape is pasted over the 4th and 5th metatarso-tarsal joints.

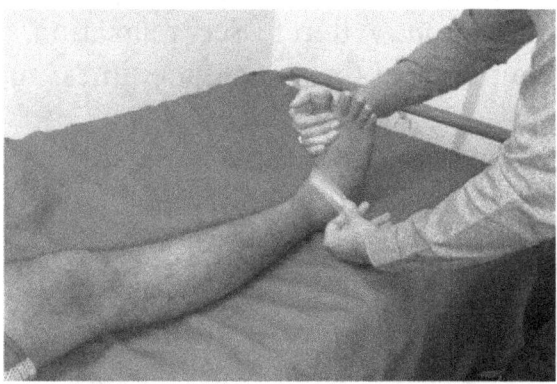

Figure 12: The end part of the tape is pasted over the lateral malleolus after the foot is taken into inversion and adduction.

(b) Proximal fibular taping:
With foot taping with inversion, adduction, the patient and therapist position for taping is the same as mentioned above; as shown in Figure 9, one end of the tape is pasted at the proximal/superior border of the fibular head, then the inferior glide slack is taken with (3-5)kg force, and additionally, the inferior glide is done with 5kg force. Then, maintaining the inferior glide, the other end of the tape is pasted over the proximal lateral surface of the fibula.

(c) Distal fibular taping:
After (a) foot inversion, adduction, and (b) proximal fibular corrective tape, as shown in Figure 10. patient's position for treatment is the same as the assessment position as explained above; one end of the tape is pasted at the fibular styloid, and then inferior slack is taken at the proximal/superior border of the fibular head with (3-5)kg force. Additionally, 5kg force is applied for the inferior glide. Then, the foot is inverted and adducted to reinforce the inferior glide of the fibula further, followed by the other end of the tape being pasted along the plantar surface of the mid-lateral foot border.

**iv) Sustained glide:** The patient's position for treatment is the same as the assessment position, as explained previously. As shown in Figure 7, along with the corrective tapes, the therapist takes up inferior fibular slack with (3-5)kg force with the inverted, adducted foot, and additionally, 5kg force is applied to maintain the fibula's inferior glide for 2-5 min, depending on the condition and tolerance of the patient.

## 5. Fibular inferior:

**Spring test:** [As shown in figure 13]

<u>Position of the patient:</u> The patient should be on the side-lying, and the pillow should be placed between the two legs; the affected right PTF joint is to be examined, and the knee and hip are about $30^0$ flexed.

<u>Position of the therapist:</u> The therapist approaches the patient from the right side. The therapist ensures symmetry of both limbs by confirming that the knee and feet are close together and exactly adjacent.

<u>Procedure:</u> The therapist then palpates the affected fibular styloid inferior border with the thumb and compares it with another limb for symmetry. The therapist's right wrist is extended, fingers flexed, and wraps around the patient's forefoot to evert and abduct the foot, further reinforcing the fibula proximal/superior glide. Then, the therapist's left thumb is placed at the inferior border of the fibular styloid, and the superior glide slack is taken with (3-5)kg of force. Additionally, 5kg force is applied with the thumb proximally to test the spring/end feel. If it does not spring, it indicates the fibular head is inferior.

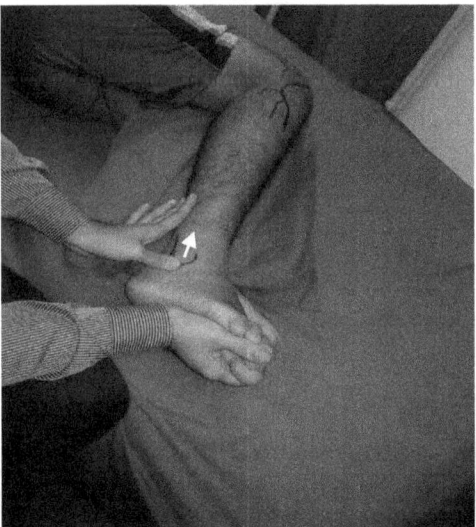

Figure 13: Spring test and treatment of fibula inferior.

**Treatment:**

**i) Mobilization:** As shown in Figure 13, the patient and therapist position for treatment is the same as the assessment position, as explained above. Additionally, the patient's foot is everted and abducted, which further reinforces the proximal/superior glide of the fibula. The fibula's superior slack is taken with 3-5kg force, and inferior to superior glides are given according to the grades of mobilization. Five glides are given three times, and a 5-second rest is given each time.

**ii) Muscle energy technique**: As shown in Figure 13, the patient and therapist position for treatment is the same as the assessment position as explained above; additionally, the patient's foot is everted and abducted, which further assists the superior/proximal glide of the fibula. The therapist's left thumb is placed at the inferior border of the fibula styloid, and superior glide slack is taken with 10kg force. The patient is asked to invert and adduct the foot, and the therapist resists simultaneously, producing an isometric contraction. After 5-Seconds relaxation, further fibular superior glide slack, and foot eversion, abduction slack is taken. Again, repeat the same three times, and a 5-second rest is given each time.

**iii) Taping:** has three parts: one on the foot, two on the inferior fibular, and three on the proximal fibula.

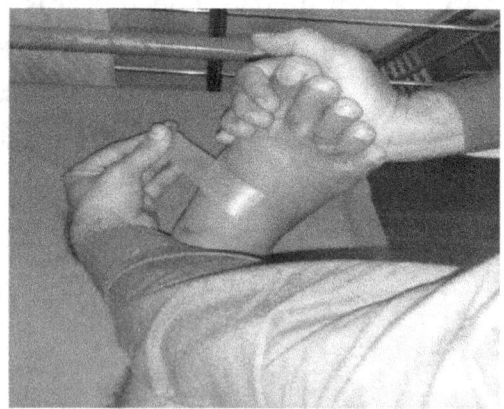

Figure 14: Part one- taping for eversion and foot abduction. The initial one end of the tape is pasted at the medial and middle cuneiform.

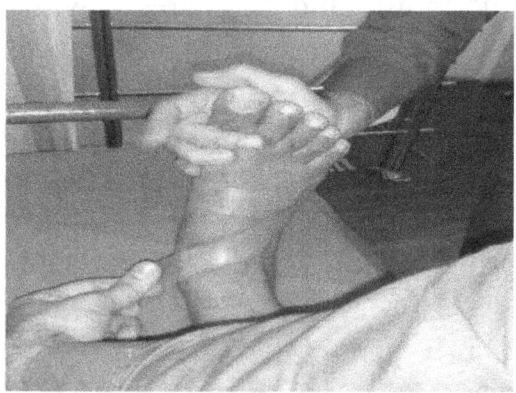

Figure 15: Part one-taping for eversion and abduction of the foot. The other end of the tape is pasted at the medial styloid.

One- eversion and abduction taping of the right foot: [As shown in figures 14&15] <u>Position of the patient:</u> The patient is supine, and the therapist approaches from the right side. <u>Procedure:</u> One end of the tape is pasted at the medial and middle cuneiform dorsum and wrapped around the foot from the medial plantar side to reach the midfoot lateral side. Then, the foot eversion and abduction barrier are reached; another end of the tape is wrapped on the dorsum of the foot to be pulled and pasted at the medial tibial styled to maintain eversion and abduction of the foot.

Two- inferior fibular styloid taping of right foot: [As shown in figures 16&17] as mentioned above, everted and abducted foot corrective tape on, patient's position for treatment is same as explained above; initial one end of the tape is pasted on the lateral plantar calcaneum surface. Following that, the foot is everted abducted to further reinforce the superior glide of the fibula. The therapist's thumb is placed at the inferior border of the fibular styloid, and the superior glide slack is taken with (3-5)kg force. Additionally, 5kg force is applied to reinforce the superior glide further. Then, the other end of the tape is pasted along the lower fibular lateral surface.

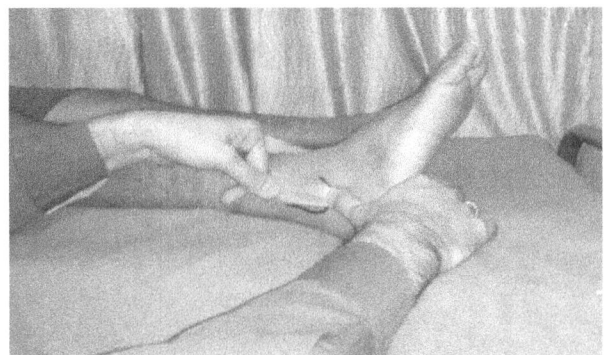

Figure 16: Part two- superior glide taping of the fibula: Initial first end of the tape is pasted at the lateral plantar calcaneum surface.

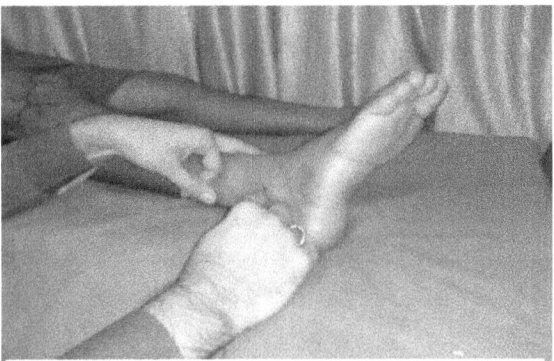

Figure 17: Part two- superior glide taping of the fibula. The other end of the tape is pasted at the lateral styloid.

Three- Superior fibular taping of the right foot: As shown in figure 18, as explained above, part one and part two of corrective tape are on; the patient's position for treatment is the same as explained above; one end of the tape is pasted on the proximal lateral surface of the fibula, then the therapist right thumb is placed on the inferior border of fibular styloid. Following the superior glide, slack is taken with (3-5)kg force, and additionally, 5kg force is applied to reinforce the superior glide further; then, another end of the tape is pasted over the lateral surface of the knee.

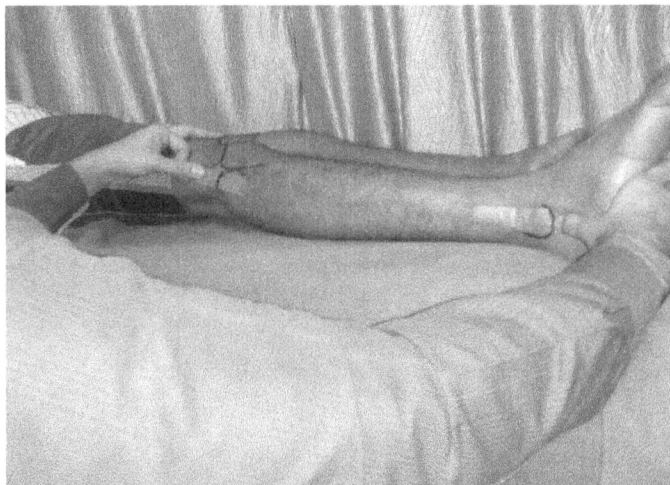

Figure 18: Part three-superior glide taping of the fibula.

**iv). Sustained glide:** The patient's position for treatment is the same as the assessment position, as explained above. As shown in Figure 18, along with the corrective tapes, the therapist's right thumb is placed on the inferior border of the fibular styloid and superior glide slack is taken with (3-5)kg force, and additionally, further sustained superior glide is applied with 5kg force for 2-5 min, depending on the condition and tolerance of the patient.

## 6. Fibular inferior and superior glide loss:

**Spring test and treatment:** both spring tests, that is, fibular dysfunctions of 4 and 5 mentioned above, are included, as we need to test the inferior and superior glide of the fibula. If spring tests are positive, the treatment follows the following: fibular dysfunctions 4 and 5.

**References:**

1. Bressler H, Deltoff M. Proximal tibiofibular joint dysfunction: an overlooked diagnosis.*Chirop Sports Med,* 1988; 2(2).
2. Ogden JA. Subluxation and dislocation of the proximal tibiofibular joint. *J Bone Joint Surg,* 1974; 56:145-54.
3. Schafer RC. *Knee and Leg Trauma.* 1997.
4. O'Leary K, Vorpahl KA, Heiderscheit B. Effect of cushioned insoles on impact forces during running. *J Am Podiatr Med Assoc*, Jan/Feb 2008; 98(1).
5. Quinn E. Checklist for Running Overuse Injuries. About.com: Sports Medicine.
6. Ahmad R, Case R. Dislocation of the fibular head in an unusual sports injury: a case report. *J Med Case Reports* 2008; 2:158.
7. Hatzokos I, Drakou A, Christodoulou A, et al. Inferior subluxation of the fibular head following tibial lengthening with a unilateral external fixator. *J Bone Joint Surg*, 2004; 86:1491-6.
8. https://www.youtube.com/watch?v=gd82b7WM4to
9. James R. Beazell, et al,. Treatment of Lateral Knee Pain by Addressing Tibiofibular Hypomobility in a Recreational Runner, N Am J Sports Phys Ther. 2009 Feb; 4(1): 21–28.
10. https://www.youtube.com/watch?v=lWtVcdw869s.
11. Ronna H. Semonian, et al,. Proximal Tibiofibular Subluxation Relationship to Lateral Knee Pain: A Review of Proximal Tibio-fibular Joint Pathologies.
12. *Manuel Duarte*, et al. Proximal Tibiofibular Joint Dysfunction; http://www.dynamicchiropractic.com/mpacms/dc/article.php?id=54496
13. https://www.youtube.com/watch?v=WvBMfe3EV1U; Assessment and Treatment of the Superior Tib-Fib Joint - Ann Porter Hoke

# CHAPTER 13
## The Soft Tissue of the Knee: Palpation and Treatment

Soft tissue palpation itself is one of the important assessments[1-3].
The detailed pathomechanics of soft tissue dysfunction and examination can be referred to in Chapter 5. Important assessment[4-6] of soft tissue dysfunction and treatment of knee joint complexes as follows:
Important soft tissues to be considered around the knee joint complex;

### I). Anterior, medial and lateral side of the knee:

**The anterior and lateral sides of the knee**

1. Patellar tendon
2. Quadriceps tendon
3. Lateral joint line/lateral meniscus
4. Lateral patellar retinaculum
5. Ilio-tibial band
6. Biceps femoris
7. Lateral collateral ligaments

**The medial side of the knee**
1. Medial meniscus
2. Medial collateral ligament
3. Pes anserinus tendon and bursa
4. Medial patellar retinaculum

### II). Posterior side of the knee:
**a) Superficial layer:**
1. Hamstrings: Medial hamstrings- bicep femoris; Lateral hamstrings- semimembranosus and semitendinosus
2. Calf: Medial calf- gastrocnemius, medial head; Lateral calf- gastrocnemius, lateral head

**b) Intermediate layer:**
1. Soleus
2. Plantaris
3. Popliteus

**c) Deep layer:**
1. Posterior medial meniscus,
2. Posterior lateral meniscus,
3. Anterior cruciate ligaments,
4. Posterior cruciate ligaments

## PALPATION: KNEE[8, 9]

Accurate palpation of knee joint landmarks in standing and sitting can sometimes be difficult due to muscular response to gravity. In standing, the knee joint posture can be influenced by biomechanical dysfunction above and below the knee. Palpation of the landmarks in supine and prone lying may yield more accurate information about the isolated tibiofemoral, patella-femoral, and tibiofibular joint structures as the upper and lower body influence is reduced. Evaluation should also include palpation of all soft tissues, especially muscles, tendons, and ligaments. A distinction needs to be made between positional dysfunction and movement dysfunction. Positional dysfunction describes how it is positioned; movement dysfunction describes how it cannot move. Evaluation and treatment that rely on position alone are, at best, speculative. Putting a patient's knee in several positions during palpation is wise. For example, meniscal cysts are best positioned at 45-degree knee flexion, whereas joint lines are palpated at 90 degrees of knee flexion. When palpating, the examiner looks for abnormal tenderness, swelling, adhesions/nodules, or abnormal temperature.

The purpose of palpating an injured patient is to acquire a feel for the underlying structures, including bony landmarks and soft tissue, as well as to attempt to identify the severity of the injury[7]. Palpation, in some cases, will cause the reproduction of pain to be measured on a general pain scale and also allow the physiotherapist to recognize the amount of inflammation present regarding the cardinal signs of inflammation, tightness, and adhesions. Palpation may also identify certain deformities within the local area of injury as well as crepitus within a joint, which may signify additional underlying conditions.

Specific structures to be palpated surrounding the knee are listed below:
**Knee soft tissue mobilization[23]:**
Soft tissue dysfunctions are mainly because of the adhesions and tightness. The important technique used for breaking adhesions of the soft tissue is **DTF-deep transverse friction:**

**Note-** knee dysfunctions involve arthrokinematic and soft tissue dysfunction or only soft tissue dysfunction. Arthrokinematic dysfunctions always involve soft tissue dysfunctions. Another way, soft tissue dysfunctions may or may not always involve arthrokinematic dysfunction of the knee. If there are no findings of arthroknematic dysfunctions, then there must be only soft tissue dysfunctions (tightness and adhesions) contributing to the knee joint dysfunction. Therefore, dysfunctions start with soft-tissue involvement and follow the joint dysfunction.

**DTF**[24]: The massage should be deep, i.e., to take up the soft tissue slack and reach specific targeted tissues and must be applied transversely to the specific tissue involved, unlike the superficial massage given in the longitudinal direction parallel to the vessels, which enhances the vessels circulation and return of fluids[5]. Before friction massage can be performed successfully, the correct structure must be found through proper evaluation procedures. The distinction must be made between contractile structures such as the muscle belly, musculo-tendinous junction, tendon, and tendon-periosteal junction. The therapist should know the given tissue fibre alignment, whether horizontal, vertical or obliquely directed at a given area. So that deep friction can be applied perpendicular to the tissue fibre to break the adhesions[10-13]

Force transducers can measure the force of deep friction, for example, a MicroFET muscle testing device (Hoggan Health Industries, Draper, UT, USA). The handheld instrument measures the amount of force the clinician applies. After taking up the slack in the soft tissue, the clinician can apply an additional force if required. Both sides are compared. The clinician can measure pre and post-treatment force. Most force transducers used in the clinic describe force in pounds or kilograms, although the force described in Newton's (N) accounts for the influence of gravity. Force in Newton and kg is mentioned to benefit the interdisciplinary audience. An additional force for deep transverse friction can be applied to take up the slack of soft tissue, averaging 29.3N (3 kg) and up to 52.8N (5 kg).

The force needed may vary from person to person depending on the superficial to a deep level of involvement in soft tissue[14,15]. The above averages serve as a guideline for developing the skill of applying to test the adhesions and treat /break them. The appropriate amount of force is the least amount that yields useful information without increasing pain. On average, three to five to and fro glides with a 1cm distance at a given point on the soft tissue is appropriate.

# I. Anterior, medial and lateral side of the knee: Soft tissue palpation and method of deep friction

## Soft tissue palpation[8,9] and method of Deep friction: Anterior and lateral knee

### 1. Patellar tendon:

**Palpation-** [as shown in figure 1] Palpate is the length of the patellar tendon from its insertion at the tibial tuberosity to the inferior aspect of the patella. The patellar tendon normally feels broad and ropelike. A chronic dysfunction often results in palpable nodules/adhesions within the mass of the tendon.

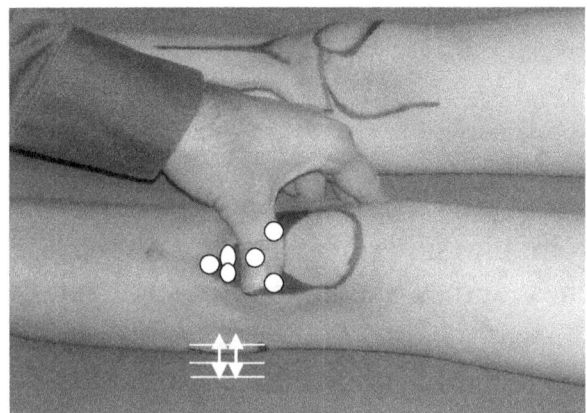

Figure 1: Palpation with the thumb: The patellar tendon is divided into three rows, and each row is again divided into points with a distance of 1cm so that the entire affected portion of the tendon will be covered for the deep friction. Horizontal lines represent the patellar tendon fibre alignment. Bilateral vertical arrow lines represent the application of deep friction.

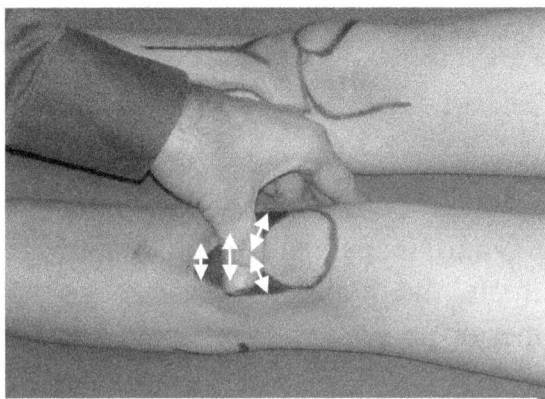

Figure 2: Deep transverse friction massage is applied transversely to the tissue. The area of the affected patellar tendon tissue is divided into three rows. A glide of 1cm distance of deep friction can be given at a given point.

Figures 1 and 2 show that the patellar tendon Area is divided into three rows[17]. Each row should cover the total length of the horizontal portion of the tissue by dividing it into points at a distance of 1cm on the tissue; likewise, three rows should cover the entire patellar tendon. The patellar tendon is covered by 3 points representing the proximal row, 2 points representing the middle row, and 1 point representing the distal row.

**Deep friction-**Therapist can give deep friction either with the thumb (figure 1 and 2) or/the olecranon of the elbow (Figure 3) according to convenience and experience. The therapist should place the thumb at one end and a particular divided point. Then, take up the slack with 1-5kg force to reach the desired tissue, according to the patient's condition and tolerance. Deep transverse friction glides are given on either side of the tissue about 1/2cm from the targeted point by maintaining the same force. Three to five glides are given for 3times per session. Each time, 5 Sec rest is given.

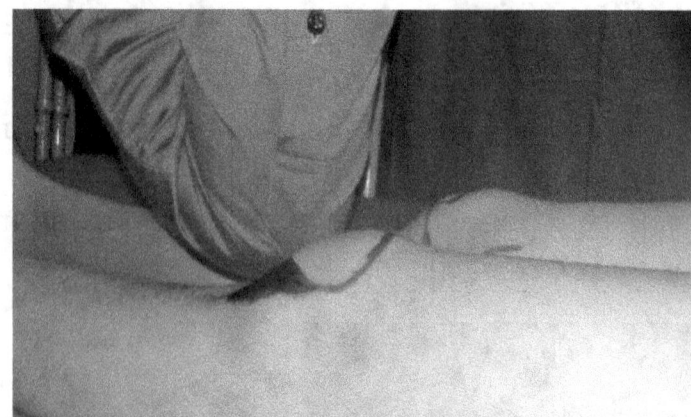

Figure 3: Showing deep friction technique with olecranon.

**2. Quadriceps tendon:** Palpation[18,19]- From the superior aspect of the patella, palpate the quadriceps tendon as it attaches across the length of the patella's superior pole.

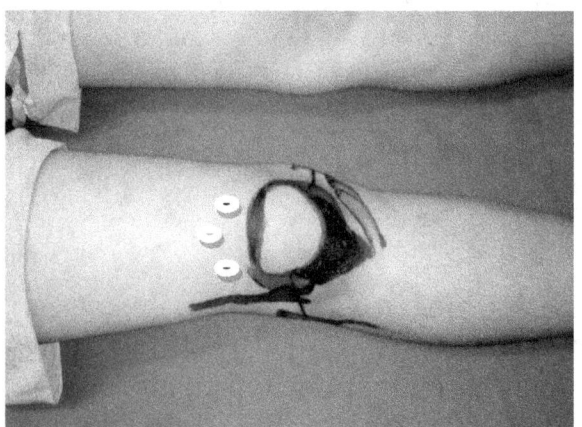

Figure 4: 3 dots indicating locators for deep friction on quadriceps tendon.

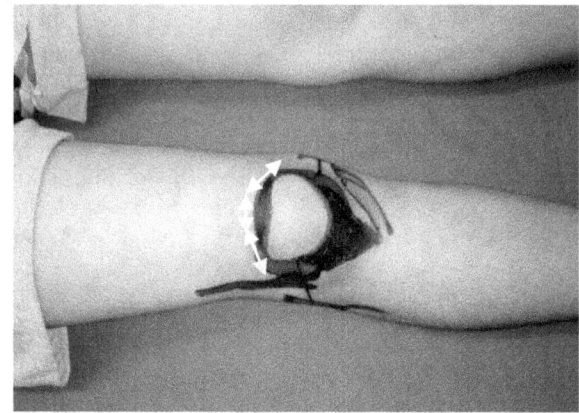

Figure 5: Arrow lines indicating deep friction glides' to and fro direction.

**Deep friction-** As shown in Figure 4, the quadriceps tendon area is divided into one row. The row should cover the total length of the quadriceps tendon portion by dividing it into three points represented by 3dots. The distance between the two dots is about 1cm on the tissue to covers the patellar tendon. The therapist can give deep friction either with thumb/olecranon, according to convenience. The therapist should place the thumb at one end over a particular divided point. Then, take up the slack with 1-5kg force to reach the desired tissue. As shown in Figure 5, deep friction glides are given on either side about 1/2cm from the targeted point by maintaining the same force. Three to five glides are given 3 times per session, according to the patient's condition and tolerance. Each time, 5 Sec rest is given.

### 3. Lateral Joint line/lateral meniscus:

**Palpation-** The position of the patient should be either supine or side-lying. Position the knee at least 20-45 degrees of flexion to locate the anterio-lateral joint line. Begin palpating the joint line lateral to the patellar tendon and progress posteriorly. Pain and palpable knot/adhesion along the joint line may indicate meniscal pathology. Internally rotating the tibia makes the lateral meniscus more palpable.

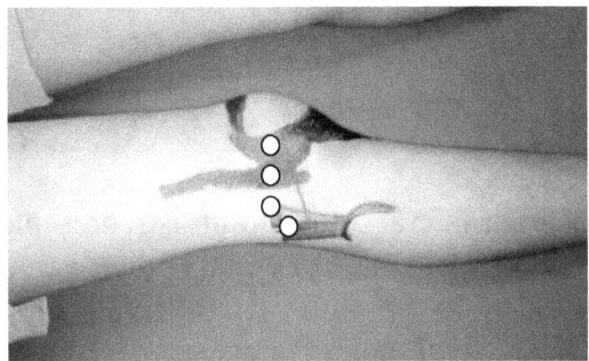

Figure 6: The dots indicate points for deep friction on the Lateral joint line.

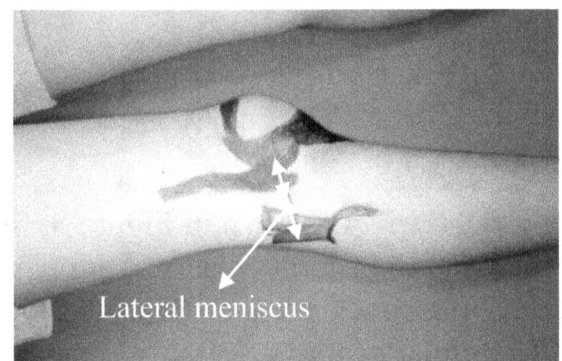

Figure 7: Arrow lines indicate deep friction glides' to and fro direction.

**Deep friction-** As shown in Figure 6, the lateral joint line/lateral meniscus area is divided into one line (the lateral joint line is the space between the femur and tibia bone). The total length of the joint line is covered by dividing it into 3 to 4 points, shown as red colour dots at a distance of 1cm. The therapist can give deep friction either with a thumb/olecranon, according to the convenience/experience. The therapist should place the thumb at one end and a divided point. Then, take up the slack with 1 to 5 kg force to reach the desired tissue, and as shown in Figure 7, by maintaining the same force, to and fro deep friction glides are given on either side about 1/2cm from the targeted point. Three to five glides are given 3 times per session, according to the patient's condition and tolerance. Each time, 5 Sec rest is given.

## 4. Lateral patellar retinaculum:

**Palpation**- lateral retinaculum consists of two layers;
- Superficial oblique layer; extends from the Iio-Tibial band to the lateral border of the patella and patellar tendon;
- Transverse retinaculum: extends from the undersurface of the Ilio-Tibial band to the lateral patellar border.

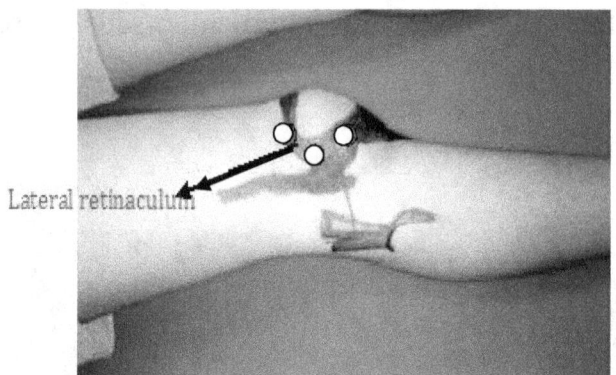

Figure 8: 3 dots indicating points for deep friction on lateral retinaculum.

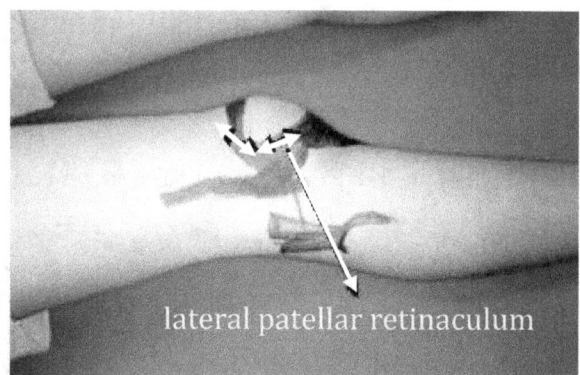

Figure 9: Arrow lines indicating the to and fro directions of deep friction glide.

**Deep friction**- As shown in Figure 8, the patellar lateral retinaculum is represented at lateral to the lateral border of the patella. The total tissue covered is divided into three points; each point is at a distance of 1 cm on the entire lateral retinaculum. The therapist can give deep friction either with the thumb/olecranon, according to the patient's convenience and tolerance. The therapist should place the thumb at one end and a particular divide point. Then, take up the slack with 1-5kg force to reach the desired tissue. As shown in Figure 9, by maintaining the same force, to and fro deep friction glides are given on either side about 1/2cm from the targeted point. Three to five glides are given 3 times per session, according to the patient's condition and tolerance. Each time, 5 Sec rest is given.

## 5. Iliotibial band:
**Palpation**- Palpate the IT band located anterior to the biceps femoris tendon at its insertion on Gerdy's tubercle, just lateral to the tibial tuberosity. The IT band becomes more identifiable during resisted flexion past 30 degrees. Palpate the IT band upward to the tensor fasciae Latae, noting any increased sensitivity adhesions, especially as it passes over the lateral femoral condyle, possibly indicating ilio-tibial band friction syndrome.

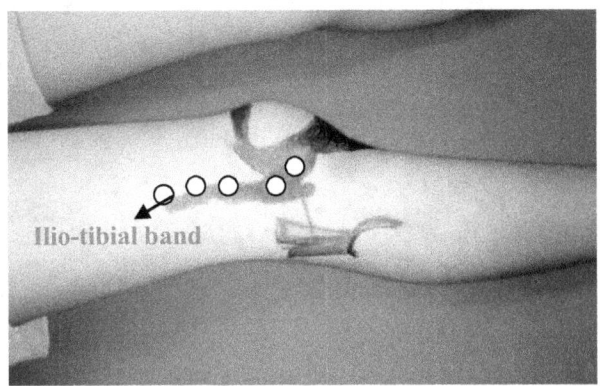
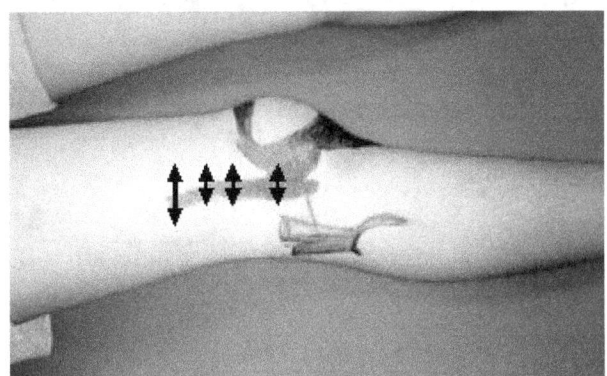

Figure 10: 5 dots indicate points of deep friction on ilio-tibial band.

Figure 11: Arrow lines indicating deep friction glide to and fro directions.

**Deep friction-** As shown in Figure 10, the IT-band area is divided into 5 points at a distance of 1cm each. According to his convenience, the therapist can give deep friction either with the thumb/olecranon. The therapist should place the thumb at one end and a particular divided point. Then, take up the slack with 1-5kg force to reach the desired tissue. As shown in Figure 11, deep friction glides are given to and fro with a distance of 1/2cm from the targeted point by maintaining the same force. Three to five glides are given 3 times per session, according to the patient's condition and tolerance. Each time, 5 Sec rest is given.

## 6. Biceps femoris:

**Palpation-** as shown in Figure 12, the position of the patient is supine lying; flex the knee to 25 degrees and ask the patient to externally rotate the lower leg to make the biceps tendon easily palpable (note that as the tendon crosses the joint line, it may become confused with the IT band). The biceps femoris tendon is inserted on the fibular head, posterior to the insertion of the LCL. Continue palpating the biceps femoris tendon to its muscular belly for adhesions and tenderness.

**Deep friction-** As shown in Figure 12, the bicep femoris is divided into three black colour points at a distance of 1cm each. According to his convenience, the therapist can give deep friction either with the thumb/olecranon. The therapist should place the thumb at one particular divided point and then take up the slack with 1-5kg force to reach the desired tissue. As shown in Figure 14, deep transverse glides are given to and fro with a distance of 1/2cm from the targeted point by maintaining the same force. Three to five glides are given 3 times per session, according to the patient's condition and tolerance. Each time, 5 Sec rest is given.

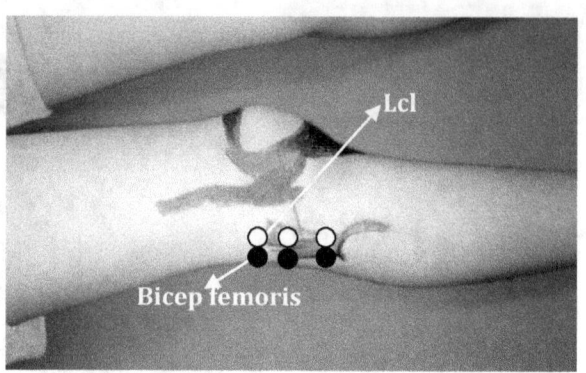

Figure 12: white dots indicating LCL and black dots indicating bicep femoris.

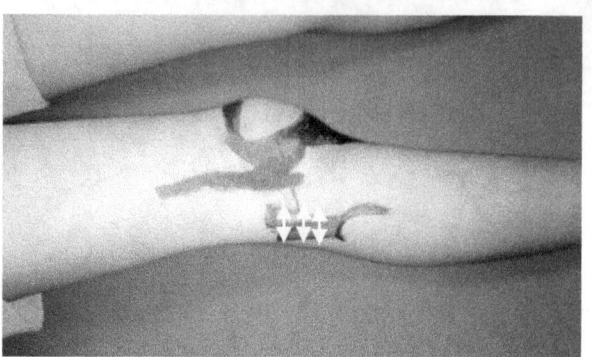

Figure 13: Arrow lines indicating the direction of to and fro deep friction glides perpendicular to LCL.

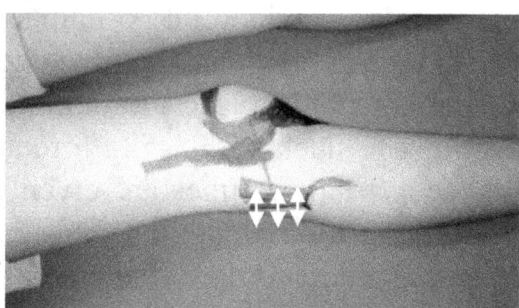

Figure 14: Arrow lines indicate the direction of to and fro glides, which are given perpendicular to the bicep femoris.

## 7. Lateral collateral ligament (LCL):

**Palpation**- the position of the patient can be prone or supine. If prone-lying, place the knee in 20 degrees of flexion and externally rotate and abduct the hip (i.e., cross the ankle of the involved leg over the opposite leg) to make the LCL more identifiable. Because it is a separate structure from the joint capsule, the LCL is easily identified as it arises from the fibular head and courses to the lateral femoral condyle. Or it can be palpated in supine lying by internally rotating the leg, as shown in Figure 12.

**Deep friction**- As shown in Figure 12, LCL is divided into three white points at a distance of 1 cm each. The therapist can give deep friction either with thumb/olecranon according to his convenience. The therapist should place the thumb at one particular divided point and then take up the slack with 1-5kg force to reach the desired tissue. As shown in Figure 13, deep friction glides are given to and fro with a distance of 1/2cm from the targeted point by maintaining the same force. Three to five glides are given 3 times per session, according to the patient's condition and tolerance. Each time, 5 Sec rest is given.

## Soft tissue palpation and method of Deep friction: Medial knee

### 1. Medial meniscus /medial Joint line:

**Palpation-** The patient is supine; place the affected hip in flexion, abduction and external rotation about $30^0$, and the knee in at least 45 degrees of flexion to locate the joint lines. Palpate on the medial side of the proximal aspect of the patellar tendon until the indentation formed by the femur and tibia is located. Palpate medially and posteriorly along the joint line, noting any crepitus/adhesions/and pain that may indicate possible meniscal, ligamentous or capsular trauma. Externally rotating the tibia makes the border of the medial meniscus more palpable.

**Deep friction-** The patient is supine; Figures 15 and 17 show that the medial meniscus is divided into four dots with a 1 cm distance each (figure 17). According to the convenience, the therapist can give deep friction. The therapist should place the thumb at one particular divided point and then take up the slack with 1-5kg force to reach the desired tissue. As shown in Figure 17, horizontal to and fro glides are given along the joint line with a distance of 1/2cm from the targeted point by maintaining the same force. Three to five glides are given 3 times per session, according to the patient's condition and tolerance. Each time, 5 seconds of rest is given.

### 2. Medial collateral ligament (MCL):

**Palpation-** The patient's position is the same as explained above. Many sprains of the MCL occur at the origin or insertion of the ligament. Palpate the length of the MCL from its origin on the medial femoral condyle, just below the adductor tubercle, progressing inferiorly to its insertion on the medial tibial flare that can be located up to 7 cm distal to the joint line. The MCL covers the medial portion of the joint line. Note the close relationship between the tendons of the pes anserine group and the MCL.

**Deep friction-** As shown in figures 15 and 16, three white dots with a 1 cm distance cover medial MCL; the direction of deep friction is perpendicular to MCL, represented with arrow lines. According to the convenience, the therapist can give deep friction either with the thumb/olecranon. The therapist should place the thumb at one particular divided point and then take up the slack with 1-5kg force to reach the desired tissue. As shown in Figure 16, by maintaining the same force, perpendicular to and fro deep friction glides are given along the MCL with a distance of ½ cm from the targeted point. Three to five glides are given 3 times per session, according to the patient's condition and tolerance. Each time, 5 Sec rest is given.

### 3. Pes anserine tendon and bursa:

**Palpation-** Patient position is the same as explained above; locate the medial tibial flare, the site of attachment for the gracilis, Sartorius, and semitendinosus muscles. Palpate is the common insertion of these tendons located just medial to the tibial tuberosity. Direct blows, overuse, or tibiofemoral dysfunctions may cause these structures and the overlying pes anserine bursa to inflame. The pes anserine bursa may be more easily identified midway between the tibial tuberosity and the anterior aspect of the medial joint line if the tibia is slightly internally rotated.

**Deep friction**[16]- As shown in figures 15 and 16, four black dots with a 1 cm distance cover the pes-anserine tendons; the direction of deep friction is perpendicular to soft tissue, represented by an arrow line. According to the convenience, the therapist can give deep friction either with the thumb/olecranon. The therapist should place the thumb at one particular divided point and then take the slack with 1-5kg force to reach the desired tissue. As shown in Figure 16, by maintaining the same force, perpendicular to and fro, deep friction glides are given along the pes-anserine tendon, a distance up to 1/2cm from the targeted point. Three to five glides are given 3 times per session, according to the patient's condition and tolerance. Each time, 5 Sec rest is given.

### 4. Medial patellar retinaculum:

**Palpation-** the patient's position is the same as explained above. It is a fibrous capsule of the knee and serves as the insertion of the vastus medialis on the tibia. It can be palpated medially along the medial patellar border. The patella can be pushed laterally to expose the medial patellar retinaculum.

**Deep friction-** As shown in Figures 15 and 16, white triangular dots in two rows with a 1 cm distance cover the medial retinaculum along the medial patellar border. The direction of deep friction is tangential to the patellar medial border, as shown in Figure 16 and represented with arrow lines. The therapist should place the thumb at one particular divided point and then take up the slack with 1-5kg force to reach the desired tissue. As shown in Figure 16, by maintaining the same force, to and fro deep friction glides are given along the medial retinaculum, a distance up to 1/2cm from the targeted point. Three to five glides are given 3 times per session, according to the patient's condition and tolerance. Each time 5 Sec rest is given.

Figure 15: Representing the palpatory landmarks of the medial retinaculum, medial meniscus, MCL and pessaries (a unit of three tendons) indicated by arrows.

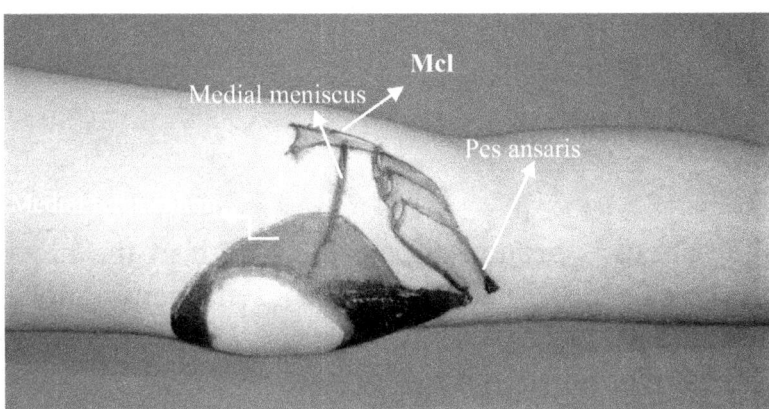

Figure 16: triangular dots represent the medial retinaculum, dark dots indicate pessaries and white dots indicate medial collateral ligaments. Dots represent the deep friction points. Arrow lines indicate the direction of deep friction.

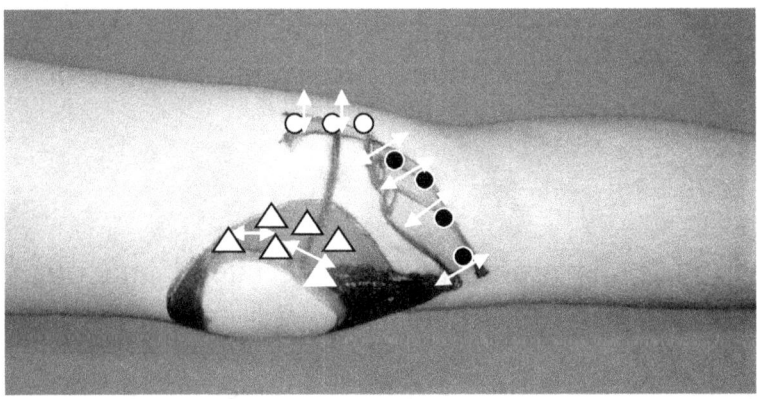

Figure 17: 4 dots indicate the medial meniscus/medial joint line. Arrow lines indicate the direction of deep friction.

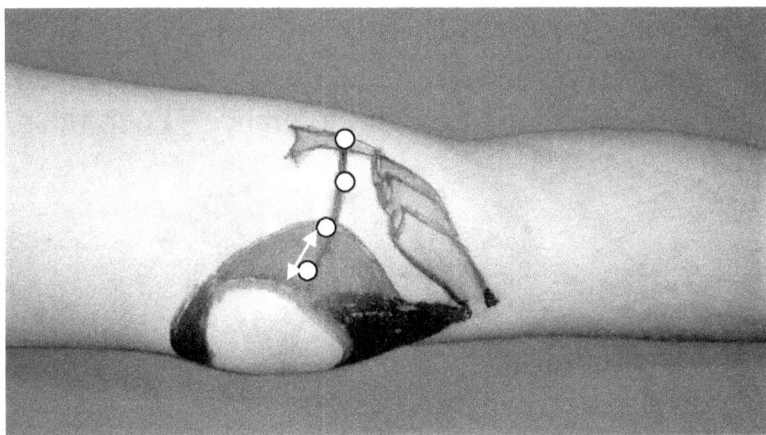

## II. Soft tissue palpation and method of deep friction: Posterior knee

Tissues are divided into superficial, middle, and deep layers based on the concept of giving deep friction

### a) Superficial layer:

### 1. Hamstrings:

**Palpation**[20]- The position of the patient is prone; palpate the length of the biceps femoris on the lateral aspect of the knee and the semimembranosus, semitendinosus muscles on the medial side of the knee as shown in Figure 18, noting for points of tenderness, spasm, or adhesions.

**Deep friction**[20,21]- as shown in Figure 18, all black dots with an average distance of 1cm represent medial and lateral hamstrings. The direction of deep friction is represented by arrow lines perpendicular to the tissue. The therapist should place the thumb/olecranon at one divided point, then the slack with 1-5kg force to reach the desired tissue. By maintaining the same force, to and fro deep friction glides are given perpendicular to the fibres of the hamstrings, a distance up to 1/2cm from the targeted point. Three to five glides are given 3 times, according to the patient's condition and tolerance. Each time, 5 Sec rest is given.

### 2. Calf: gastrocnemius:

**Palpation**- The position of the patient is prone; palpate the lateral and medial heads of the gastrocnemius muscle, as shown in Figure 18.

**Deep friction**[22]: as shown in Figure 18, all white dots with an average distance of 1cm represent medial and lateral gastrocnemius. The therapist should place the thumb/olecranon at one particular divided point and then take up the slack with 1-5kg force to reach the desired tissue. By maintaining the same force, to and fro deep friction glides are given a distance up to ½ cm from the targeted dot perpendicular to the fibres of the gastrocnemius. Three to five glides are given 3 times per session, according to the patient's condition and tolerance. Each time, 5 Sec rest is given.

# Chapter 12: Proximal Tibio-Fibular Joint: Biomechanics, Pathomechanics and Treatment

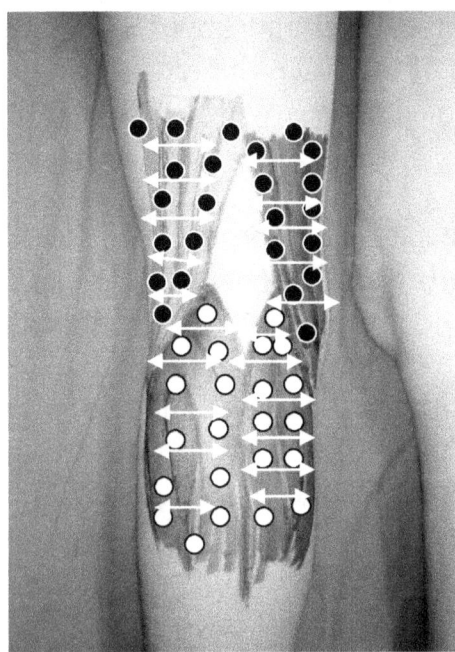

Figure 18: Black dots represent deep friction points on medial and lateral hamstrings. White dots represent the deep friction points on the medial and lateral gastrocnemius. Arrow lines indicate the direction of deep friction.

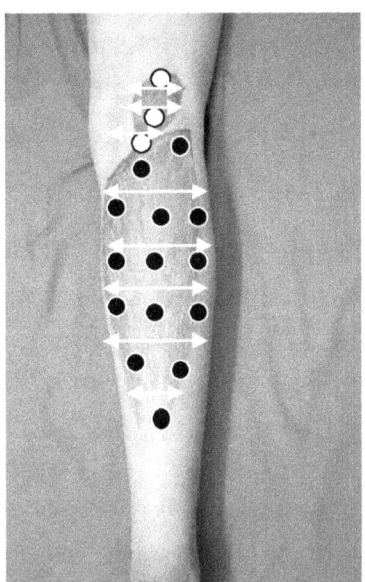

Figure 19: Black dots represent the deep friction points on the soleus, and white dots for planters.

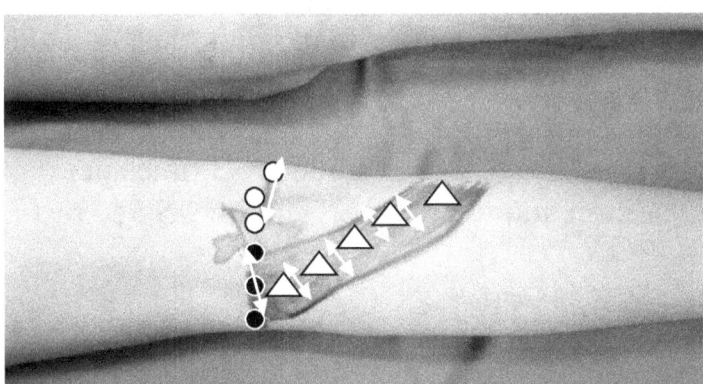

Figure 20: white triangular dots for popliteus, white dots for posterior medial meniscus, and black dots for posterior lateral meniscus. Dots represent the respective deep friction points of soft tissue. Arrow lines indicate the direction of deep friction.

### b) Intermediate layer

**1. Soleus:** Origin is from the posterior surface of the head and upper 1/3 of the shaft of the fibula; Middle 1/3 of the medial border of the tibia, the tendinous arch between the tibia and fibula. It was inserted into the calcaneus with gastrocnemius by way of the Achilles tendon.

**Palpation and deep friction-** The position of the patient is prone; deep to the gastrocnemius, it will be found soleus, as shown in Figure 19. This muscle can be found by palpating down the distal lateral aspect of the posterior leg. While the patient plantar flexes his foot, this muscle should become easily palpable and prominent. As shown in Figure 19, all black dots with an average distance of 1cm represent Soleus. The therapist should place the thumb/olecranon at one divided dot, then take the slack with 3-5kg force to reach the desired tissue. Maintaining the same force, to and fro glides are given perpendicular to the Soleus fibres, a distance up to 1/2cm from the targeted point. Three to five glides are given 3 times per session, according to the patient's condition and tolerance. Each time, 5 Sec rest is given.

**2. Plantaris:** Origin is the lateral supra-condylar ridge of the femur and inserted into the calcaneus via the Achilles tendon.
**Palpation and deep friction-** Position the patient in a prone, note origin and insertion; as it is a deeper muscle, slack should be taken with more force. Figure 19 shows three white dots with an average distance of 1 cm, representing plantaris. The therapist should place the thumb/olecranon at one divided point, then take the slack with 3-7kg force to reach the desired tissue. Maintaining the same force, to and fro glides are given a distance up to ½ cm from the targeted point perpendicular to the plantaris fibres. Three to five glides are given 3 times per session, according to the patient's condition and tolerance. Each time, 5 Sec rest is given.

**3. Popliteus:** Origin is the lateral condyle of the femur and inserted into the posterior proximal tibia.
**Palpation and deep friction-** The position of the patient is prone; note origin and insertion, and as it is a deeper muscle, slack has to be taken with more force. As shown in Figure 20, five white triangular dots with an average distance of 1 cm represent popliteus. The therapist's thumb/olecranon is placed on the desired tissue and then takes up the slack with 3-7kg force to reach the desired tissue. Maintaining the same force, to and fro glides are given a distance up to 1/2cm from the targeted point perpendicular to the fibres of the popliteus. Three to five glides

are given 3 times per session, according to the patient's condition and tolerance. Each time, 5 Sec rest is given.

**Note:** Origin and insertion are mentioned for Soleus, Plantaris, Popliteus, and Posterior cruciate ligaments for palpation, as they cover a smaller area

### c). Deep layer:

### 1. Posterior medial meniscus/medial posterior Joint line:

**Palpation-** The position of the patient is prone, as shown in Figure 20; three white dots with an average distance of 1cm represent the posterior medial joint line. Place the knee in at least 45 degrees of flexion to locate the joint line. Palpate with more force to locate the posterior aspect of the medial joint line. Noting any crepitus or pain may indicate possible meniscal trauma.
**Deep friction-** The therapist can screen out the possible lesions/adhesions of soft tissue from superficial to deep by gradually increasing the force. The therapist's thumb/olecranon is placed on the desired tissue and then takes up the slack with 5-10kg force to reach the desired tissue. As shown in Figure 20, by maintaining the same force, to and fro deep friction, glides are given a distance of up to 1/2cm from the targeted point along the joint line/to the fibres of the medial meniscus (three white dots). Three to five glides are given 3 times per session, according to the patient's condition and tolerance. Each time, 5 Sec rest is given.

### 2. Posterior lateral meniscus/lateral posterior joint line:

**Palpation-** The position of the patient is prone. Figure 20 shows three black dots with an average distance of 1 cm, representing the posterior lateral joint line. Place the knee in at least 45 degrees of flexion to locate the joint line. Palpate with more force to locate the posterior aspect of the lateral joint line, noting any crepitus/adhesions or pain that may indicate possible lateral meniscal trauma. The therapist can screen out the possible lesions/adhesions of soft tissue from superficial to deep by gradually increasing force.

**Deep friction-** The therapist's thumb/olecranon is placed on the desired tissue and then takes up the slack with 5-10kg force to reach the desired tissue. As shown in Figure 20, by maintaining the same force, to and fro deep friction, glides are given a distance up to 1/2 cm from the targeted point along the joint line/ to the fibres of the posterior lateral meniscus (three black dots). Three to five glides are given 3 times per session, according to the patient's condition and tolerance. Each time, 5 Sec rest is given.

## 3. Anterior cruciate ligaments:

**Palpation-** The position of the patient is prone; the ACL originates from the medial and anterior aspect of the tibial plateau and runs superiorly, laterally, and toward its insertion on the lateral femoral condyle. It is composed of the anterio-medial and posterior-lateral bundles.

Only posterior-lateral bundles can be palpable at the lateral femoral condyle. It is represented in a dark dot on the femur area, as shown in Figure 21; arrow lines indicate the direction of the deep friction point of ACL.

**Deep friction-** The therapist's thumb/olecranon is placed on the desired tissue, and then slack is taken with 5-10kg force to reach the desired tissue. As shown in Figure 21, by maintaining the same force, to and fro deep friction glides are given over ACL (black dot) distance up to 1/2cm from the targeted point. Three to five glides are given 3 times per session, according to the patient's condition and tolerance. Each time, 5 Sec rest is given.

## 4. Posterior cruciate ligaments:

**Palpation-** PCL is approximately twice as strong and twice as thick as the normal ACL (therefore less commonly injured).
**Origin:** PCL originates from the anterior-lateral aspect of the medial femoral condyle in the area of the intercondylar notch;
**Insertion:** tibial attachment is not intra-articular, but over the back of the tibial plateau, it is approximately 1 cm distal to the joint line;
The position of the patient is in the prone position; only the tibial attachment of PCL can be palpable. As shown in Figure 21, the triangular shape at the tibial plateau represents the palpable PCL, and two dark green dots represent the deep friction points on PCL.

**Deep friction-** The therapist's thumb/olecranon is placed on the desired tissue, and slack is taken with 5-10kg force to reach the desired tissue. As shown in Figure 21, by maintaining the same force, to and fro deep friction glides are given over PCL (two white dots), a distance up to 1/2cm from the targeted point. Three to five glides are given 3 times per session according to the patient's condition and tolerance. Each time, 5 Sec rest is given.

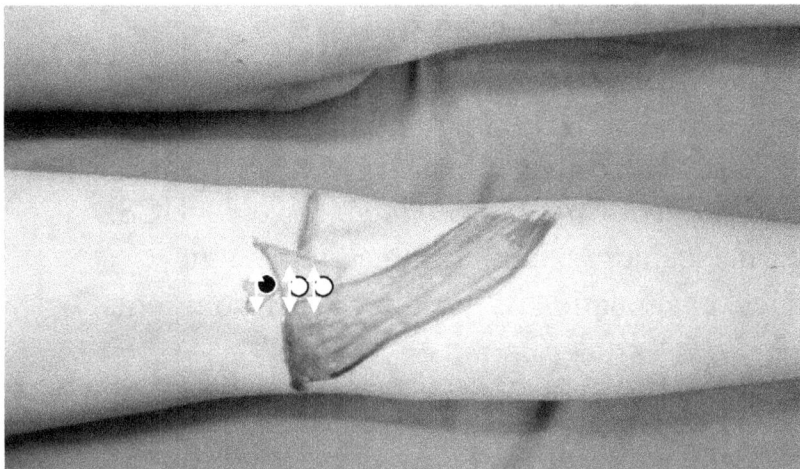

Figure 21: A black dot on the femur represents the palpable and deep friction points of ACL, and two white dots on the tibia represent the palpable and deep friction points of PCL.

**References:**

1. https://www.youtube.com/watch?v=ONA_y0znCoU
2. www.youtube.com/watch?v=-b_MAq6Rkwk
3. https://www.youtube.com/watch?v=ZNzfJCIEkQI
4. Knee Examination,http://www.osceskills.com/e-learning/subjects/knee-examination/
5. Charlie Goldberg, M.D., *A Practical Guide to Clinical Medicine,* UCSD School of Medicine,https://meded.ucsd.edu/clinicalmed/joints.htm
6. Roberto Rossi, et al., Clinical examination of the knee: know your tools for diagnosis of knee injuries,https://bmcsportsscimedrehabil.biomedcentral.com/articles/10.1186/1758-2555-3-25
7. Starkey & Ryan; examination of orthopedics and athletic injuries, 3red edition, 2010
8. Saurab Sharma, knee joint palpation; https://www.slideshare.net/saurabsharma/6-knee-joint-palpation
9. Orthopedic Evaluation of the Knee- Palpation and Special Testshttp://webcache.googleusercontent.com/search?q=cache:http://www.meorthopedicseminars.com/wp-content/uploads/2014/03/M-Lab-1-Orthopedic-evaluation-of-the-knee-palpation-and-special-tests.pdf&gws_rd=cr&ei=yMfhWPyIGsmr0gT60Z6ICg
10. J Rehabil Res Dev.et al, The effects of tibial rotation on the patellofemoral joint: assessment of the changes in in situ strain in the peripatellar retinaculum and the patellofemoral contact pressures and areas.Continuing Education Program. 2001 Sep-Oct; 38(5):463-9.
11. John Winslow, Treatment of Lateral Knee Pain Using Soft Tissue Mobilization in Four Female Triathletes,Int J Ther Massage Bodywork. 2014 Sep; 7(3): 25–31.https://www.ncbi.nlm.nih.gov/pmc/articles/PMC4145001/
12. Gregory s johson, chapter 30, soft tissue mobilization. http://andoaston.com/files/pdf/STM_IPA.pdf
13. Mike Robertson, self myofacial release, purpose, methods, and technique: http://robertsontrainingsystems.com/downloads/SMR-manual.pdf
14. Hunter G, Specific soft tissue mobilization in the management of soft tissue dysfunction. Man Ther. 1998 Feb; 3 (1): 2-11 https://www.ncbi.nlm.nih.gov/pubmed/11487295
15. Starkey & Ryan; examination of orthopedics and athletic injuries, 3red edition, 2010
16. https://www.youtube.com/watch?v=Wy7kT59T49k
17. https://www.youtube.com/watch?v=W_IrZOtWqpg

18. http://www.dwsportsmassage.com/blog/2014/06/soft-tissue-release
19. https://www.youtube.com/watch?v=1hsfNXDqUE0
20. https://www.youtube.com/watch?v=noNuNGp7QGA
21. https://www.youtube.com/watch?v=JPIFStDea0M
22. https://www.youtube.com/watch?v=BlVwvBadzPw
23. Janet McMurray, ATC, LAT, MEd • McMurry University and University of Idaho; Scott Landis, ATC, LAT, MA, LMT • King University and University of Idaho; Kris Lininger, ATC, MS • College of the Siskiyous and University of Idaho; Russell T. Baker, DAT, ATC, LAT, Alan Nasypany, EdD, ATC, LAT, and Jeff Seegmiller, EdD, AT • University of Idaho. A Comparison and Review of Indirect. Myofascial Release Therapy, Instrument- Assisted Soft Tissue Mobilization, and Active Release Techniques to Inform Clinical Decision Making.30,September 2015 international journal of Athletic Therapy & training
24. . Salvi Shah1*, Akta Bhalara2 1Lecturer, SPB Physiotherapy College, Ugat-Bhesan Road, Surat, Gujarat 2Lecturer, Shree Swaminarayan Physiotherapy College, Khambhaliya highway, Jamnagar. Myofascial Release. International Journal of Health Sciences & Research (www.ijhsr.org) 69 Vol.2; Issue: 2; May 2012.

# CHAPTER 14
## Ankle and Foot: Biomechanics, Pathomechanics, and Treatment

Postural stability and dynamic movement begin with the gait cycle. Foot posture and alignment are the critical first link in the kinetic chain. Understanding these postural deficiencies will greatly enhance manual therapy management. The use of stabilizing orthotics can also provide the patient with specific support in their subluxation-based care plan.

Within the normal **gait cycle**, pronation[1] and supination are essential for proper momentum and balance. Upon heel strike, the foot is slightly supinated. As the foot moves through the heel strike, pronation at the ankle and knee flexion absorb most of the impact. This rolling action, from supination to pronation, also compensates for irregularities in the striking surface. The foot then shifts into supination and acts as a fixed lever, which allows for a strong push-off. This supinated motion also occurs at the subtalar joint, allowing for efficient and strong support at the toe-off.

The excessively supinated[1,2] foot cannot move easily into pronation at heel strike. [2] The rigid foot posture results in a more stressful heel strike and a less accommodating foot on irregular terrains. As these impacts are translated through the biomechanical chain, other structures are affected by the increased shock. Pes cavus is viewed as a contributing component in the development of idiopathic scoliosis at the spine[3] and genu varum at the knee. The rigid, supinated foot[5] is more unstable than an overpronated or normally aligned foot, and there is a greater risk for inversion ankle injuries due to this instability. On the other hand, the excessively pronated foot cannot go easily into supination at toe-off. The soft, unlocked foot posture results in a more stressful toe-off phase. Excessively pronated foot results in a decreased arch and internal rotation of the tibia, resulting in genu valgum at the knee.

The most common foot dysfunctions are shown in figures (**a**) and (**b**):
a. Foot: plantar-flexed, adducted, and inverted – figure (**a**)
b. Foot: plantar-flexed, abducted, and everted – figure (**b**)

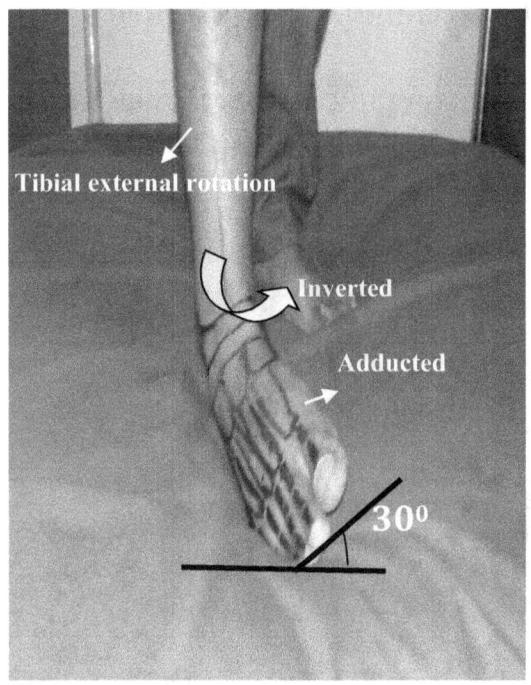 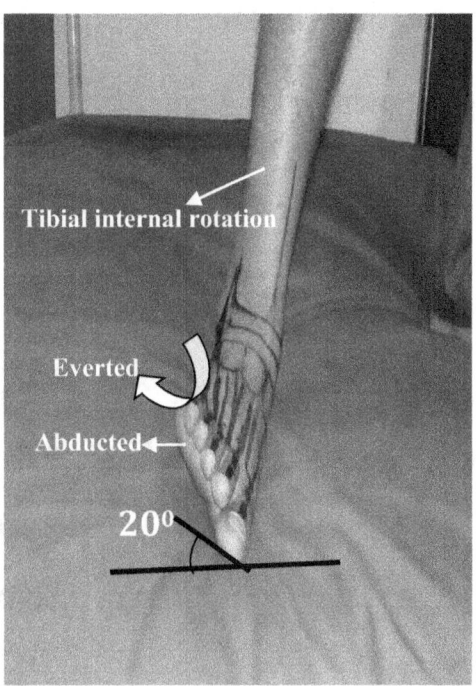

Figure a: Foot- Plantar flexed, adducted and internally rotated, depicting the supinated foot where the arch is exaggerated. Showing foot internal rotation of 30°

Figure b: Foot- Plantar flexed, abducted and everted. Depicting the pronated foot where the arch is decreased. Showing foot eversion of 20°

**Ankle and Foot:** are below knee kinetic chain which influences normal mechanics of the knee

The foot has two main dysfunctions which influence the tibial rotation, which in turn affects the knee's normal mechanics, i.e. one is plantar-flexed, everted, abducted (pronated foot), and the second is plantar-flexed, inverted, adducted (supinated foot)

From the perspective of knee dysfunctions, foot mechanics mainly depend on tibio-talar and inter-tarsal mechanics. Therefore, assessment and treatment of foot dysfunctions are divided into two levels:

1. Tibio-talar (ankle)
2. Inter-tarsal

The primary contributory factor for foot dysfunction is tibio-talar joint, and secondarily, the abnormal mechanical force follows into inter-tarsal joints, tarsometatarsal and phalangeal joints.

Note: as tarso-metatarsal and the phalangeal joints are covered in basic physiotherapy courses, they are not dealt with in detail in this book.

## Important Surface anatomy and palpatory bony landmarks of the foot:

As shown in figures 1, 2, and 3, roughly depicting the surface anatomy and palpatory landmarks of the foot, mainly tibio-talar and inter-tarsal joints[11]

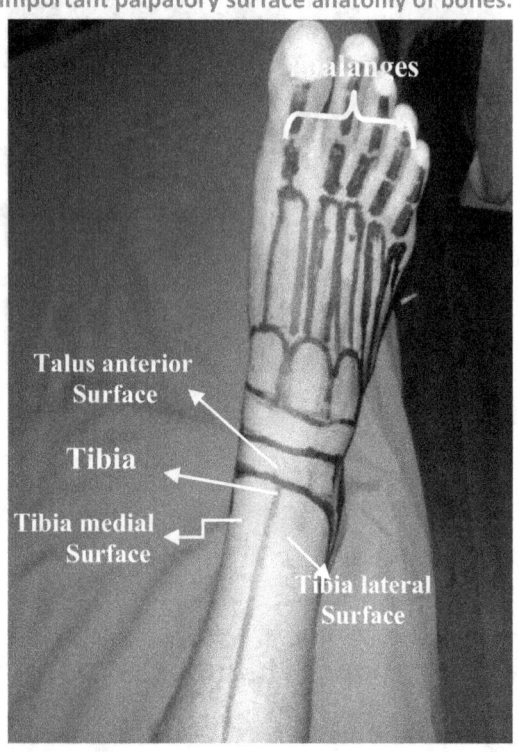

Figure 1: Anterior view of a foot depicting important palpatory surface anatomy of bones.

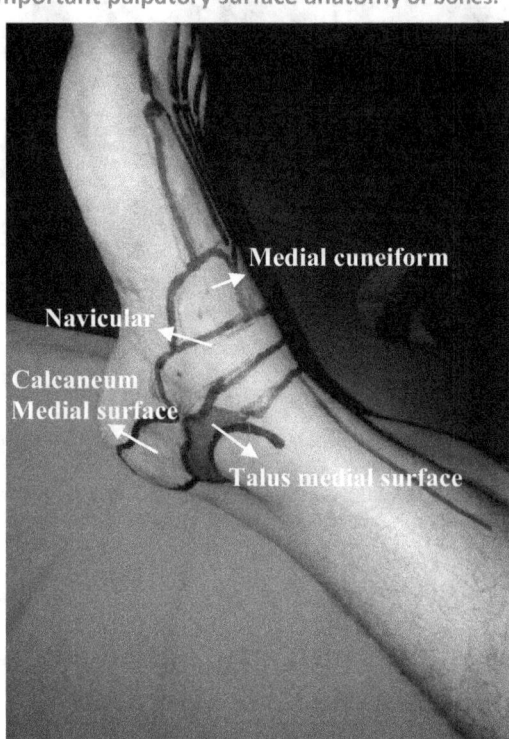

Figure 2: Medial view of a foot depicting important palpatory surface anatomy of bones.

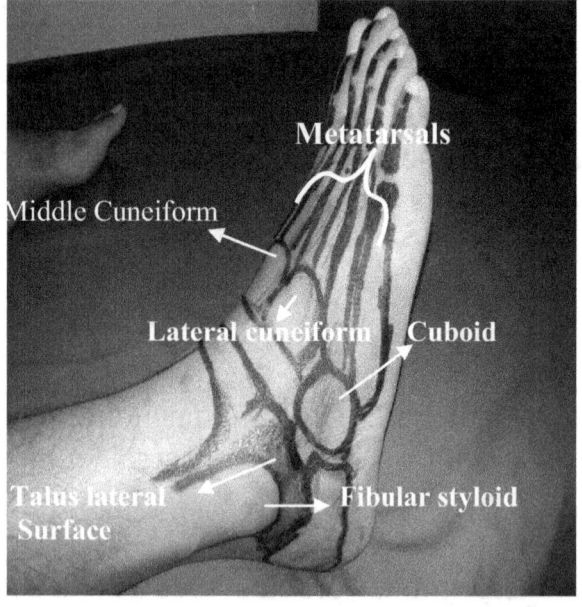

Figure 3: Lateral view of a foot depicting important palpatory surface anatomy of bones.

# Chapter 14: Ankle and Foot – Biomechanics, Pathomechanics and Treatment

**Normal mechanics of Tibio-talar (ankle) and Intertarsal joints:**
Movement of the foot is in three planes[6]:
Sagittal plane – dorsi-flexion and plantar flexion
Transverse plane - inversion and eversion
Frontal plane - adduction and abduction

- A lateral glide of the talus occurs during inversion and adduction. A medial glide of the talus occurs during eversion and abduction.
- External rotation of the distal tibia occurs during inversion and adduction of the foot.
- Internal rotation of the distal tibia occurs during eversion and adduction of the foot.
- Inversion of the foot always follows adduction, and eversion of the foot follows abduction.
- Supination of the foot involves some movement into plantar flexion, adduction, and inversion.
- Pronation of the foot involves some movement into dorsi-flexion, abduction, and eversion.

Adducted and inverted foot: Calcaneum, Navicular, and Cuboid are inverted. Cuneiforms are dorsal (arch increases).
Abducted and Everted foot: Calcaneum, Navicular, and Cuboid are Everted. Cuneiforms are plantar (arch decreases).

**Foot dysfunctions**[1, 2, 9]:
-Foot dysfunctions are mostly extended: the foot is in plantar flexion.
-Dorsi-flexion is always limited; there is a rare limitation of plantar flexion.
-Dorsi-flexion limitations are Extended Type II dysfunctions of the tibio-talar joint. The ankle is stuck plantar-flexed (Extended) and cannot flex (dorsiflex).
-The positional diagnosis is always extended.

Therefore, possible dysfunctions of the foot:

**1. Plantar flexed/ flexion lag with inverted and adducted foot.**

**2. Plantar flexed / flexion lag with everted and abducted foot.**

**3. Plantar flexed/flexion lag with both inversion and adduction plus eversion and abduction loss.**

**Possible foot dysfunctions:**
Foot Joint dysfunction: involvement of tibio-talar and inter-tarsal joints

## 1. Plantar flexed/flexion lag with inverted and adducted foot: Supinated foot.

i) Tibio-talar joint: Talus anterior and lateral
   Distal tibia externally rotated

ii) Inter-tarsal: Calcaneum-inverted, Navicular-inverted, Cuniform- dorsal, cuboid-inverted.

## 2. Plantar flexed/flexion lag with everted and abducted foot: Pronated foot.

i) Tibio-talar joint: Talus anterior and medial
   Distal tibia internally rotated

ii) Inter-tarsal: Calcaneum-everted, Navicular-everted, cuniform-plantar, cuboid-everted.

## 3. Plantar flexed/flexion lag with both inversion and adduction plus eversion and abduction loss.

i) Tibio-talar joint: Talus lateral to medial and medial to lateral glide loss, plus talus anterior.
   Distal tibia external and internal rotation loss

ii) Inter-tarsal: Calcaneum-inversion and eversion loss, Navicular-inversion and eversion loss, Cuniform-dorsal to plantar and plantar to dorsal glide loss, cuboid–inversion and eversion loss.

**Note:** Once an ankle (talo-crural) joint is corrected, inter-tarsal joint dysfunctions are automatically corrected. Basic assessment and treatment with mobilisation of tarso-metatarsal, inter-metatarsal, metatarso-phalangeal joints, and inter-phalangeal joints are beyond the scope of the book, as they are covered in the basic physiotherapy syllabus.

## Specific spring test (assessment) and treatment of foot dysfunctions:

### 1. Dysfunction (supinated foot): Plantar flexed/flexion lag with inverted and adducted foot

These dysfunctions are divided into two parts, one at the talo-crural/tibio-talar joint and the second at the inter-tarsal joints[3,4].

There are two ways of applying the spring test: one is osteo-kinematic (gross), and another is Arthro-kinematic (specific)

As is already discussed, the most efficient way of applying the spring test between the two ways of tests is Arthro-kinematic (specific) test. Therefore, arthro-kinematic (specific) spring test is applied to assess dysfunctions.

**Spring test**:
**Dysfunction: Plantar flexed/flexion lag with inverted and adducted foot (figure 4):**
The foot is stuck: Extended (plantar flexed), adducted, and internally Rotated (inverted).
The movement barrier: the foot cannot flex (dorsiflex), Abduct and externally Rotate (evert).
The position of assessment and treatment is the same as the movement barrier:

### i) Tibio-talar joint: Talus lateral and anterior
###       Distal tibia externally rotated
### ii) Inter-tarsal: Calcaneum- inverted, Navicular- inverted,
###   Cuneiform- dorsal, cuboid- internally rotated.

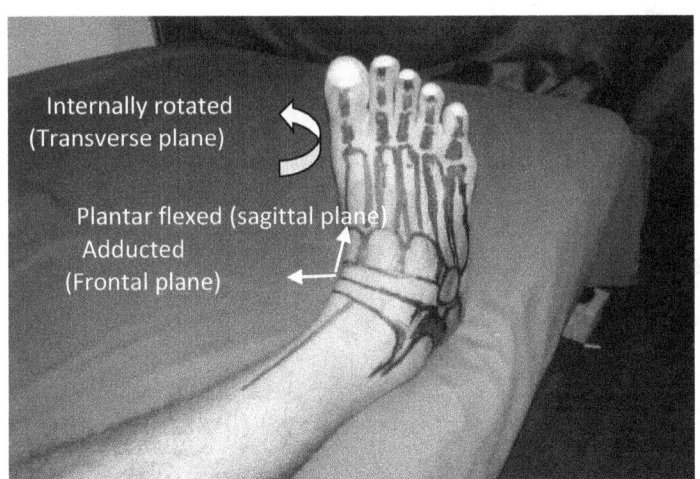

Figure 4: Foot Dysfunction 1: The foot is adducted (frontal plane), inverted (transverse plane) and plantar flexed (sagittal plane)

## i) Dysfunctions of Tibio-talar joint:

Talus (covered and uncovered) stuck in lateral and anterior
Distal tibia externally rotated.
For accurate diagnosis, Specific spring glides that need to be performed after taking the slack are as follows

**a) Talus (covered and uncovered) – lateral to medial glide**
**b) Talus – anterior to posterior glide**
**c) Distal tibia – internal rotation glide**

**Note:** The fibular styloid process covers some part of the upper/proximal lateral surface of the Talus; in the same way, some part of the upper/proximal medial surface of the talus is covered by a tibial styloid process; these parts are called covered talus. This upper/proximal part of the talus articulates with talo-crural joint. Some parts of the talus's lower/distal medial and lower/distal lateral surfaces, which are not covered by the tibial styloid, are called the uncovered part of the talus. This lower part of the talus articulates with tarsal joints. Therefore, for accurate diagnosis and treatment of talus dysfunction, both covered/proximal and uncovered/distal parts of the talus spring test and treatment should be included.

### a) Uncovered/distal Talus - lateral to medial glide

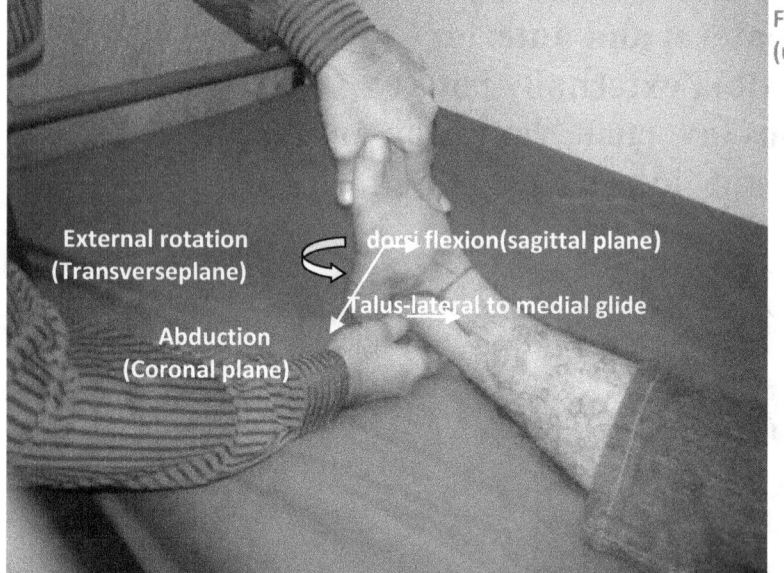

Figure 5: Spring test- distal talus (uncovered) lateral to medial glide.

**Spring test:**
**Position of the patient:** As shown in Figure 5, the patient is lying supine, and the left foot is to be examined.
**Position of the therapist and procedure:** The therapist approaches the patient from the left side. The left hand of the therapist holds the patient's forefoot. Then,

the therapist passively abducts (coronal plane), everts (transverse plane), and dorsi-flexes (sagittal plane) to reach an inter-barrier zone. Simultaneously, the therapist's right thumb is placed on the talus's uncovered/distal lateral surface just below the lateral malleolus and takes the medial glide slack with 5kg force. Additionally, 3kg force is applied to feel the spring/end feel. If it doesn't spring- it indicates dysfunction.

**Treatment:**
**Mobilization:** The patient and therapist position for treatment is the same as the assessment position, as explained above. After reaching the movement barrier in three planes, talus medial slack is taken with 5kg force; then, talus medial glides are done according to the grades of mobilisation. 5 glides of mobilization are given 3 times in one session. Each time, 5 seconds of rest is given.
**Muscle energy technique**: As shown in Figure 5, patient and therapist positions are the same as explained above; after reaching the movement barrier in three planes, talus medial glide slack is taken with 5kg force with the thumb. Then, the patient is asked to plantar-flex the foot, and simultaneously, the therapist resists producing an isometric contraction. After 5 Sec relaxation, a further new movement barrier zone in three planes of the foot is reached, and further new talus medial glide slack is taken. Again, repeat the same 3 times per session. Each time, 5 seconds of rest is given.
**Taping:** As shown in Figure 6, the patient is supine, has a right foot to be treated, and the therapist approaches the patient from the right side of the patient.

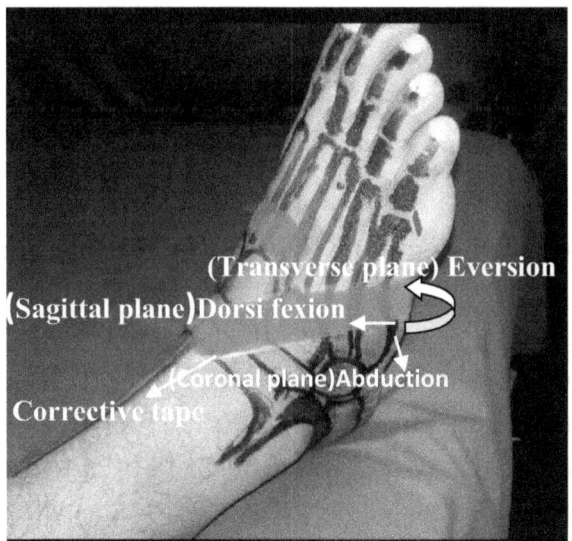

Figure 6: Taping to correct adducted, inverted and dorsi flexed of the foot.

Taping is to correct adducted, inverted, and plantar-flexed feet. One end of the tape is pasted on the dorsal surface of the 1$^{st}$, 2$^{th}$metatarsal head, and then the foot is abducted (coronal plane), everted (transverse plane), and dorsiflexed (sagittal plane) to reach a movement-barrier zone. Following that, the talus lateral to medial slack is taken with 5kg force, and the medial glide is applied with 3kg force. The foot is wrapped with tape from the plantar surface to the lateral side of the foot, and the other end of the tape is pasted at the lower end of the medial surface of the styloid process of the tibia, as shown in the figure.

**Sustained glide**: The patient is lying on the right side, and the hip and knee are flexed to 450-900, and the right foot is to be treated. With corrective tape on, as mentioned above, further sustained lateral to medial glide of uncovered/distal talus is achieved either passively by the therapist or with a specially made talus stand, as shown in Figure 7.

The stand with the pointed edge is placed just below the lateral malleolus on the uncovered lateral surface of the talus. It is kept for a duration of 2 to 5 min, according to patient tolerance and the condition of the problem.

<u>Description of the Stand</u>: The stand consists of a circular base with a radius of 6 cm, 1.5cm thickness, and a rounded cylindrical central projection with a height of 8.5 cm with a .5cm radius, as shown in Figure 7.

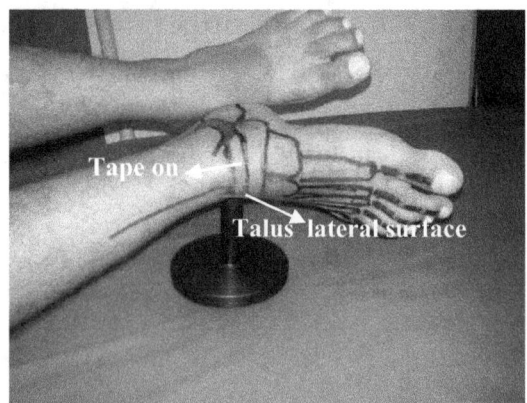

Figure 7: Talus stand is kept on talus lateral uncovered surface (with corrective tape on) to give sustained medial glide.

**Covered/proximal- talus: Spring test and mobilization from lateral to medial**
**Spring test:**
**Position of the patient:** As shown in Figure 8, the patient is supine.
**Position of the therapist and procedure:** left leg to be treated. The left hand of the therapist holds the patient's forefoot. Then the therapist passively abducts (coronal plane), everts (transverse plane), and dorsi-flexes (sagittal plane) to reach three planar movement-barrier zones. Simultaneously, the therapist's right hand's thumb is placed on the lateral malleolus. Then (covered/proximal) talus medial slack is taken with 5kg force, and additionally, 3kg force is applied medially to test the spring/end feel. If it does not, spring indicates dysfunction.

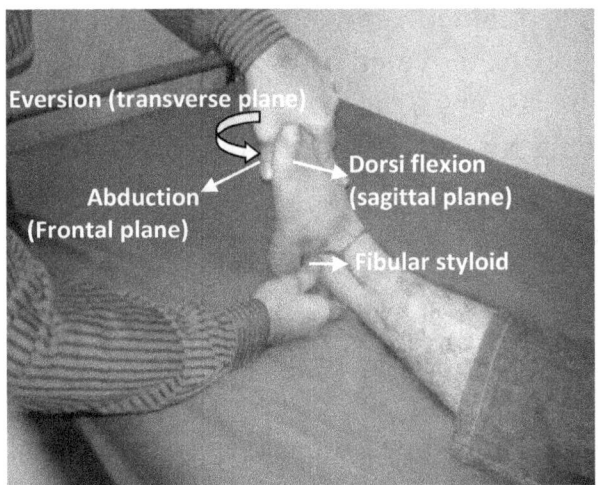
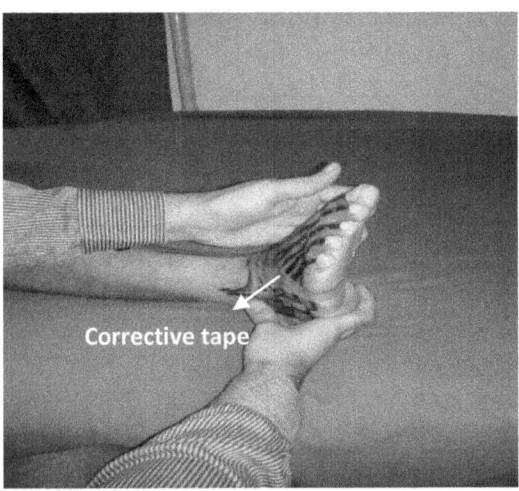

Figure 8: Spring test and mobilization of (covered/proximal) talus from lateral to medial glide through fibular styloid.

Figure 9: Taping to correct inverted, adducted and dorsi flexed foot and simultaneously, (covered) talus lateral to medial glide mobilization.

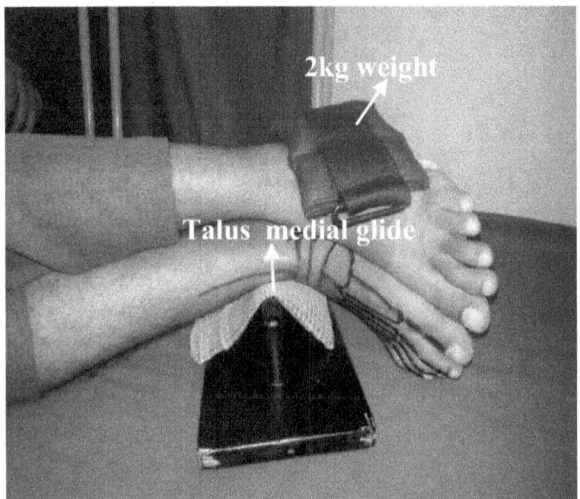

Figure 10: Sustained glide of covered/proximal talus from lateral to medial glide through fibular styloid on the stand.

## Treatment:

**Mobilization:** As shown in Figure 8, the patient position for treatment is the same as the assessment position as explained above; after reaching the movement barrier in three planes simultaneously, covered/proximal talus medial glide slack is taken with 5kg force. Then, talus medial glides are done according to the grades of mobilisation. 5 glides are given 3 times in one session. Each time 5 seconds of rest is given.

**Muscle energy technique**: as shown in Figure 8, the patient and therapist position is the same as the assessment position as explained above; after reaching the movement barrier in three planes simultaneously, covered/proximal talus medial glide slack is taken with 5kg force. Then, the patient is asked to plantar-flex, and simultaneously, the therapist resists producing an isometric contraction. After 5 Sec relaxations, a further new movement barrier in three planes, eversion, abduction, and dorsi-flexion is reached, and further covered talus medial glide slack is taken. Again, repeat the same 3 times per session.

**Taping:** As shown in figure 6 and 9, the patient and therapist position is the same as the assessment position explained above; taping is to correct adduction, inversion, and plantar flexion- i.e., one end of the tape is pasted on the dorsal surface of 1$^{st}$, 2$^{nd}$ metatarsal head, then the foot is abducted (coronal plane), everted (transverse plane) and dorsi-flexed (sagittal plane) to reach the inter barrier zone. Simultaneously, covered talus medial glide slack is taken with 5kg force, and additionally, 3kg force is applied to glide medially. Then, the foot is wrapped with tape from the plantar surface to the lateral side of the foot, and the other end of the tape is pasted at the lower end of the medial surface of the tibia.

**Sustained glide**: As shown in figure 10, the patient is on the right side-lying with hip and knee flexed to 90$^0$. As mentioned above, with the correction tape on, further sustained lateral to medial glide of the covered talus is achieved by placing the stand on the lateral surface of the fibular styloid. The above procedure gives the sustained medial glide with other leg weight. Sustained glide can be given for 2 to 5 min, according to patient tolerance and the condition of the problem.
Dimensions of stand: a rectangular base (15 cm × 39 cm); a rectangular projection (6cm × 25cm); and the thickness of the base and projection are about 1.5 cm.

**b) Talus: anterior to posterior glide:**
**Spring test:**
**Position of the patient:** is supine, left leg to be treated.
**Position of the therapist and procedure**: as shown in Figure 11, the therapist approaches from the left side, the left hand of the therapist hold the forefoot of the patient, then abducts (coronal plane), everts (transverse plane), and dorsi-flexes (sagittal plane) to reach inter-barrier zone. Simultaneously, the Therapist's right thumb is placed on the anterior surface of the talus at the ankle mortise and takes posterior glide slack with 5kg fore, and additionally, 3kg force is applied to test the spring/end feel. If it does not, spring indicates dysfunction.

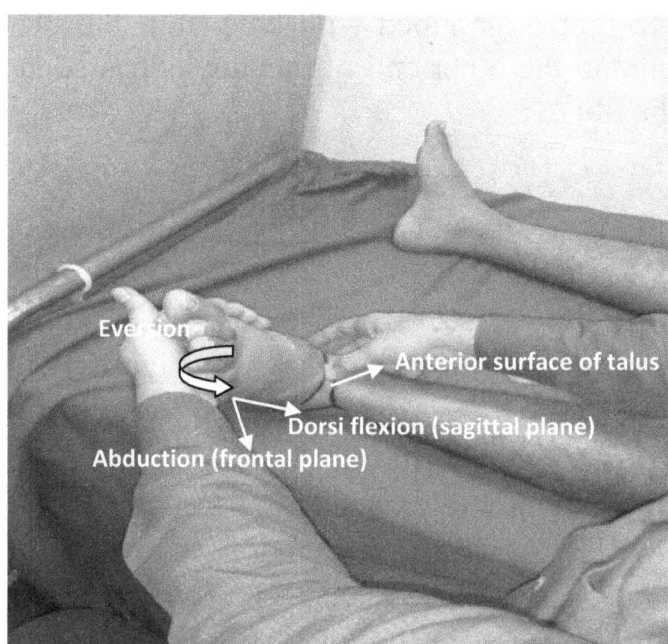

Figure 11: With corrective tape on, the talus anterior to posterior glide is done from the anterior surface of the talus.

**Treatment:**
**Mobilization:** As shown in Figure 11, the patient and therapist position for treatment is the same as the assessment position as explained above; after reaching the movement barrier in three planes of the foot, simultaneously, talus posterior glide slack is taken with 5kg force and posterior glides are done according to the grades of mobilisation. 5 glides are given 3 times in one session. Each time, 5 seconds of rest is given.

**Muscle energy technique**: As shown in Figure 11, the patient and therapist position for treatment is the same as the assessment position explained above; after reaching the movement barrier in three planes of the foot, simultaneously, talus posterior glide slack is taken with 5kg force, and the patient is asked to plantar-flex, and simultaneously therapist resists, producing an isometric contraction. After 5 Sec of relaxation, a further new movement barrier in three planes of the foot is reached, and the talus's new posterior glide is reached. Again, repeat the same 3 times per session.

**Taping:** As shown in Figure 6, the patient and therapist position is the same as the assessment position as explained previously; taping is to correct adduction, inversion, and plantar flexion- i.e., one end of the tape is pasted on the dorsal surface of 1st, 2nd metatarsal head, then the foot is abducted (coronal plane), everted (transverse plane) and dorsi-flexed (sagittal plane) to reach the inter barrier zone. Simultaneously, talus posterior glide slack is applied with 5kg force, and 3kg force is applied to glide further. Then, the foot is wrapped with tape from the plantar surface to the lateral side of the foot, and the other end of the tape is pasted at the lower end of the medial surface of the tibia.

**Sustained glide**:

**Position of the patient:** As shown in Figures 12**a** and **b**, the position of the patient is prone, with the knee flexed to $30^0$.

**Procedure:** As mentioned above, with the correction tape on, a further sustained posterior glide of the talus is achieved with a stand, as shown in Figure 12a. The talus stand is placed on the anterior surface of the talus; if needed, weight can be added (figure 12b) to reinforce the posterior glide further. Sustained glide can be given for 2 to 5 min, according to the patient's tolerance and the condition of the problem. The advantage is that the glide is gradual and causes less pain to the patient, and the therapist's time and energy will be saved. Or it can be done in supine lying by the therapist, as shown in Figure 11, but the therapist needs to hold the sustained posterior glide of the talus for 2-5 min passively.

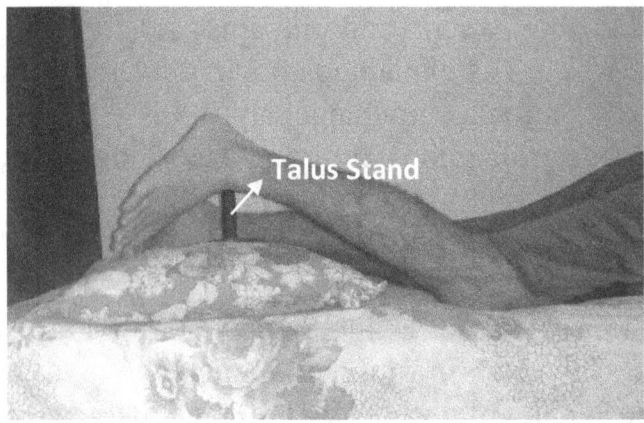

Figure 12a: Talus anterior to posterior sustained glide with talus stand.

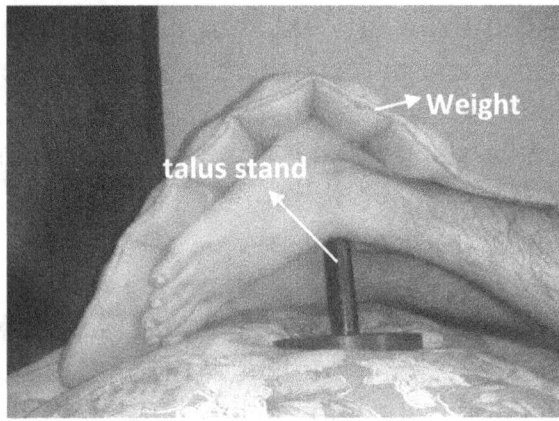

Figure 12b: Talus anterior to posterior sustained glide with talus stand with weight.

**c) Distal tibia: external rotation to internal rotation**

**Spring test:**

**Position of the patient**: is supine, right leg to be treated.

**Position of the therapist and procedure**: as shown in Figure 13, the therapist approaches from the right side of the patient, the right hand of the therapist hold the forefoot, then abducts (coronal plane), everts (transverse plane), and dorsi-flexes (sagittal plane) to reach three planar inter barrier zone. Simultaneously, the therapist's left thumb (figure13)/olecranon (figure14) is placed on the lower lateral surface of the tibia closest to the midline and then takes the internal rotation slack with 5kg force. Additionally, 3kg force is applied to test the spring/end feel. If it does not, spring indicates dysfunction.

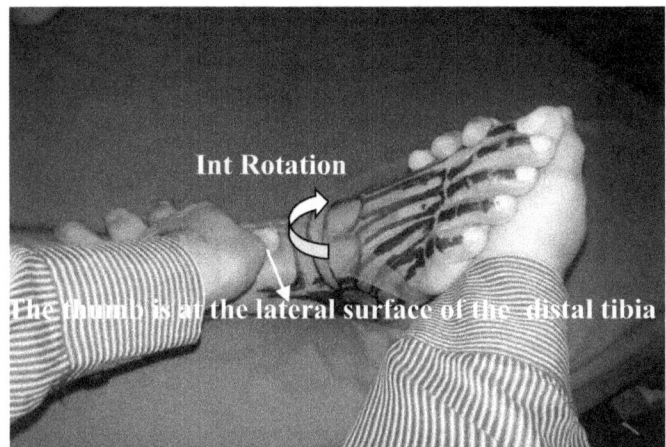

Figure 13: externally rotated distal tibia spring test and internal rotation mobilisation with the thumb.

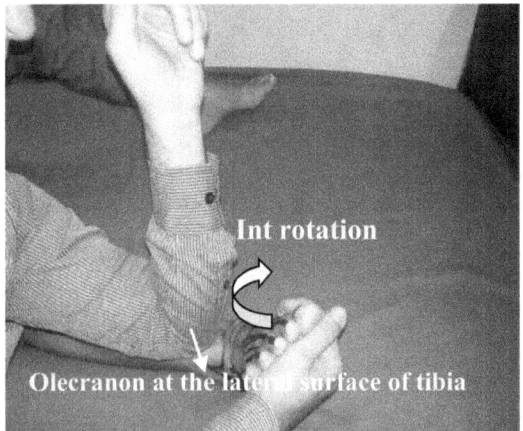

Figure 14: externally rotated Distal tibia spring test and internal rotation mobilsation with olecranon.

## Treatment:

**Mobilization**: As shown in figures 13 and 14, the patient and therapist's position for treatment is the same as the assessment position as explained above after reaching the movement barrier in three planes of the foot; the therapist's left thumb/olecranon is placed on the lower lateral surface of the tibia, and internal rotation slack is taken with 5kg force. Further internal rotation glides are done according to the grades of mobilisation. 5glides are given 3 times in one session. Each time, 5 seconds of rest is given.

**Muscle energy technique**: As shown in Figures 13 and 14, the patient and therapist position for treatment is the same as the assessment position as explained above; after reaching the movement barrier in three planes of the foot, the distal tibia internal rotation slack is taken with 5kg force as mentioned above. Then, the patient is asked to plantar-flex, and simultaneously, the therapist resists producing an isometric contraction. After 5 Sec of relaxation, a further new movement barrier in three planes of the foot and further distal tibia internal rotation glide is reached. Again, repeat the same 3 times per session.

**Taping:** to correct the right foot's adduction, inversion, and plantar flexion. The same steps are followed as mentioned in Figure 6 of taping; additionally, to increase and maintain internal rotation of the distal tibia, as shown in Figure 15, the therapist approaches from the patient's right side. One end of the tape is pasted on the lower lateral surface of the tibia. Then, internal rotation slack is taken with 5kg force. Additionally, 3kg force is applied to glide the distal tibia into further internal rotation. Another end of the tape is pasted obliquely on the medial plantar surface of the calcaneum.

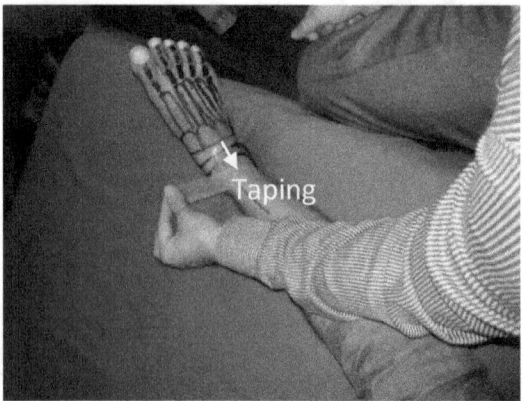

Figure 15: Taping to correct external rotation of the distal tibia.

## ii) Dysfunctions of inter-tarsal joints: (Dysfunction: supinated foot- Plantar flexed/ flexion lag with inverted and adducted foot)
a) **Calcaneum- inverted,** b) **Navicular- inverted,** c) **Cuneiform- dorsal,**
d) **cuboid- inverted**

Spring test/assessment and treatment of inter-tarsal Joints are:

### a) Calcaneum-inverted:

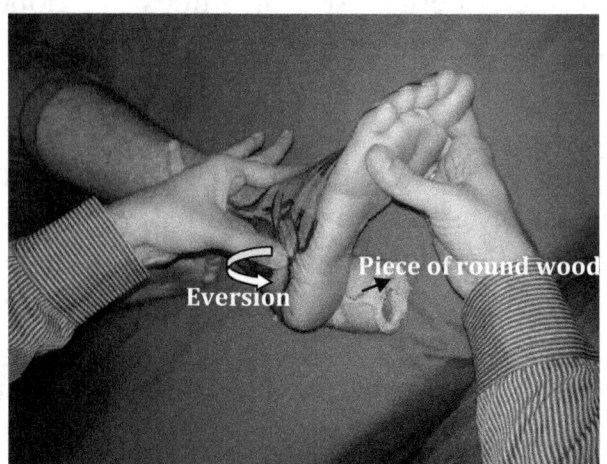

Figure 16: Spring test and mobilisation of calcaneum into eversion with the thumb.

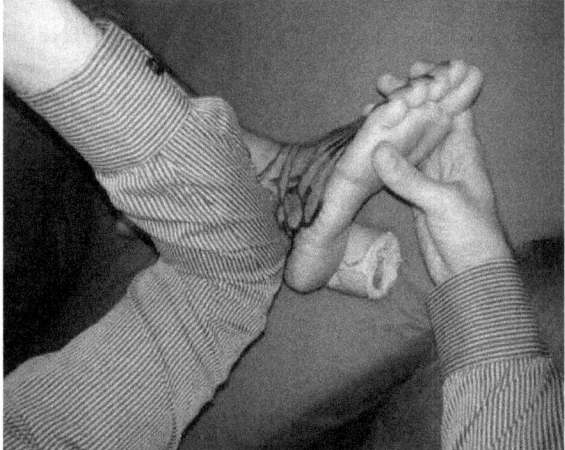

Figure 17: Spring test and mobilisation of calcaneum into eversion with olecranon of the elbow.

## Spring test:
**Position of the patient:** is in the side-lying, right foot to be assessed, right hip and knee of the patient are flexed to $45^0$-$90^0$, as shown in figures 16 and 17. A rounded log is placed under the calcaneum obliquely for better grip of the foot and to reinforce the eversion of the calcaneum.

**Position of the therapist and procedure:** The right hand of the therapist holds the forefoot of the patient, then abducts (coronal plane), everts (transverse plane), and dorsi-flexes (sagittal plane) to reach three planar inter-barrier zones. Simultaneously, the therapist's left thumb/olecranon is placed on the lateral surface of the calcaneum just below the cuboid and takes the eversion glide slack with 5kg force, and additionally, 3kg force is applied to test the spring/end feel. If it does not, spring indicates dysfunction.

**Treatment:**

**Mobilization:** As shown in figures 16 and 17, the patient position for treatment is the same as the assessment position as explained above; after reaching the movement barrier in three planes, simultaneously, the left thumb/olecranon of the therapist is placed on the lower lateral surface of the calcaneum just below cuboid and takes the eversion glide slack with 5kg force. Further eversion glides are given according to the grades of mobilization. 5 glides are given 3 times in one session. Each time, 5 seconds of rest is given.

**Taping:** has three parts; one part is to correct inverted, adducted, and plantar-flexed foot, and the second is to correct inverted calcaneum. The third part is to correct distal tibial external rotation, which is connected pathomechanically.

Part one: to correct adduction, inversion, and plantar flexion of the right foot. the same steps are to be followed, as mentioned in Figure 6.

Part two: The patient position for treatment is the same as the assessment position as explained above; one end of the tape is pasted over the medial surface of the calcaneum, and eversion glide slack is taken with 5kg force. An additional 3kg force is applied to evert the calcaneum. The other end of the tape is pasted over the lateral surface of the cuboid, as shown in Figures 18a and 18b, and it can be extended up to the dorsum of the 4th and 5th base of the metatarsals.

Part three: The therapist approaches the patient's right side to achieve and maintain internal rotation of the distal tibia, as shown in Figure 15. One end of the tape is pasted on the lower lateral surface of the tibia. Then, the internal rotation slack is taken with thumb/olecranon, and the other end of the tape is pasted obliquely over the calcaneum's medial and plantar surface.

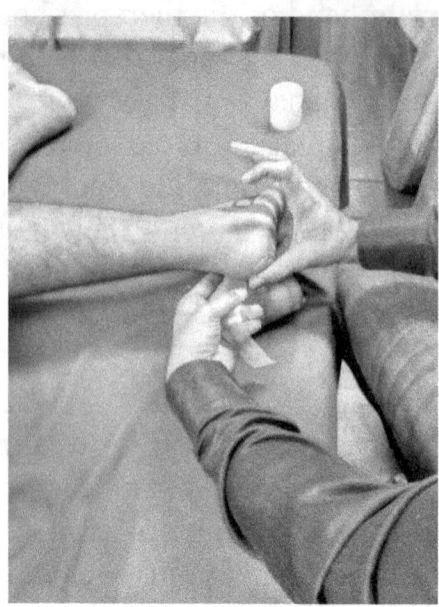

Figure 18a: Taping to correct inversion of the calcaneum- initially, one end of the tape is pasted over the medial surface of the calcaneum.

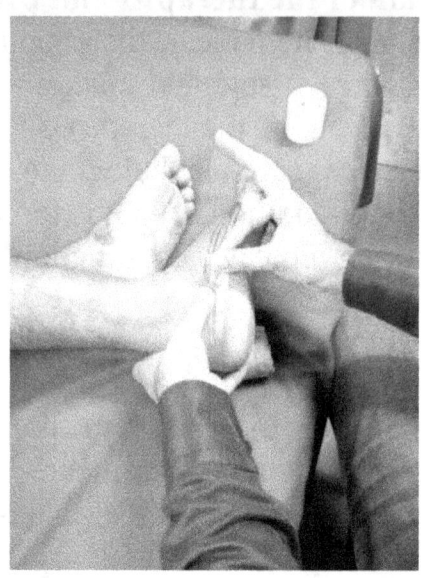

Figure 18b: Taping to correct inversion of the calcaneum- another end of the tape is pasted over the lateral surface of the cuboid and 4th and 5th Meta-Tarsal.

**Muscle energy technique:** As shown in figures 16 and 17, the patient and therapist's position for treatment is the same as the assessment position as explained after reaching the movement barrier in three planes of the foot; simultaneously, the left thumb/olecranon of the therapist is placed on the lateral surface of calcaneum just below the cuboid and takes the eversion glide slack with 5kg force. Then, the patient is asked to plantar-flex, and simultaneously, the therapist resists producing an isometric contraction. After 5 Sec of relaxation, a further new movement barrier in three planes of the foot and new calcaneum eversion glide slack is taken. Again, repeat the same 3 times per session.

**Sustained glide:**

**Position of the patient:** The patient is on the right side, lying with bilateral hip and knee flexed to $90^0$. As mentioned above, with the correction tape on, further sustained eversion of the right calcaneum is achieved by a therapist or with a stand, as shown in Figure 19.

**Procedure:** the stand with the pointed edge is placed just below the cuboid on the lateral surface calcaneum just below the cuboid. It is kept for a duration of 2 to 5 min, according to the patient's tolerance and the condition of the problem.

Description of the stand: The stand consists of a circular base with a radius of 6 cm and 1.5cm thickness and a rounded cylindrical central projection with a height of 8.5 cm and a .5cm radius.

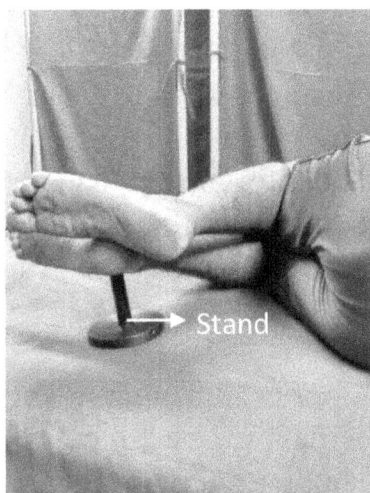

Figure 19: Sustained glide of the calcaneum into eversion.

## b) Navicular: inverted

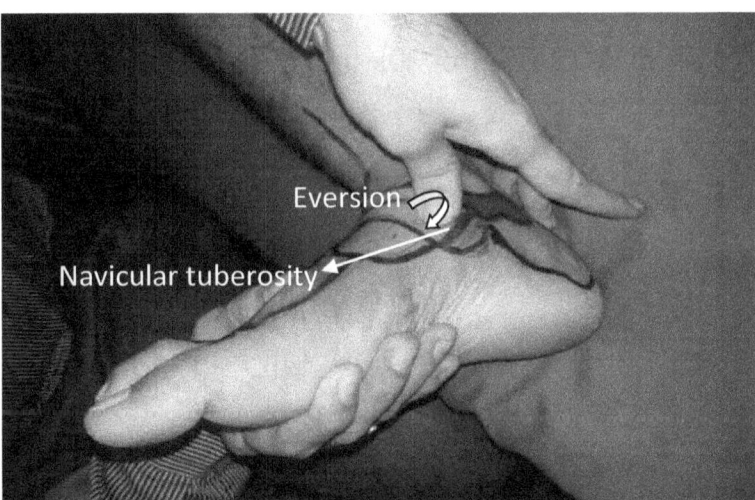

Figure 20: Spring test and external rotation/eversion mobilization of navicular with the thumb.

**Spring test:**
**The patient's position** is side-lying, the right foot is to be treated, and the hip is abducted, flexed, and knee flexed about $30^0$.
**Position of the therapist and procedure:** therapist approaches from the right side, as shown in Figure 20; right hand of the therapist hold the forefoot, then abducts (coronal plane), everts (transverse plane), and dorsi-flexes (sagittal plane) to reach a movement-barrier zone in three planes. Simultaneously, the left thumb/olecranon of the therapist is placed above the navicular tuberosity to take the eversion slack with 5kg force, and additionally, 3kg force is applied to test the spring/end feel. If it doesn't, spring indicates dysfunction.

**Treatment:**
**Mobilization:** As shown in Figure 20, the patient and therapist position for treatment is the same as the assessment position as explained above; after reaching the movement barrier in three planes, simultaneously, the left thumb/olecranon of the therapist is placed above the navicular tuberosity to take the eversion slack with 5kg force, and further eversion glides are done according to the grades of mobilization. 5glides are given 3 times in one session. Each time, 5sec rest is given.

**Taping:** Navicular inversion correction occurs when the foot is adducted, inverted, and plantar-flexed. In order to correct it, the same steps have to be followed, as mentioned in Figure 6, and then added to achieve and maintain internal rotation of the distal tibia; as shown in Figure 15, the therapist approaches from the right side of the patient. One end of the tape is pasted on the lower lateral surface of the tibia, then internal rotation slack is taken with thumb/olecranon, and the other end of the tape is obliquely pasted over the medial surface of the calcaneum.

**Muscle energy technique:** As shown in Figure 20, the patient and therapist's position for treatment is the same as the assessment position as explained above; after reaching the movement barrier in three planes, simultaneously, the left thumb/olecranon of the therapist is placed above the navicular tuberosity to take the eversion slack with 5kg force. Then, the patient is asked to plantar-flex, and simultaneously, the therapist resists producing an isometric contraction. After 5 Sec of relaxation, a further movement barrier in three planes of foot and a new navicular eversion glide is reached. Again, repeat the same 3 times per session.

**Sustained glide:** The therapist can do it manually as it is a small bone.
As shown in Figure 20, the Patient and therapist position for treatment is the same as the assessment position as explained above. After reaching the movement barrier in three planes of the foot, the left thumb/olecranon of the therapist is placed above the navicular tuberosity, then the navicular eversion slack is taken with 5kg force, and additionally, 3kg force is applied for 2- 5 min according to the patient's condition and tolerance.

### c) Cuneiform- dorsal
**Spring test:**
**Position of the patient:** The patient is supine, with the right foot to be treated and hip and knee flexed $30^0$, as shown in Figure 21.
**Position of the therapist and procedure:** The therapist approaches the patient from the right side, and the right hand of the therapist holds the patient's forefoot.

Then abducts (coronal plane), everts (transverse plane), and dorsiflexes (sagittal plane) the foot to reach three planar inter-barrier zones. Then, the left thumb/olecranon of the therapist is placed on cuneiform (medial, middle, and lateral as shown in figures 21, 22, 23 with thumb and 24, 25, 26 with olecranon) and takes the planter to glide slack with 5kg force. 3kg force is also applied to test the spring/end feel. If it does not, spring indicates dysfunction.

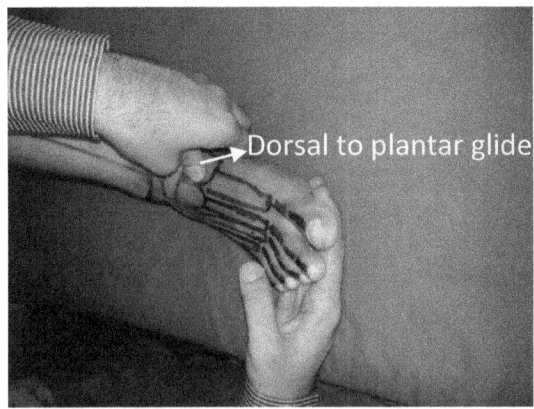

Figure 21: Spring test and mobilization of medial cuneiform from dorsal to plantar with the thumb.

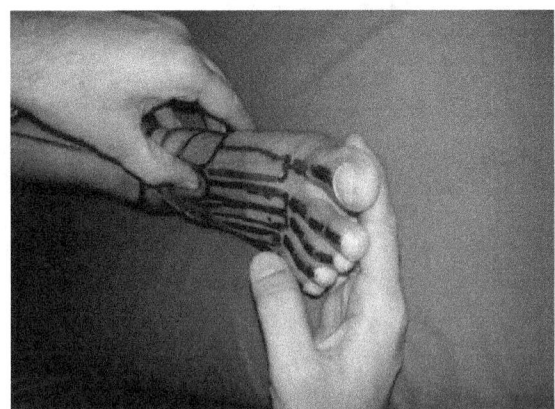

Figure 22: Spring test and mobilization of middle cuneiform from dorsal to plantar with the thumb.

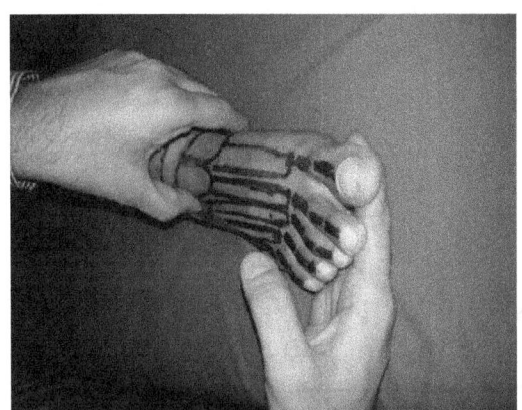

Figure 23: Spring test and mobilization of lateral cuneiform from dorsal to plantar with the thumb.

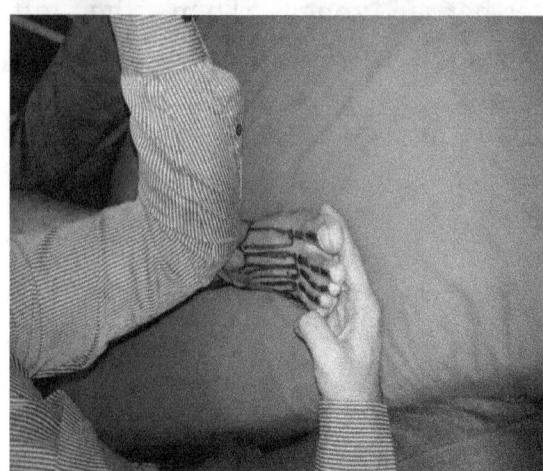

Figure 24: Spring test and mobilization of medial cuneiform from dorsal to plantar with olecranon of the elbow.

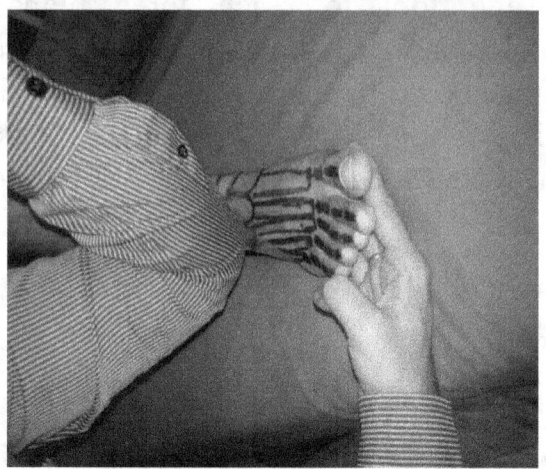

Figure 25: Spring test and mobilization of middle cuneiform from dorsal to plantar with olecranon of the elbow.

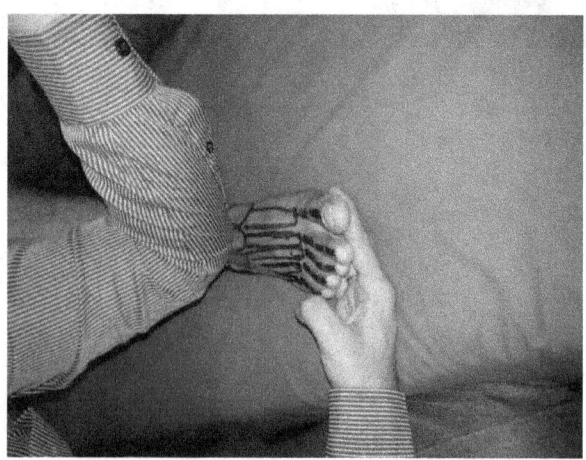

Figure 26: Spring test and mobilization of lateral cuneiform from dorsal to plantar with olecranon of the elbow.

## Treatment:

**Mobilization:** The patient and therapist's position for treatment is the same as the assessment position as explained above; after reaching the movement barrier zone in three planes, the left thumb/olecranon of the therapist is placed on the dorsal surface of respective cuneiforms and takes the plantar glide slack with 5kg force. And further plantar glides are done according to the grades of mobilization. 5 glides are given 3 times in one session. Each time, 5-sec rest is given.

**Taping:** to correct the right foot's adduction, inversion, and plantar flexion. The same steps are to be followed as mentioned in Figure 6 then additionally, to achieve and maintain internal rotation of the distal tibia, as shown in Figure 15, the therapist approaches from the right side of the patient; one end of the tape is pasted on the lower lateral surface of the tibia. Then, internal rotation slack is taken with the thumb/olecranon, and the other end of the tape is obliquely pasted over the calcaneum's medial and plantar surface. Cuneiforms automatically (based on the biomechanics) become more plantar in this taping. Therefore, the arch is decreased.

**Muscle energy technique:** As shown in Figure 21, the patient and therapist position for treatment is the same as the assessment position, as explained above. After reaching the movement barrier in three planes, the therapist's left thumb/olecranon is placed on the respective cuneiform, and plantar glide slack is taken with 5kg force. Then, the patient is asked to plantar-flex, and simultaneously, the therapist resists producing an isometric contraction. After 5 seconds of relaxation, a further new movement barrier in three-foot and cuneiform plantar glide planes is reached. Again, repeat the same 3 times per session.

**Sustained glide**:
**Position of the patient**: As shown in Figure 27a, the position of the patient is prone, the right foot is to be treated, and the knee is flexed to 30 degrees.
**Procedure**: The stand is placed below the cuneiform (a pillow can be placed under the stand to increase the height ). It is kept for about 2-5 min, according to the patient's tolerance and condition of the dysfunction. If required, weight should be added over the plantar surface of the foot to reinforce the plantar glide, as shown in Figure 27b.

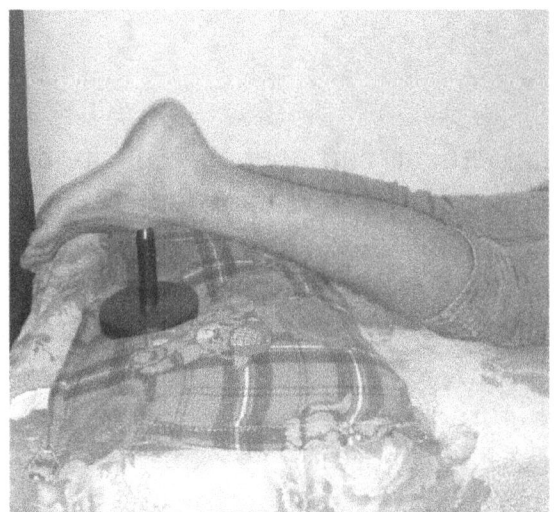
Figure 27a: Sustained plantar glide of cuneiform with the stand.

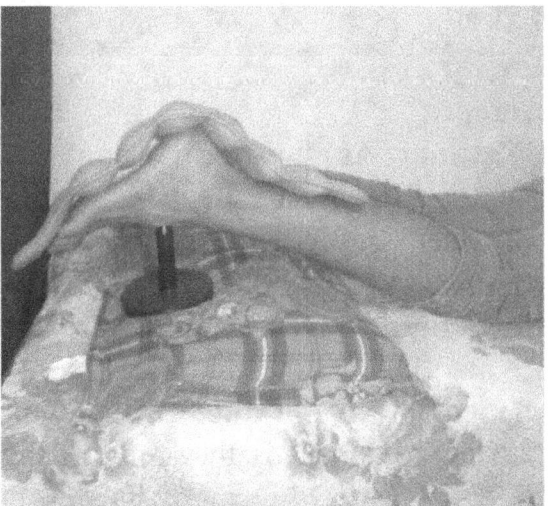
Figure 27b: Sustained plantar glide of cuneiform with the stand and weight is added.

### d) Cuboid – Internally rotated
**Spring test:**
**Position of the patient**: is supine, right foot to be treated, as shown in Figure 28.
**Position of the therapist and procedure:** therapist approaches the patient from the right side; the left hand of the therapist holds the forefoot, then abducts (coronal plane), everts (transverse plane), and dorsi-flexes (sagittal plane) to reach three planar inter barrier zone. Then, the right thumb/olecranon of the therapist is placed on the medial border of the cuboid, and the eversion slack is taken with 5kg of force. 3kg force is also applied to test the spring/end feel. If it does not, spring indicates dysfunction.

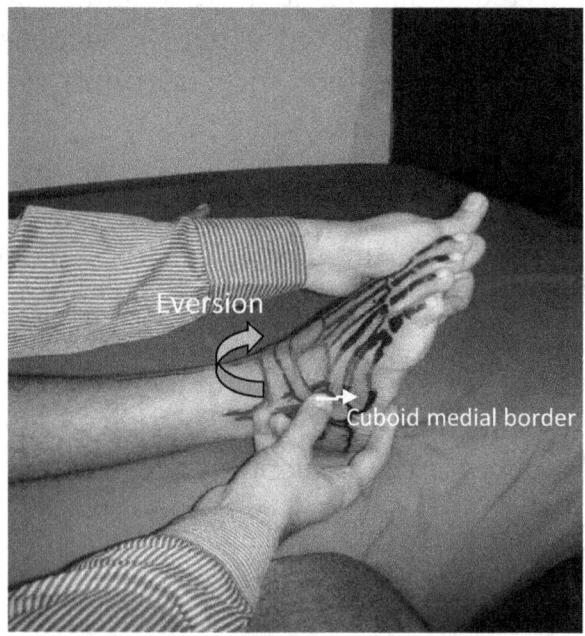

Figure 28: Spring test and mobilization of the cuboid into eversion.

### Treatment:
**Mobilization:** As shown in Figure 28, the patient and therapist position for treatment is the same as the assessment position as explained above after reaching the movement barrier in three planes; the right thumb/olecranon of the therapist is placed on the medial border of the dorsal cuboid, and eversion slack is taken with 5kg force. Further eversion glides are done according to the grades of mobilization. 5glides are given 3 times in one session. Each time, a 5-sec rest is given.

**Muscle energy technique:** As shown in Figure 28, the patient and therapist's position for treatment is the same as the assessment position as explained above; after reaching the movement barrier in three planes, simultaneously, the right thumb/olecranon of the therapist is placed on the medial border of the cuboid to take the eversion glide slack with 5kg force. Then, the patient is asked to plantar-flex, and simultaneously, the therapist resists producing an isometric contraction.

After 5 Sec of relaxation, a further new movement barrier in three planes of foot and cuboid eversion glide is reached. Again, repeat the same 3 times per session.

**Taping**: It has two parts. One part of taping to correct adduction, inversion, and plantar flexion is the same as already explained and shown in Figure 6, and another part of taping is to correct lower/distal tibial external rotation is same as already explained and shown in Figure 15. With these two parts of taping and based on the biomechanics of the foot, cuboid eversion takes place.

**Sustained glide:** The therapist can do it manually as it is a small bone.

As shown in Figure 28, the patient and therapist position for treatment is the same as the assessment position, as explained above. After reaching the movement barrier in three planes of the foot, the right thumb/olecranon of the therapist is placed on the medial border of the dorsal cuboid, and eversion slack is taken with 5kg force, and additionally, 3kg force is applied further to maintain the glide for 2-5min, according to patients tolerance and dysfunction.

### Orthotics: For supinated foot- plantar-flexed/ flexion lag with inverted and adducted foot[10]

Note: If initial dysfunction is not diagnosed early and treated, then the above dysfunction may end up as a supinated foot. If the initial stage of supinated foot sets in, a therapist can advise suitable orthotics for gradual correction along with manual therapy techniques. As we know from the kinetic chain of pathomechanics of the lower limb, if the supinated foot is not diagnosed early and treated, it will lead to gradual genu varum of the knee. That is, the patient walks with the lateral border of the foot. Therefore, for genu varum, correction of footwear would be a lateral raise, as shown in Figures F1 and F2. Lateral wedge can be ranged from $2^0$ to $6^0$

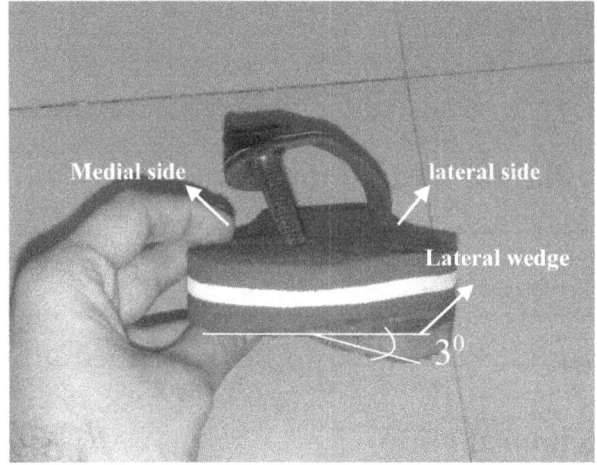

Figure F1: frontal view- Lateral raise of left foot wear with $3^0$ wedge.

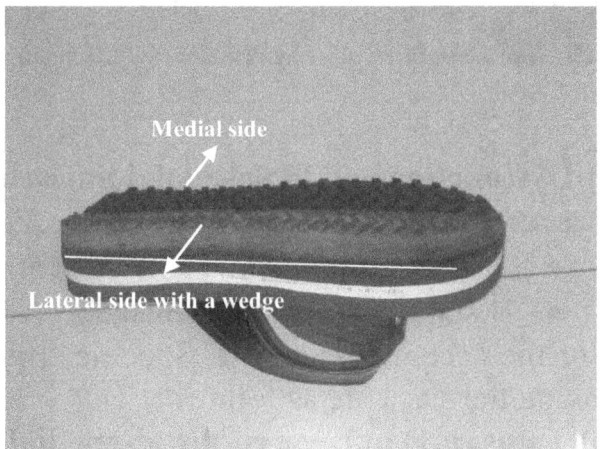

Figure F2: plantar view- Lateral raise of left foot wear with $3^0$ wedge.

**Progressive strengthening:** is advised according to the patient's condition.

## 2. Dysfunction: pronated foot- Plantar flexed/Dorsi-flexion lag with everted, abducted.

These dysfunctions are further divided into two parts: i) talo-crural/tibio-talar joint and ii) inter-tarsal joints.

Dysfunction: Plantar flexed/dorsi-flexion lag with everted and abducted foot (figure 29)

The foot is stuck in Extended (plantar flexed), Abducted and externally Rotated (everted).

The movement barrier: the foot cannot flex (dorsi-flex), Adduct, and internally rotate (invert).

The position of assessment and treatment is the same as the movement barrier:

**i) Tibio-talar joint: Talus medial and anterior
                     Distal tibia internally rotated**
**ii) Inter-tarsal joint: Calcaneum- everted, Navicular- everted, Cuneiform- plantar, cuboid- everted.**

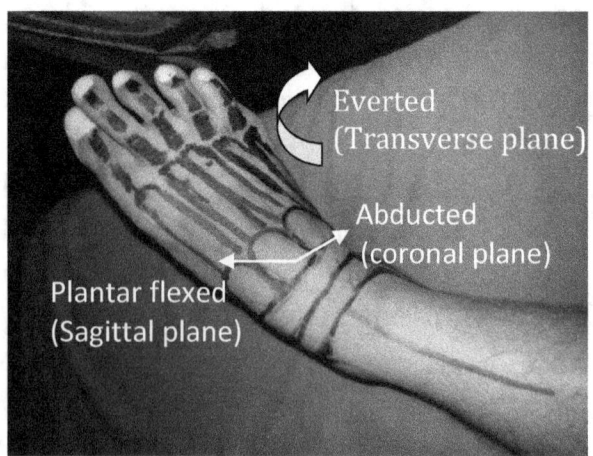

Figure 29: foot dysfunction- Dorsi flexion lag with everted and abducted.

**i) Dysfunctions of Tibio-talar joint are: (Plantar flexed/ dorsi-flexion lag with everted and abducted foot -figure 29)**
- Talus stuck in medial and anterior
- Distal tibia internally rotated.

For the accurate diagnosis, Specific spring glides that need to be performed after taking the slack are as follows

**a) Talus: a.1) uncovered/distal- medial to lateral glide
            a.2) proximal/covered- medial to a lateral glide**
**b) Talus- anterior to posterior glide**
**c) Distal tibia- external rotation glide**

### a) : a.1 Distal/Uncovered Talus: medial to a lateral glide

**Spring test:**

**Position of the patient:** in supine, as shown in Figures 30a and 30b, the patient's right leg is to be treated, hip is flexed, abducted, externally rotated, and knee flexed to $30^0$ to expose the medial side of the foot.

**Position of the therapist and procedure:** The therapist approaches from the right side of the patient. The right hand of the therapist holds the forefoot of the patient, then adducts (coronal plane), inverts (transverse plane), and dorsi-flexes (sagittal plane) to reach the movement barrier zone. The left thumb/olecranon is placed just below the medial malleolus, on the medial surface of the uncovered/distal talus, and takes the lateral slack with 5kg force, and 3kg force is applied to test the spring/end feel. If it does not, spring indicates dysfunction.

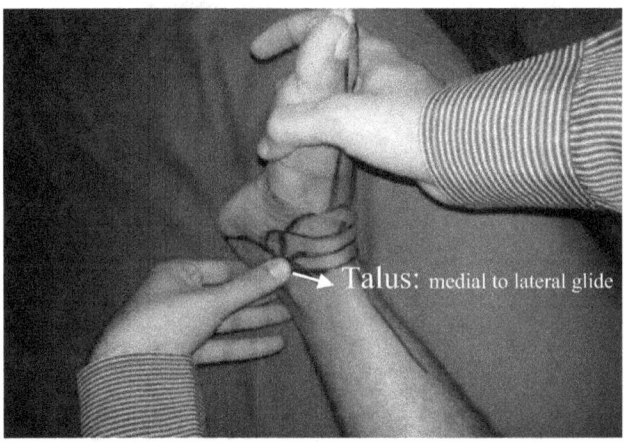

Figure 30a: Spring test and treatment of uncovered/distal talus from medial to lateral glide with the thumb.

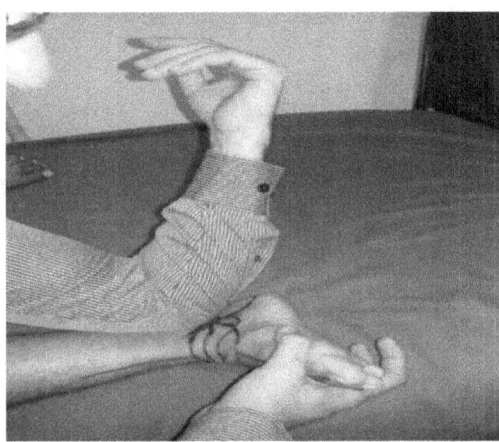

Figure 30b: Spring test and treatment of uncovered/distal talus from medial to lateral glide with the elbow.

### Treatment[4]:

**Mobilization:** As shown in Figures 30a and 30b, the patient and therapist position for treatment is the same as the assessment position as explained above, after taking up the slack with 5kg force; uncovered-talus lateral glide is done according to the grades of mobilization. 5 glides are given 3 times in one session. Each time 5sec rest is given.

**Muscle energy technique:** As shown in figures 30a and 30b, the patient and therapist position for treatment is the same as the assessment position as explained above. After taking up the uncovered/distal talus lateral glide slack with 5kg force, the patient is asked to plantar-flex, and simultaneously, the therapist resists producing an isometric contraction. After 5 Sec of relaxation, a further new movement barrier in three planes, that is, an inversion, adduction, and dorsi-flexion of the foot, is reached. Simultaneously, a new talus lateral glide barrier is reached. Again, repeat the same 3 times per session.

**Taping:**

**Position of the patient:** is supine and right leg to be treated. As shown in Figures 31a and 31b, taping is to correct abduction, eversion, and plantar flexion of the foot so that the talus automatically glides laterally.

**The position of the therapist and procedure:** one end of the tape is pasted over the dorsal surface of the cuboid and base of the 4$^{th}$, and 5$^{th}$ metatarsal, then the foot is adducted (coronal plane), inverted (transverse plane), and dorsi-flexed (sagittal plane) and another end of the tape comes over the dorsum of the foot and is pasted at the lower end of the lateral fibular styloid.

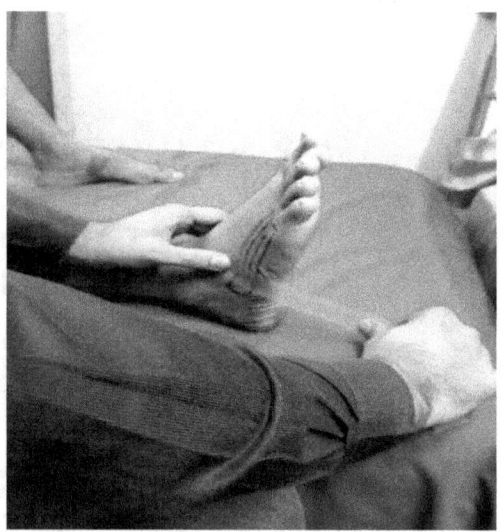

Figure 31a: Taping to correct foot abduction, eversion and Dorsi flexion- Starting part

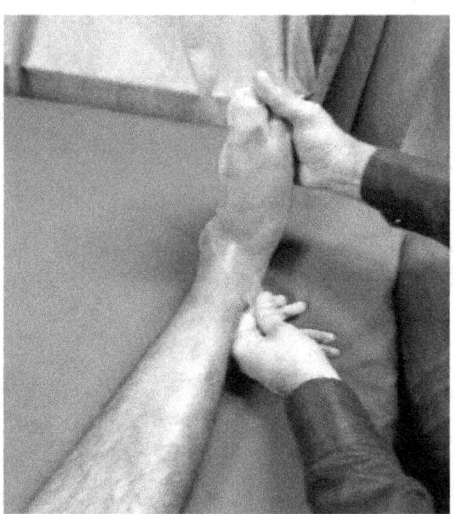

Figure 31b: Taping to correct foot abduction, eversion and dorsi flexion- Ending part

**The sustained glide of talus from medial to lateral:**

As shown in figure 32, with the correction tape on, the patient should be on the left side, with the left leg hip and knee flexing about 30 degrees. The right leg to be treated is 90 degrees flexed at the hip and knee. The talus-stand with the pointed edge is placed on the medial surface of the distal/uncovered-talus in order to apply the medial to lateral glide. The pillow can be placed under the stand to increase the height. Sometimes, weight can be added to the lateral surface of the foot to increase lateral glide force, according to dysfunction and the patient's tolerance. Slow and sustained glide is kept for 2 to 5 min.

# Chapter 14: Ankle and Foot – Biomechanics, Pathomechanics and Treatment

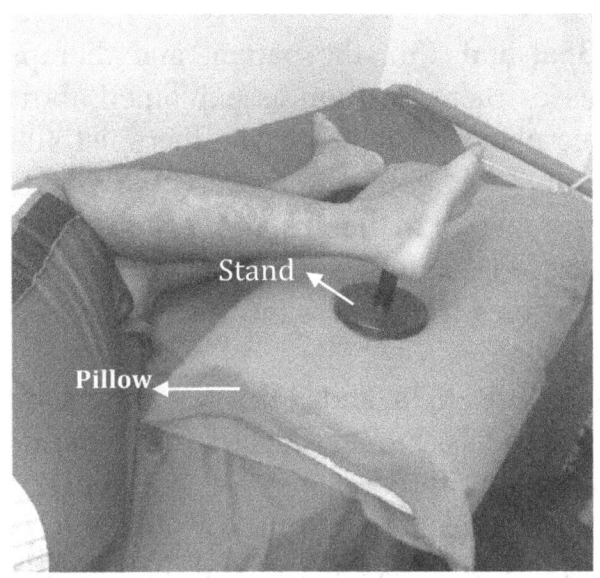

Figure 32: sustained glide of uncovered talus from medial to lateral glide.

### a) : a.2 Proximal/Covered Talus: Medial to lateral glides
**Spring test:**
**The position of the patient:** is supine, as shown in figures 33a, 33b, patient's right leg is to be treated, the hip is flexed, externally rotated, abducted, and the knee is flexed to $30^0$ to expose the medial side of the foot.

**Position of the therapist and procedure:** The therapist approaches from the right side of the patient. The right hand of the therapist holds the forefoot of the patient, adducts (coronal plane), inverts (transverse plane), and dorsi-flexes (sagittal plane) to reach the movement-barrier zone. Then, the therapist's left thumb/olecranon is placed on the medial malleolus/tibial styloid to reach the medial surface of the proximal talus and take the lateral slack with 5kg force and additionally, 3kg force is applied to test the spring. If it does not, spring indicates dysfunction.

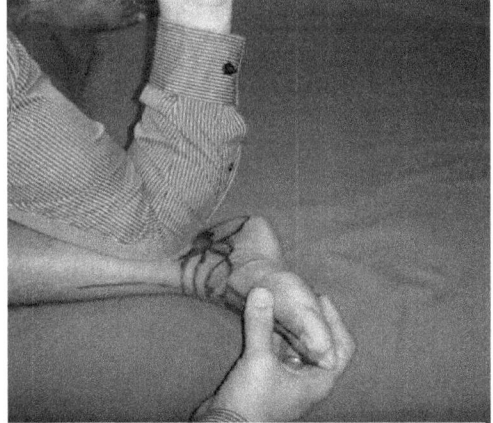

Figure 33a: Proximal/Covered talus medial to lateral glide spring test and treatment with olecranon through tibial styloid.

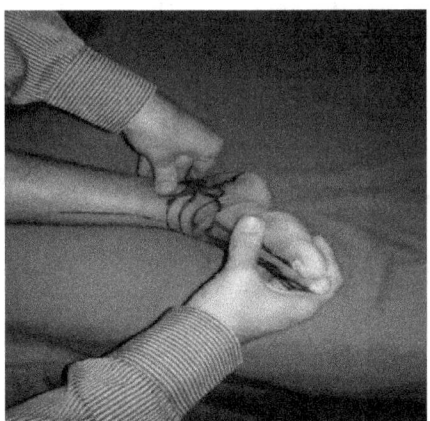

Figure 33b: Proximal/Covered talus medial to lateral glide with thumb through tibial styloid.

**Treatment:**
**Mobilization:** As shown in the figures 33a, and 33b, the patient and therapist position for treatment is the same as the assessment position as explained above; after reaching the movement barrier in three planes of the foot, the therapist's left thumb/olecranon is placed on the medial malleolus to reach the medial proximal/covered surface of the talus through medial malleolus and take the lateral glide slack with 5kg force. And lateral glides of the talus are done according to the grades of mobilization. 5 glides are given 3 times in one session. Each time 5-sec rest is given.

**Muscle energy technique**: As shown in figures 33a and 33b, the patient and therapist position for treatment is the same as the assessment position as explained above. After reaching the movement barrier in three planes of the foot, the therapist's left hand of the thumb/olecranon is placed on the medial malleolus to take the lateral glide slack of the proximal talus with 5kg force, and the patient is asked to plantar-flex, and simultaneously, therapist resists producing an isometric contraction. After 5 sec of relaxation, further new movement barrier in three planes of the foot is reached, and proximal/covered talus new lateral glide slack is taken. Again, repeat the same 3 times per session.

**Taping**: It has two parts. The position of the patient is supine; the therapist approaches from the right side.

Part one: As shown in Figures 31a and 31b, taping to correct abduction, eversion, and plantar flexion. One end of the tape is pasted over the dorsal surface of the cuboid and base of the 4th and 5th metatarsal, and then the foot is adducted (coronal plane), inverted (transverse plane), and dorsi-flexed (sagittal plane). And the other end of the tape comes over the dorsum of the foot and is pasted at the lower end of the lateral fibular styloid.

Part two: as shown in figure 34, distal tibia internal rotation to external rotation correction. One end of the tape is pasted on the lower medial surface of the tibia, and the external rotation glide barrier is reached with the thumb of therapist. Then further external rotation slack with 5kg force is taken, and the other end of the tape is pasted obliquely below the lateral malleolus of the foot.

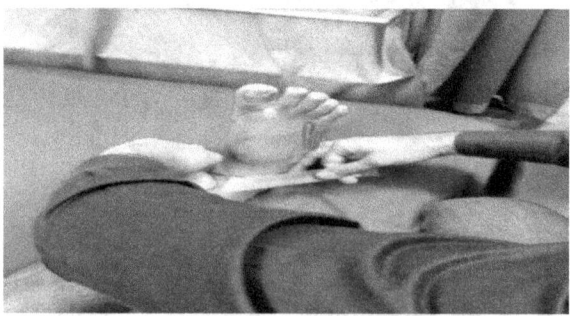

Figure 34: taping of the distal tibia from internal rotation to external rotation.

With above mentioned two parts of the taping, the talus can be laterally shifted.

**Sustained glide**: with the correction tape on, as mentioned above, the sustained lateral glide of covered-talus is employed with a special stand as shown in Figures 35a and 35b.

**The position of the patient and procedure:** The patient should be on the side-lying, the right leg to be treated, right hip and knee should be flexed to 90 degrees. The stand with a pointed rectangular projection is placed on the medial malleolus in order to glide proximal/covered talus from medial to lateral (figure 35a). Sometimes weight can be added to increase the glide according to dysfunction and the patient's tolerance, as shown in figure 35b.

Description of stand: a rectangular base (15 cm X 39 cm) and a rectangular projection (6cm x 25cm), and both have a thickness of about 1.5 cm.

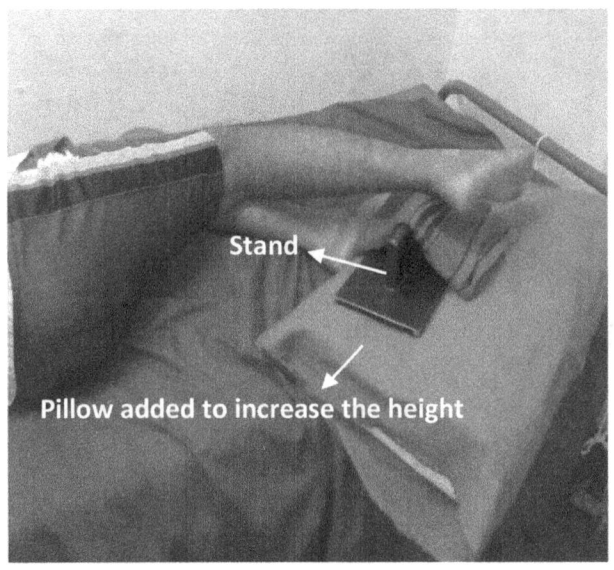

Figure 35a: Sustained lateral glide of proximal/covered-talus) on the stand through tibial styloid.

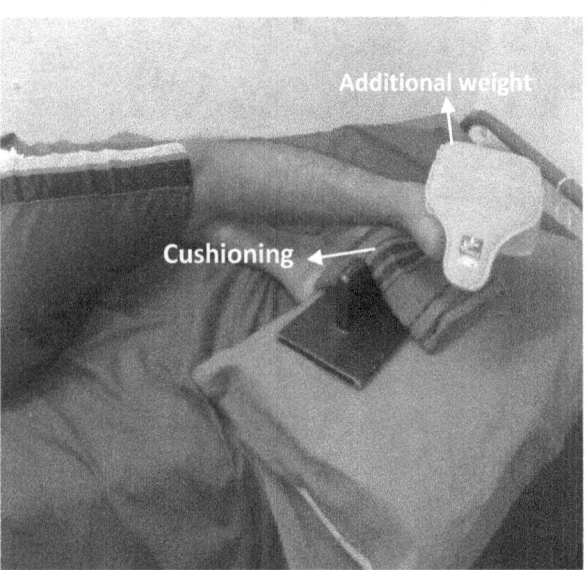

Figure 35b: Sustained lateral glide of proximal/covered-talus on the stand through tibial styloid. If required additional weight can be added.

**b) Talus- anterior:**

**Spring test:**

**The position of the patient:** is in supine, patient's right foot to be treated.

**The position of the therapist and procedure:** therapist approaches from the right side of the patient, as shown in figure 36. The therapist holds the forefoot of the patient with the right hand, then adducted (coronal plane), inverted (transverse plane), and dorsi-flexed (sagittal plane) to reach three planar movement-barrier zones. Then therapist's left thumb is placed on the anterior surface of the talus at the ankle mortise and takes the posterior slack with 5kg force, and additionally, 3kg force is applied to test the spring/end feel. If it does not, spring indicates dysfunction.

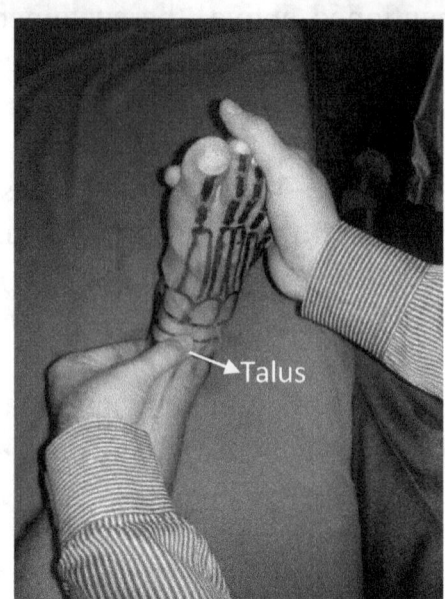

Figure 36: spring test and treatment- talus anterior to posterior glide with the thumb.

**Treatment:**

**Mobilization:** As shown in Figure 36, the patient and therapist's position for treatment is the same as the assessment position as explained above. After taking up the talus slack into the posterior glide with 5kg force, posterior glides are done according to the grades of mobilization. 5 glides are given 3 times in one session. Each time 5-sec rest is given.

**Muscle energy technique**: As shown in figure 36, the patient and therapist position for treatment is the same as the assessment position as explained above. After taking up the talus posterior glide slack with 5kg force, the patient is asked to plantar-flex, and simultaneously, the therapist resists producing an isometric contraction. After 5 sec of relaxation, a further new movement barrier in three planes is an inversion, adduction, and dorsi-flexion of foot reached, and the talus's further posterior glide barrier is reached. Again, repeat the same 3 times per session.

**Taping:** It has two parts. The position of the patient is supine, and the therapist approaches from the right side of the patient. The right foot is to be treated.
<u>Part one:</u> as shown in figures 31a and 31b, taping to correct abduction, eversion, and plantar flexion, one end of the tape is pasted over the dorsal surface of the cuboid and base of the 4$^{th}$, 5th metatarsal, then the foot is adducted (coronal plane), inverted (transverse plane) and dorsi-flexed (sagittal plane). Then, the other end of

the tape is wrapped from the plantar surface over the dorsum of the foot and is pasted at the lower end of the lateral fibular styloid.

Part two: distal tibia internal rotation to external rotation.

One end of the tape is pasted on the distal medial surface of the tibia, and the external rotation glide barrier is reached; then, further external rotation slack with 5kg force is taken. The other end of the tape is pasted obliquely below the lateral malleolus of the foot, as shown in figure 34.

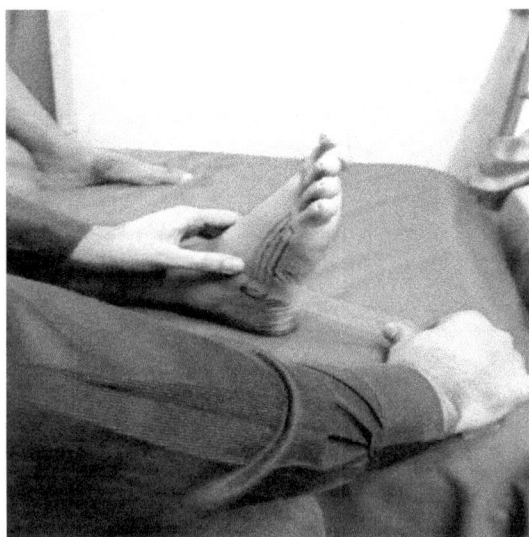

Figure 31a: Taping to correct foot abduction, eversion and dorsi flexion - Initial one end of the tape.

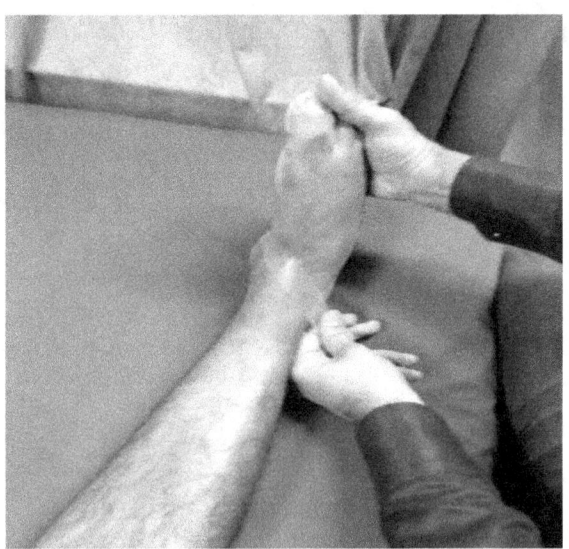

Figure 31b: Taping to correct foot abduction, eversion and dorsi flexion -Terminal end of the tape.

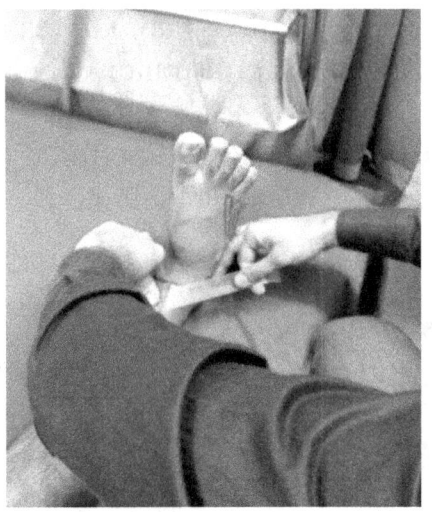

Figure 34: Taping of the distal tibia from internal rotation to external rotation.

## Sustained glide:

**Position of the patient:** With the correction tape on, as mentioned above, the Position of the patient is prone, and the right foot is to be treated.

**Procedure**: As shown in Figure 37a, the knee is flexed to 30 degrees. The foot is plantar-flexed, and the stand is placed below the anterior surface of the talus surface. Weight can be added over the posterior surface of the heel to further reinforce the posterior glide, as shown in figure 37b. It should be kept for about 2-5min according to the patient's tolerance and condition of the dysfunction.

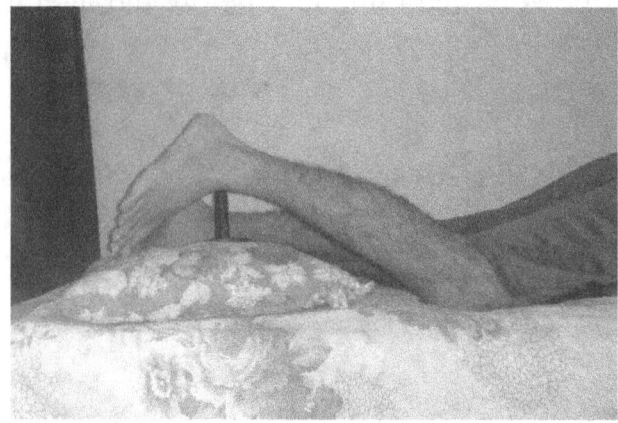
Figure 37a: Sustained posterior glide of talus with talus stand.

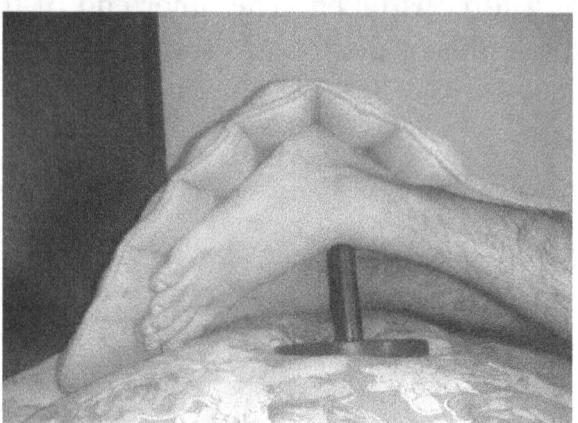
Figure 37b: Sustained posterior glide of the talus with talus stand and additional weight can be added to reinforce the glide.

### c). Distal tibia – Internally rotated
**Spring test:**
**The position of the patient** is supine, as shown in Figures 38a and 38b. The right foot is to be treated.
**Position of the therapist and procedure:** The therapist approaches from the right side of the patient. The right hand of the therapist holds the forefoot and adducts (coronal plane), inverts (transverse plane), and dorsi-flexes (sagittal plane) to reach the movement barrier zone. Then, the left thumb (figure 38a)/olecranon (figure 38b) is placed on the lower medial surface of the tibia. Then, the distal tibia external rotation slack is taken with 5kg force, and additionally, 3kg force is applied to test the spring/end feel. If it does not, spring indicates dysfunction.

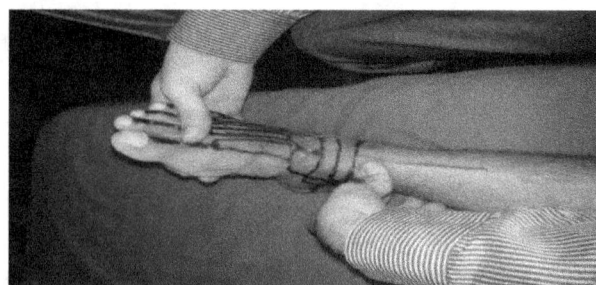
Figure 38a: Distal tibia- external rotation spring test and treatment with the thumb.

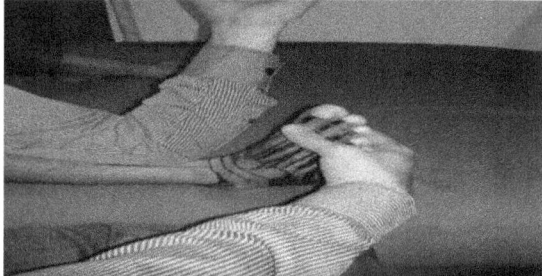
Figure 38b: distal tibia- external rotation spring test and treatment with olecranon.

# Chapter 14: Ankle and Foot – Biomechanics, Pathomechanics and Treatment

**Treatment:**

**Mobilization:** As shown in Figures 38a and 38b, the patient's position for treatment is the same as the assessment position, as explained above. After reaching the movement barrier in three planes, the therapist's left thumb/olecranon is placed on the lower medial surface of the tibia and takes the external rotation slack with 5kg force. Then, further distal tibia external rotational glides are applied according to the grades of mobilization. 5 glides are given 3 times in one session. Each time 5-sec rest is given.

**Muscle energy technique:** As shown in Figures 38a and 38b, the position of the patient for treatment is the same as the assessment position as explained above. After reaching the movement barrier in three planes, as mentioned above, simultaneously, the therapist's left thumb/olecranon is placed on the lower medial surface of the tibia and takes the external rotation slack with 5kg force. Then the patient is asked to plantar-flex, and simultaneously, the therapist resists (5 grams force; unidirectional/uniplanar resistance; 6 seconds resistance), producing an isometric contraction. Followed by 5 sec of relaxation, further new movement barrier in three planes, that is, an inversion, adduction, and dorsiflexion of the foot is reached, and distal tibia external rotation new glide barrier is reached. Again, repeat the same 3 times per session. Each time, 5sec rest is given.

**Taping:** It has two parts.
<u>Part one:</u> As shown in figures 31a and 31b, taping to correct abduction, eversion, and plantar flexion, one end of the tape is pasted over the dorsal surface of the cuboid and base of the $4^{th}$, 5th metatarsal, then the foot is adducted (coronal plane), inverted (transverse plane) and dorsiflexed (sagittal plane) and another end of the tape is wrapped from the plantar surface to over the dorsum of the foot, and the terminal end of the tape is pasted at the lower end of the lateral fibular styloid.
<u>Part two:</u> distal tibia internal rotation to external rotation
One end of the tape is pasted on the lower medial surface of the tibia, and an external rotation glide barrier is reached. Then further external rotation slack with 5kg force is taken, and the other end of the tape is obliquely pasted, as shown in figure 34, below the lateral malleolus of the foot.

ii) **Inter-tarsal joint: Calcaneum- everted, Navicular- everted, Cuneiform- plantar, cuboid- everted.**

**Dysfunction/pronated foot: Plantar flexed/dorsi-flexion lag with everted and abducted foot.**

Spring test and treatment of Inter-tarsal dysfunctions: **a) Calcaneum- everted, b) Navicular- everted, c) Cuneiform- plantar, d) cuboid- everted**

**a) Calcaneum- everted**
**Spring test:**
**Position of the patient:** in side-lying, right foot to be examined, right hip and knee of the patient is flexed about $45^0$.
**Position of the therapist:** approaches patient from the left side, as shown in figure 39, the left hand of the therapist holds the forefoot of the patient, and a log wrapped with pink crepe bandage is placed obliquely under the calcaneum lateral surface. Then the foot is adducted (coronal plane), inverted (transverse plane), and dorsi-flexed (sagittal plane) to reach the movement-barrier zone. The right thumb/olecranon of the therapist is placed on the medial surface of calcaneum just below the medial surface of the talus, then inversion slack is taken with 5kg force, and additionally, 3kg force is applied to test the spring/end feel. If it does not, spring indicates dysfunction.

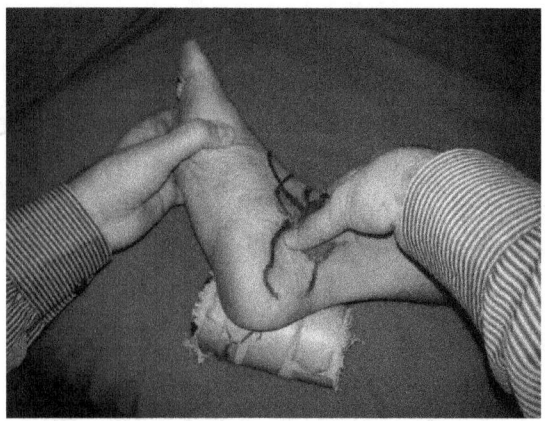

Figure 39: Spring test and treatment of everted calcaneum with thumb.

**Treatment:**
**Mobilization:** As shown in figure 39, the patient position for treatment is the same as the assessment position as explained above; after reaching the movement barrier in three planes, the right thumb/olecranon of the therapist is placed on the lower medial surface of the calcaneum just below the medial surface of the talus. Then calcaneum inversion slack is taken with 5kg force, and additionally, inversion glides of calcaneum are given according to the grades of mobilisation. 5 glides are given 3 times in one session. Each time 5sec rest is given.

**Muscle energy technique**: As shown in figure 39, the patient position for treatment is the same as the assessment position as explained above. After reaching the movement barrier in three planes, simultaneously, the therapist's left thumb/olecranon is placed on the lower medial surface of the calcaneum just below the medial surface of the talus and takes the inversion slack with 5kg force. Then the patient is asked to plantar-flex, and simultaneously therapist resists (5 grams force; unidirectional/uniplanar resistance; 6 seconds resistance.), producing an isometric contraction. Followed by 5 sec of relaxation, then further movement barrier in three planes, that is, an inversion, adduction, and dorsi-flexion of the foot is reached, and further calcaneum inversion glide barrier is reached. Again, repeat the same 3 times per session. Each time 5sec rest is given.

**Taping:** It has three parts

Part one: as shown in figure 31a and 31b, to correct abduction, eversion, and plantar flexion of foot-one end of the tape is pasted on the dorsal surface of cuboid and lateral cuneiform, then the foot is adducted (coronal plane), inverted (transverse plane) and dorsi-flexed (sagittal plane) to reach three planar inter movement barrier zone. And additionally, the left hand of the thumb/olecranon of the therapist is placed on the medial surface of the calcaneum just below the medial surface of the talus and takes the inversion slack with 5kg force. Then the other end of the tape comes over from the plantar surface to the dorsum of the foot and is pasted at the lower end of the lateral fibular styloid.

Part two: As shown in Figures 40a and 40b, to correct calcaneum eversion- one end of the tape is pasted on the dorsal lateral surface of the calcaneum, and, as mentioned above, three planar inter barrier zone is reached. Then calcaneum inversion slack with 5kg force is taken as mentioned above, and the other end of the tape is pasted on the medial dorsal surface of the medial cuneiform.

Part three: Correction of distal tibia internal rotation; one end of the tape is pasted on the lower medial surface of the tibia, and distal tibia external rotation glide movement barrier is reached. External rotation slack with 5kg force is taken, and a further 3kg force is applied. Then the other end of the tape is pasted obliquely below the lateral malleolus of the foot, as shown in figure 34.

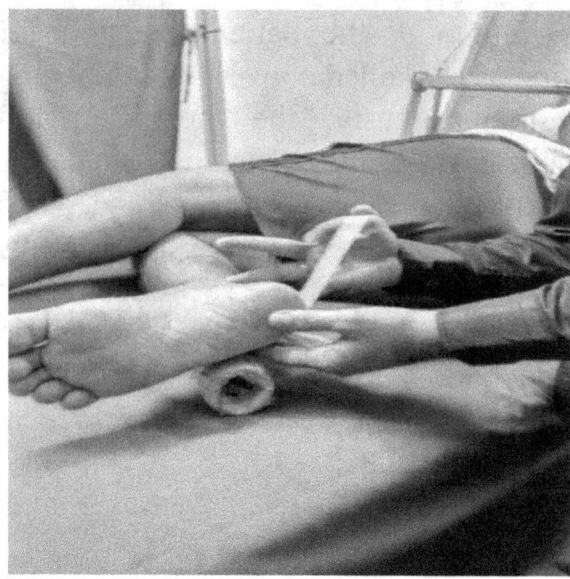

Figure 40a: calcaneum inversion taping. The initial end of the tape.

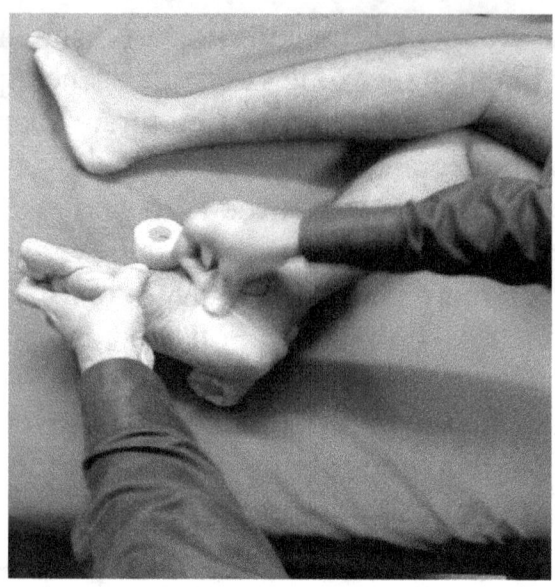

Figure 40b: calcaneum inversion taping. Another end of the tape.

**Sustained glide:**

**Position of the patient:** As shown in figure 41, the right foot is to be treated, the patient is on the left side-lying, right hip and knee are flexed about 45 degrees.

**Procedure:** pointed edge of the talus stand is placed on the medial surface of the calcaneum just below the medial surface of the talus. According to patient tolerance, weight can be added over the lateral surface of the foot to reinforce the calcaneum inversion. It can be kept for about 2-5min according to the patient's tolerance and condition of dysfunction.

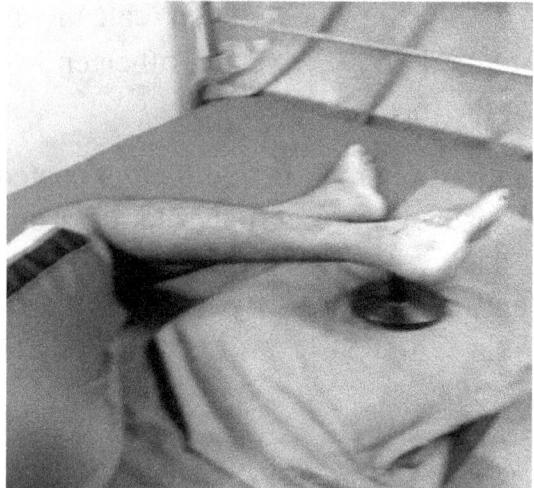

Figure 41: Sustained inversion glide of calcaneum with stand.

## b) Navicular- everted:

### Spring test:

**The position of the patient:** is on the right side-lying, right foot to be assessed and right hip is flexed, externally rotated and abducted about 30 degrees, and the knee is also flexed to $30^0$, as shown in figure 42.

**Position of the therapist and procedure:** The therapist approaches from the right side of the patient; the right hand of the therapist holds the forefoot, then adducts (coronal plane), inverts (transverse plane), and dorsi-flexes (sagittal plane) to reach an inter movement-barrier zone in three planes. Simultaneously, the left thumb/olecranon of the therapist is placed below the navicular tuberosity, and inversion slack is taken with 5kg force, and additionally, 3kg force is applied to test the spring/end feel. If it does not, spring indicates dysfunction.

Figure 42: Spring test and navicular inversion glide with the thumb.

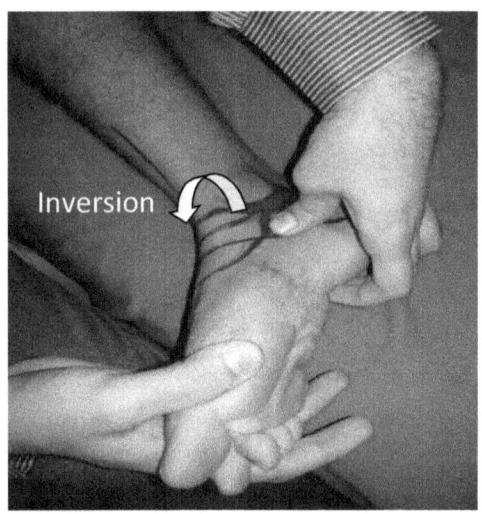

### Treatment:

**Mobilization:** as shown in figure 42, the patient position for treatment is the same as the assessment position as explained above. After reaching the movement barrier in three planes, the left thumb/olecranon of the therapist is placed below the navicular tuberosity, then the navicular inversion slack is taken with 5kg force, and additionally, further inversion glides are applied according to the grades of mobilisation. 5 glides are given 3 times in one session. Each time 5sec rest is given.

**Muscle energy technique:** as shown in figure 42, the position of the patient is the same as the assessment position as explained above. After reaching the movement barrier in three planes, simultaneously, the left thumb/olecranon of the therapist is placed below the navicular tuberosity, and then inversion slack is taken with 5kg force. Then the patient is asked to plantar-flex, and simultaneously therapist resists (5 grams force; unidirectional/uniplanar resistance; 6 seconds resistance.), producing an isometric contraction. Followed by 5 sec of relaxation, a further new movement barrier in three planes that is an inversion, adduction, and dorsiflexion of the foot is reached and a navicular new inversion glide barrier is reached. Again, repeat the same 3 times per session. Each time 5sec rest is given.

**Taping:** It has two parts

Part one: as shown in figures 31a and 31b, to correct abduction, eversion, and plantar flexion of the foot- one end of the tape is pasted on the dorsal surface of the cuboid and lateral cuneiform, and then the foot is adducted (coronal plane), inverted (transverse plane) and dorsi-flexed (sagittal plane) and the other end of the tape comes over from the plantar surface to the dorsum of the foot and is pasted at the lower end of the fibular styloid.

Part two: distal tibia external rotation taping

As shown in figure 34, one end of the tape is pasted on the lower medial surface of the tibia, and an external rotation glide barrier is reached. The further external rotation slack is taken with 5kg force, and the other end of the tape is pasted obliquely below the lateral malleolus of the foot.

**Sustained glide:** The therapist can give sustained glide as it is a small bone.

As shown in figure 42, the patient position for treatment is the same as the assessment position as explained above. After reaching the movement barrier in three planes, the left thumb/olecranon of the therapist is placed below the navicular tuberosity. Then the navicular inversion slack is taken with 5kg force, and additionally, further inversion glide is applied with 3kg force. It can be maintained for about 2-5min according to the patient's tolerance and condition of dysfunction.

## c) Cuneiform- plantar:
### Spring test:
**Position of the patient**: is on right side-lying and right foot to be treated. The patient's right hip and knee flexed about $45^0$, as shown in figure 43a.

**Position of the therapist and procedure:** The therapist approaches the patient from the patient's left side. The left hand of the therapist holds the forefoot. The foot is adducted (coronal plane), inverted (transverse plane), and dorsi-flexed (sagittal plane) to reach the inter barrier zone, and simultaneously, the right thumb of the therapist (figure 43a)/projected part of the talus stand (figure 43b) is placed on the plantar surface of the medial cuneiform. Then dorsal slack is taken with 5kg force, and additionally, 3kg force is applied to test the spring/end feel. If it does not, spring indicates dysfunction.

Same way, middle and lateral cuneiform spring tests are followed.

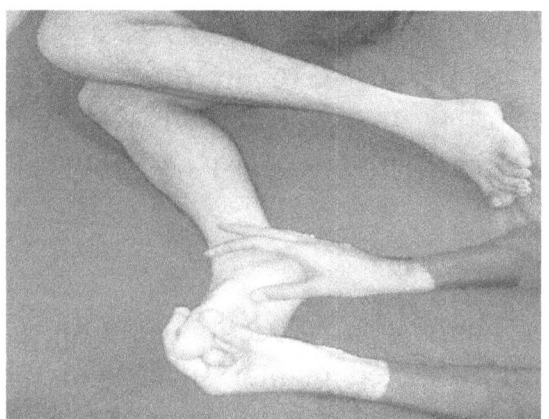

Figure 43a: Spring test and treatment of cuneiform- plantar to dorsal glide with the thumb.

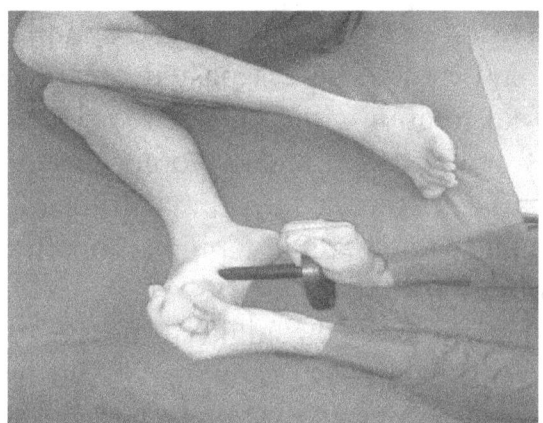

Figure 43b: Spring test and treatment of cuneiform- plantar to dorsal glide with projected part of the stand.

### Treatment:
**Mobilization:** The position of the patient is the same as the assessment position as explained above; after reaching the movement barrier in three planes, the right thumb of the therapist (figure 43a)/with the pointed edge of the talus stand (figure 43b) is placed on the respective plantar surface of cuneiform and take the dorsal slack with 5kg force. Further dorsal glides are done according to the grades of mobilization. 5 glides are given 3 times in one session. Each time 5sec rest is given.

**Muscle energy technique**: as shown in figure 43a, the position for treatment is the same as the assessment position as explained above; after reaching the movement barrier in three planes, simultaneously, the left hand of the thumb/olecranon of the therapist is placed on the respective plantar surface of cuneiform, and dorsal slack is taken with 5kg force. Then the patient is asked to plantar-flex, and simultaneously therapist resists (5 grams force; unidirectional/uniplanar resistance; 6 seconds resistance.), producing an isometric contraction. Followed by 5 sec of relaxation, further new movement barrier in three planes, which is an inversion, adduction, and dorsi-flexion of the foot, is reached, and respective cuneiform dorsal new glide barrier is reached. Again, repeat the same 3 times per session. Each time 5sec rest is given.

**Taping:** It has two parts

Part one: as shown in Figures 31a and 31b, taping to correct abduction, eversion, and plantar flexion. One end of the tape is pasted over the dorsal surface of the cuboid and base of the $4^{th}$, and 5th metatarsal, and then the foot is adducted (coronal plane), inverted (transverse plane), and dorsi-flexed (sagittal plane). The other end of the tape is wrapped from the plantar surface to reach over the dorsum of the foot and is pasted at the lower end of the lateral fibular styloid.

Part two: distal tibia internal rotation to external rotation
One end of the tape is pasted on the lower medial surface of the tibia, and an external rotation glide barrier is reached. Then further external rotation slack with 5kg force is taken, and the other end of the tape is obliquely pasted, as shown in figure 34, below the lateral malleolus of the foot.

With these two parts of taping automatically, cuneiforms become dorsal.

**Sustained glide:**

The patient is in the high sitting position in a chair with correction tape on, as shown in figure 44, right leg to be treated, the affected plantar surface of the cuneiform is placed on the projected part of the stand, and slowly about 5kg body weight force is shifted to glide the affected cuneiform into dorsal. Sustained glide is maintained for about 2-5min according to the patient's condition and tolerance.

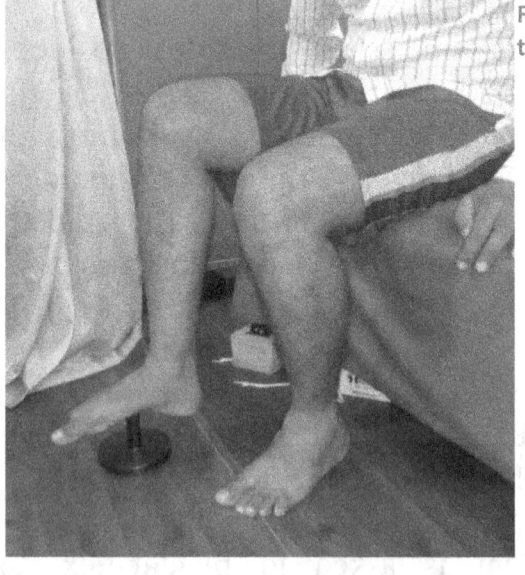

Figure 44: Sustained glide of cuneiform from plantar to dorsal.

## d) Cuboid- externally rotated

**Spring test:**

**The position of the patient:** is supine, right leg to be treated.

**Position of the therapist and procedure:** as shown in figure 45, the therapist's left hand holds the forefoot. Then the foot is adducted (coronal plane), inverted (transverse plane), and dorsi-flexed (sagittal plane) to reach an inter movement-barrier zone. Simultaneously, the right thumb/olecranon of the therapist is placed on the lateral border of the cuboid to take the inversion slack with 5kg force, and additionally, 3 kg force is applied to test the spring/end feel. If it does not, spring indicates dysfunction.

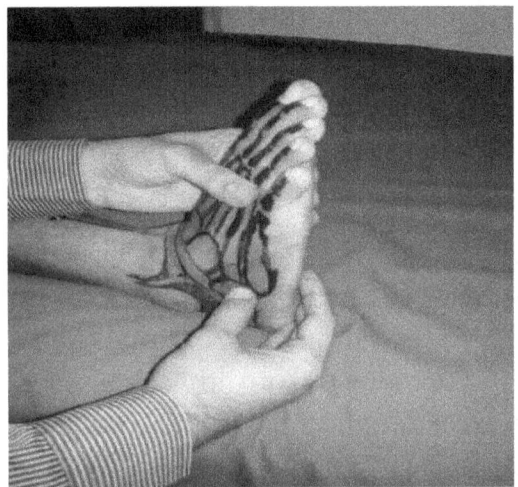

Figure 45: Spring test and treatment- cuboid inversion glide with the thumb.

**Treatment:**

**Mobilization:** As shown in figure 45, the patient position for treatment is the same as the assessment position as explained above; the therapist's left hand holds the forefoot. Then the foot is adducted (coronal plane), inverted (transverse plane), and dorsi-flexed (sagittal plane) to reach an inter movement-barrier zone. Simultaneously, the right hand of the thumb/olecranon of the therapist is placed on the lateral border of the cuboid to take the inversion slack with 5kg force. And further inversion glides of a cuboid are done according to the grades of mobilization. 3 glides are given 3 times in one session. Each time 5sec rest is given.

**Muscle energy technique:** As shown in figure 45, the position of the patient is the same as the assessment position as explained above. After reaching the movement barrier in three planes, the therapist's left thumb/olecranon is placed on the lateral border of the cuboid to take the inversion slack with 5kg force. Then the patient is asked to plantar-flex, and simultaneously therapist resists (5 grams force;

unidirectional/uniplanar resistance; 6 seconds resistance.), producing an isometric contraction. Followed by 5 sec of relaxation, a further new movement barrier in three planes, which is an inversion, adduction, and dorsi- flexion of the foot, is reached, and a further new cuboid inversion glide barrier is reached. Again, repeat the same 3 times.

**Sustained glide:** As it is a small bone, the therapist can give sustained glide. As shown in figure 45, the patient position for treatment is the same as the assessment position explained above. After reaching the movement barrier in three planes, the right thumb/olecranon of the therapist is placed on the lateral border of the cuboid to take the inversion slack with 5kg force, and additionally, 3kg force is applied. Sustained cuboid inversion glide is maintained for about 2-5min according to the patient's tolerance and condition of dysfunction.

**Taping:** It has two parts
<u>Part one:</u> as shown in figures 31a and 31b, taping to correct abduction, eversion, and plantar flexion, one end of the tape is pasted over the dorsal surface of the cuboid and base of the 4$^{th}$, 5th metatarsal, then the foot is adducted (coronal plane), inverted (transverse plane) and dorsi-flexed (sagittal plane). The other end of the tape is wrapped from the plantar surface to reach over the dorsum of the foot and is pasted at the lower end of the lateral fibular styloid.
<u>Part two:</u> distal tibia internal rotation to external rotation
One end of the tape is pasted on the lower medial surface of the tibia, and an external rotation glide barrier is reached. Then further external rotation slack with 5kg force is taken, and the other end of the tape is obliquely pasted, as shown in figure 34, below the lateral malleolus of the foot.These two parts of taping will invert the cuboid.

**Orthotics: for pronated foot- plantar-flexed/dorsi-flexion lag with everted and abducted.**
Note: if initial dysfunction is not diagnosed early and treated, the above dysfunction may end up as a pronated foot. If the initial stage of pronated foot sets in, the therapist can advise suitable orthotics for gradual correction along with manual therapy techniques. As we know from pathomechanics of the lower limb kinetic chain, a pronated foot, if not diagnosed early and treated, will lead to the gradual valgus knee. That is, the patient walks with the medial border of the foot[7, 8]. Therefore, for the valgus knee, footwear correction would be medial raise, and as we also know, in the pronated foot, the arch of the foot decreases. Therefore,

medial arch support can be added along with medial raise[8], as shown in Figures F3 and F4. Medial wedge can range from 2°-6°

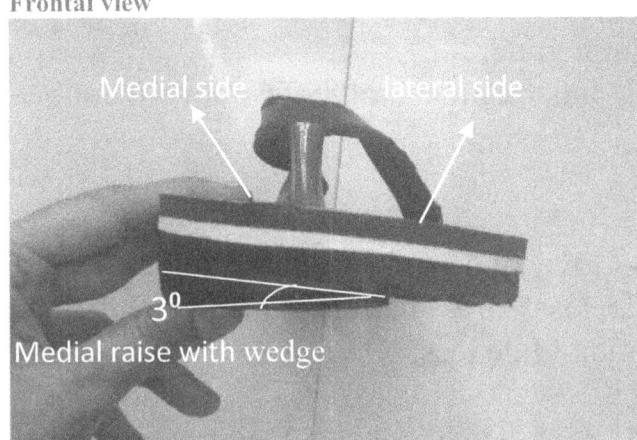

Figure F3: Medial raise of left footwear with 3° wedge. Frontal view

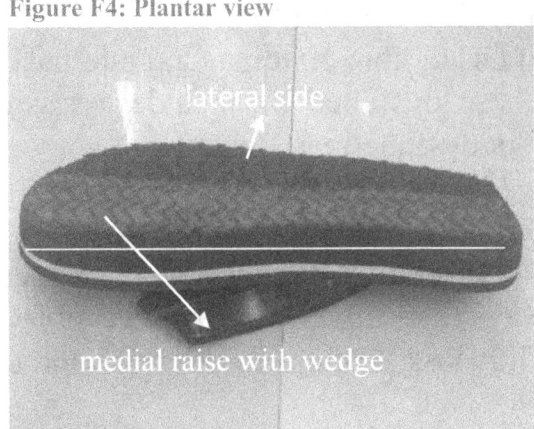

Figure F4: Plantar view

**Progressive strengthening:** is advised according to patient condition and tolerance

## 3. Dysfunction: Plantar flexed/ dorsi-flexion lag with both inversion and adduction plus eversion and abduction loss:

According to the biomechanics of the foot, inversion always goes with adduction; eversion always goes with abduction, as they are coupled movements. As in this dysfunction, both inversion and eversion are restricted. Therefore, there will be adduction and abduction loss, respectively.

**Spring test and treatment:**
Dysfunction: Plantar flexed/dorsi-flexion lag with loss of eversion, abduction and inversion, adduction of the foot:

i) **Tibio-talar joint:** talus posterior glide loss and medial to lateral as well as lateral to medial glide loss
   Distal tibia internal and external rotation loss
ii) **Inter-tarsal:** a) Calcaneum- inversion and eversion glide loss, b) Navicular- inversion and eversion glide loss, c) Cuneiform- plantar and dorsal glide loss, d) cuboid-inversion and eversion glide loss.

Main dysfunctions of
**i) Tibio-talar joints are:** Talus- medial, lateral, and posterior glide loss.
   Distal tibia- internal and external rotation glides loss.

For the accurate diagnosis and treatment, a specific spring glide that needs to be performed after taking the slack is as follows:
a) Talus- medial to lateral glide, lateral to medial glide
b) Talus- anterior to posterior glide.
c) Distal tibia- external and internal rotation glide.
These dysfunctions include assessment and treatment of both above-mentioned foot dysfunctions 1 and 2.

Similarly main dysfunctions of
**ii) Inter-tarsals are:** a) Calcaneum- inversion and eversion glide loss, b) Navicular- inversion and eversion glide loss, c) Cuneiform- plantar and dorsal glide loss, d) cuboid- inversion and eversion glide loss.

These above-mentioned dysfunctions (i and ii) assessment and treatment will follow the same steps of both foot dysfunction **1** and **2,** which are already covered. But only the orthotic part must be avoided as in this dysfunction; the foot will lose both pronation and supination.

**Pathomechanics:**
**Supinated foot dysfunction → knee joint dysfunction → Medial Knee Arthritis/"varus knee":**

---

**Foot dysfunction (1)**: Plantar flexed/ Dorsiflexion lag with inverted and adducted.(supinated foot)

⇩

**Talo-crural:** Talus- shifts to lateral and anterior.
          Distal tibia- externally rotated
**Inter-tarsal:** Calcaneum-inverted, Navicular-inverted, Cuneiform-dorsal, cuboid- inverted.

⇩

**Proximal tibia-** Externally rotated and glides/shifts lateral.
          Medial compression and lateral gapping of knee joint

⇩

**Knee dysfunction** - Knee extension lag with proximal tibia externally rotated and laterally shifted/glide

**W**eight **B**earing **A**xis of the limb shift towards medial knee

⇩

Above mentioned knee dysfunction, puts varus pressure over the knee during knee extension weight bearing phase of gait cycle, leading to **Medial Knee Arthritis/varum knee.**

---

The above flow chart shows step-by-step pathomechanics from supinated foot dysfunction to medial knee arthritis/varus knee; dorsi-flexion lag with inverted and adducted foot will lead to external rotation and lateral shift of proximal tibia with knee extension lag. This dysfunction of the knee, if not diagnosed early and treated, puts varus stress over the knee during the knee extension weight-bearing phase of the gait cycle, leading to medial knee arthritis/" varus knee".

**Pathomechanics:**
**Pronated foot dysfunction (2) → knee joint dysfunction → Lateral Knee Arthritis/ "valgus knee" :**

> **Foot dysfunction (2):** Plantar flexed/ Dorsi flexion lag with everted and abducted. (Pronated foot)

⇩

> **Talo-crural:** talus- shifts to medial and anterior.
> Distal tibia- internally rotated.
> **Inter-tarsal:** Calcaneum-everted, Navicular-everted, Cuneiform- plantar, cuboid- everted. Arch of the foot decreases

⇩

> **Proximal tibia**- internally rotated and glides/shifts medial.
> Medial gapping and lateral compression of knee joint.

⇩

> **Knee dysfunction**- extension lag with proximal tibia internally rotated and medially shifted.
> **W**eight **B**earing **A**xis of the limb shifts to lateral compartment of the knee

⇩

> Above mentioned knee dysfunction puts valgus pressure over the knee during knee extension weight bearing phase of gait cycle, leading to **L**ateral **K**nee Arthritis/ **valgus knee.**

The above flow chart shows step-by-step pathomechanics from pronated foot dysfunction to valgus knee. That is, dorsi-flexion lag with everted and abducted foot will lead to internal rotation and medial shift of proximal tibia with knee extension lag. This knee dysfunction, if not diagnosed early and treated, over the long run, puts the valgus stress over the knee during the knee extension weight-bearing phase of the gait cycle, leading to lateral knee arthritis/"valgus knee" deformity.

**Note: Pathomechanics of foot dysfunction (3):** Plantar flexed/ dorsi-flexion lag with both inversion and adduction plus eversion and abduction loss. This dysfunction of the foot doesn't lead to either medial knee arthritis/varus knee or lateral knee arthritis valgus knee as it is a neutral dysfunction, meaning the foot is neither inverted nor everted. Therefore, it will not put varus or valgus force over the knee, but there will be severe knee extension lag dysfunction and total joint compression.

**References:**

1. Dr. Nicolas campos; foot dysfunction, over pronation and over supination lead to cronic pain.
   http://webcache.googleusercontent.com/search?q=cache:http://www.drnickcampos.com/health-newsletter/FootDysfunction.html&gws_rd=cr&ei=exviWJmJKIOb0gSFkrnICQ
2. Kendrick, Overview of Foot and Ankle Disorders; Temple University School of Podiatric Medicine
3. Hyperpronation;http://webcache.googleusercontent.com/search?q=cache:http://www.hyperpronation.com/&gws_rd=cr&ei=iR_iWP3zC4K90gSogYu4Dg
4. How to correct foot pronation; https://www.youtube.com/watch?v=8TKPEmCzzkk
5. A brief discussion on pronation and supination of the foot: https://www.youtube.com/watch?v=vNmdyshqkao
6. Ankle & Subtalar Joint Motion Function Explained Biomechanic of the Foot - Pronation & Supination;https://www.youtube.com/watch?v=0R4zRSE_-40
7. How Shoes Cause Flat Feet and Over Pronation; https://www.fixflatfeet.com/how-shoes-cause-flat-feet-and-overpronation/
8. https://www.youtube.com/watch?v=c4R-5e461DU
9. Sharon, Thomas, et al., Integrative manual therapy for upper and lower extremities, 2008, p 26
10. SUPINATION; Learn more about diagnosis, treatment, and prevention.https://www.footsmart.com/health-resource-center/foot/supination
11. http://www.fisiokinesiterapia.biz/NewDownload/surfa.pdf

# CHAPTER 15
## Hip joint: Biomechanics, Pathomechanics, and Treatment

The hip joint dysfunctions affect themselves and can cause pelvic-lumbar dysfunctions above and knee joint dysfunctions below. As lumbopelvic joint dysfunctions are beyond the scope of this book, this book's main focus is on the knee complex; therefore, how hip joint dysfunctions can influence normal mechanics of the knee joint complex is elaborated.

The pathomechanics of hip joint dysfunctions which influences normal knee mechanics are as follows:

**Two major hip dysfunctions which contribute to knee dysfunctions are:**

**1. Hip extension lag with internally rotated and adducted**
**2. Hip extension lag with externally rotated and abducted.**

This is because the extension of the hip is used in weight-bearing and erect posture of activities of daily life. Hip flexion lag dysfunctions won't come into play in weight-bearing, so they affect less in day-to-day activities of life.

Type II Movement of Hips:
Hip joints are femoral/acetabular joints. Physiologic movements of the hips are flexion, extension (Sagittal plane); abduction, adduction (coronal plane); external rotation, and internal rotation (transverse plane).

Direct accessory movements of the femoral head are[1]:
- Anterior glide for extension
- Posterior glide for flexion
- Caudal glide for abduction
- Cephalad glide for adduction
- Anterior glide plus caudal glide for external rotation
- Posterior glide plus cephalad glide for internal rotation

As a biomechanical principle, internal rotation occurs with adduction, and external rotation occurs with abduction. All peripheral joints fall under type II dysfunctions.

**Hip Dysfunctions are type II[1-3] dysfunctions:**

1. **Flexion lags:** hip is extended
2. **Extension lags:** hip is flexed
3. **Extension lag and flexion lag: The** hip will be in the mid-range; that is, both terminal extension and flexion of the hip will be lost.

Type II movement dysfunctions are 3-planar Torsion dysfunctions.
**Possible Type II dysfunctions at the hip (femoral-acetabular) joint:**

**1. Flexion lag:**

a) With Adducted, Internally Rotated

b) With Abducted, Externally Rotated

c) With the loss of abduction, external rotation, and adduction, internal rotation.

**2. Extension lag:**

a) With adducted, Internally Rotated

b) With abducted, externally Rotated

c) With the loss of abduction, external rotation, and adduction, internal rotation.

**3. Both extension and flexion lag: it includes both 1 and 2 of the above hip dysfunctions**

## Essential surface anatomy and palpatory landmarks of the hip joint:

Figure 1: Anterior view of the hip joint. Important palpatory surface anatomy landmarks.

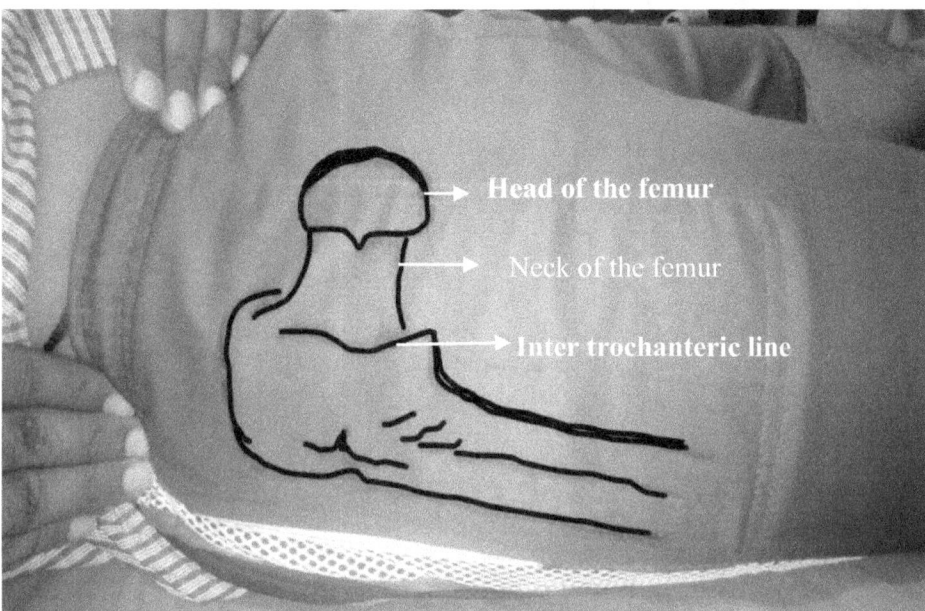

Figure 2: Posterior view of the hip joint and important palpatory and surface anatomy landmarks.

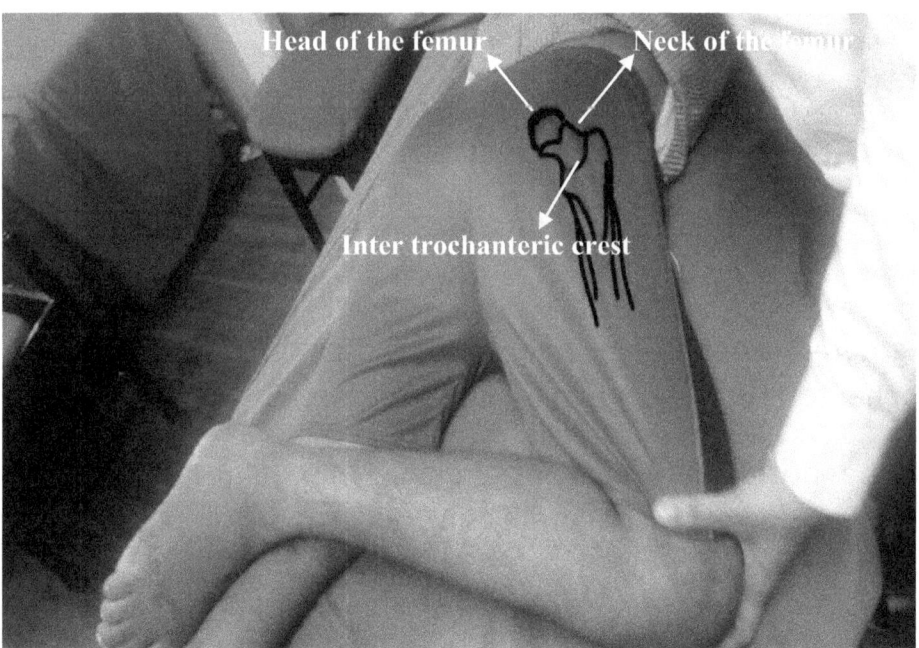

Figure 3: Important anatomical landmarks of anterior (left) and posterior views of right femur.

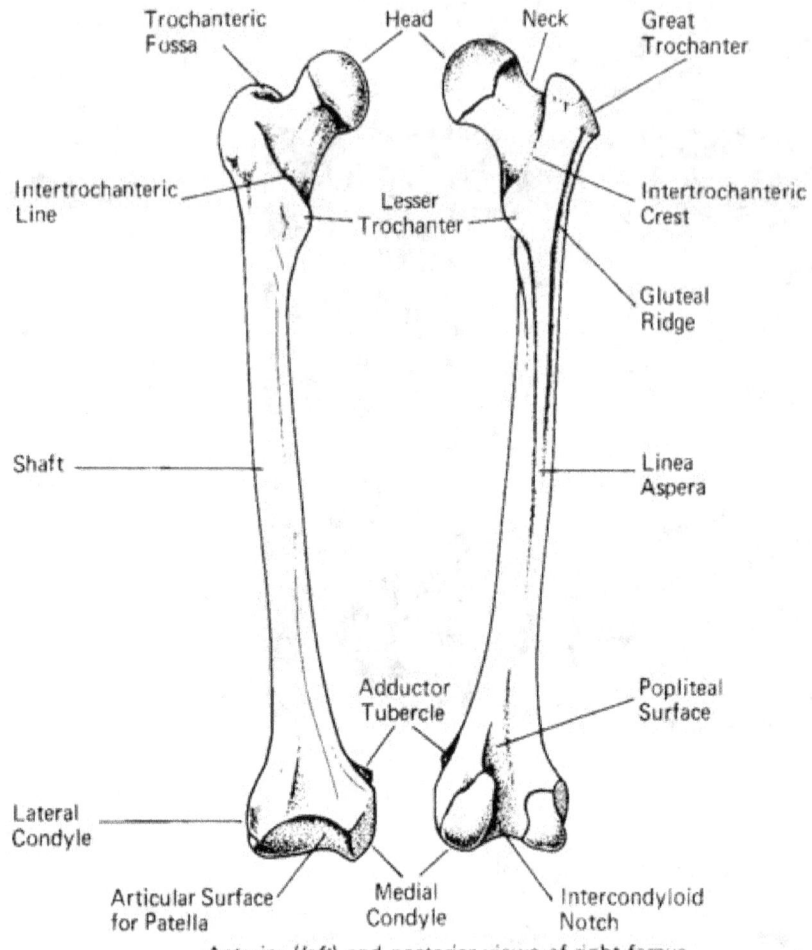

Anterior (*left*) and posterior views of right femur.

1. Palpate the glides of the femoral head during Physiologic hip flexion and extension[10].

2. Palpate at the greater trochanter: posteriorly inter-trochanteric crest, anteriorly inter-trochanteric line as shown in figure 1, 2 and 3

3. Springtest should be positive during three planar hip joint (usually the terminal) glides in flexion and extension, indicating normal hip joint.

## Spring test and treatment of hip joint flexion lag dysfunctions:

**1. Hip flexion lag:**
a) With Adducted, Internally Rotated
b) With Abducted, Externally Rotated
c) With abduction, external rotation, and adduction, internal rotation loss

**a) Hip flexion lag: with adducted and internally rotated.**
**Spring test:**
**Position of the patient:** is in long sitting as shown in Figures 4 and 5.
**Position of the therapist:** The therapist approaches from the right side of the patient, the affected right hip should be taken in external rotation (transverse plane), abduction (coronal plane), and flexion (sagittal plane) to reach an inter-barrier zone in three planes with the knee flexed about $90^0$. The therapist's left olecranon/thumb is placed on the femoral head. The upper body (trunk) has to be flexed and supported by the wall to take out the further soft tissue slack of hip flexion. The therapist's right fingers and wrist are wrapped around the affected leg's lateral side of the knee to take the hip into further flexion (sagittal plane). Then hip flexion slack (femoral head posterior glide) is taken with 12kg force, and additionally, 8kg force is applied to test the spring/end feel. If it does not, spring indicates dysfunction.

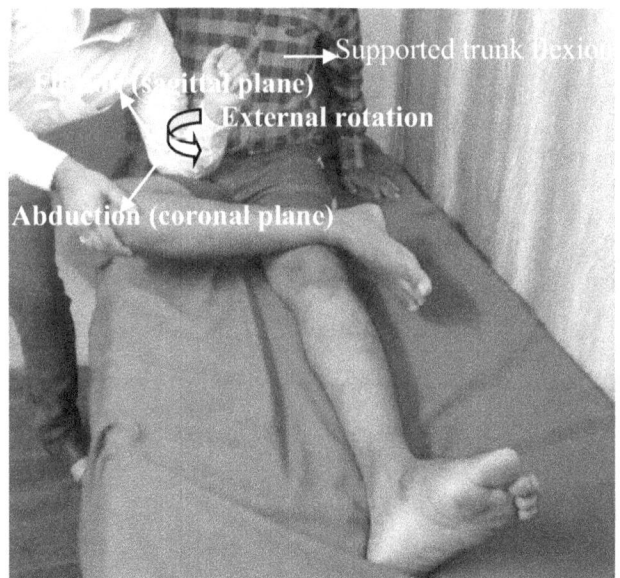

Figure 4: Spring test and treatment of hip joint dysfunction by olecranon: flexion lag with internally rotated and adducted. The wall supports trunk flexion.

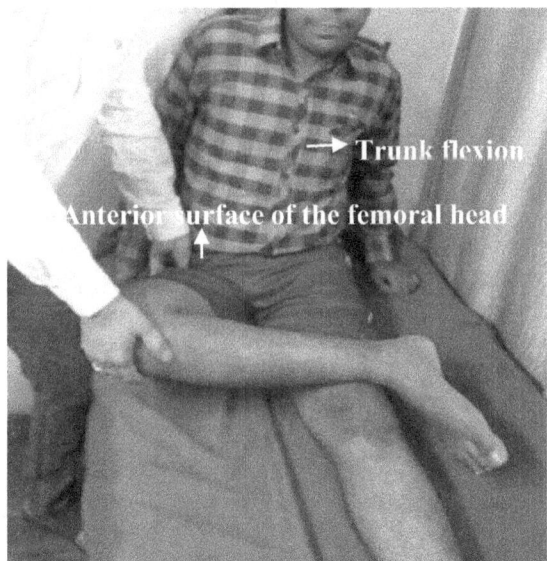

Figure 5: Spring test and treatment of hip joint dysfunction by thumb: flexion lag with internally rotated and adducted. Trunk flexion is supported by the wall.

**Treatment:**
**Mobilization:** As shown in Figures 4 and 5, the patient position for treatment is the same as the assessment position as explained above; the movement barrier in three planes is reached. Then left olecranon/thumb of the therapist is placed on the anterior surface of the femoral head, and then hip flexion slack is taken with 12kg force to glide the femoral head posteriorly. Then further glides are applied according to the grades of mobilization. 5 glides are given 3 times in one session. Each time 5-sec rest is given[4-6].

**Muscle energy technique:** As shown in figure 4 and 5, the patient position for treatment is the same as the assessment position as explained above; after reaching the movement barrier in three planes, the left olecranon/thumb of the therapist is placed on the anterior surface of the femoral head and then hip flexion slack is taken with 12kg force to glide femoral head posteriorly. Following this, the patient is asked to extend the hip, and simultaneously, the therapist resists producing an isometric contraction. After 5 sec of relaxation, a further new movement barrier in three planes: external rotation, abduction, and flexion of affected hip and femoral head posterior glide are reached. Again, repeat the same 3 times in one session.

**Sustained stretch:**
As shown in figure 6, the patient should stand on the left leg with the affected right hip should be in external rotation (transverse plane), abduction (coronal plane), and flexion (in the sagittal plane) with the lateral surface of the knee placed on the bed, then further soft tissue slack is taken by flexing the upper body and affected hip so that three planar movement- barrier zone is reached. This position of stretch can be maintained for 2-5 min, according to the patient condition and tolerance.

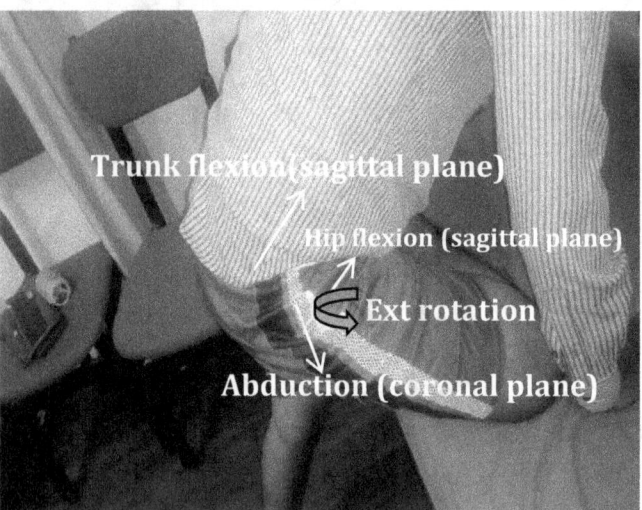

Figure 6: Sustained glide and stretch of the right hip into abduction, external rotation and flexion.

**Progressive strengthening of the hip:** is advised according to patient condition and tolerance

**b) Hip Flexion lag: with Abducted and externally rotated:**

## Spring test:

**Position of Patient**: is on left side bend, sitting with the left side of the trunk supported by the wall. The affected right side of the leg's hip and the knee is flexed, and the trunk should be bent towards the right, as shown in figure 7.

**Position of the patient and procedure:** The therapist approaches from the patient's right side. The therapist's right wrist extended and fingers flexed grab the right medial surface of the knee. Then hip adduction (coronal plane) barrier is reached by gradually trunk right side bending, the hip internal rotation (transverse plane) barrier is reached by placing the suitable height pillow or a bed sheet between the legs, and then hip flexion barrier is reached with a therapist flexing the right hip. After reaching the three planar movement barrier, the therapist's left olecranon/pisiform is placed over the head of the femur to take posterior glide slack with 12 kg force, and additionally, 8kg force is applied to test the spring/end feel. If it does not, spring indicates the dysfunction.

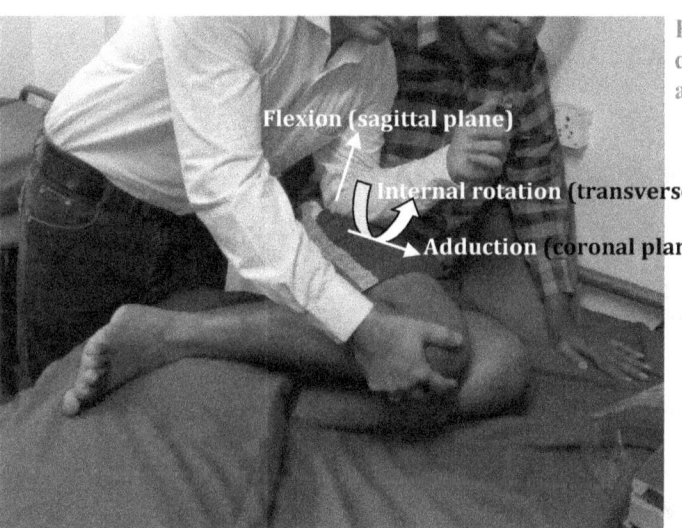

Figure 7: Spring test and treatment of hip dysfunction by olecranon- flexion lag with abducted and externally rotated.

## Treatment:

**Mobilization:** As shown in figure 7, the patient treatment position is the same as the assessment position as explained above; after reaching the movement barrier in three planes, the therapist's left pisiform/olecranon is placed on the femoral head, and posterior glide/ hip flexion slack is taken with 12 kg force. Further femoral head posterior glides are done according to the grades of mobilization. 5 glides are given 3 times in one session. Each time 5-sec rest is given.

**Muscle energy technique**: As shown in figure 7, the position of the patient for treatment is the same as the assessment position as explained above; after reaching the movement barrier in three planes, the therapist's left pisiform/olecranon is placed on the femoral head and posterior glide or hip flexion slack is taken with 12 kg force. Following this, the patient is asked to extend the hip, and simultaneously therapist resists producing an isometric contraction. After 5 sec relaxation, further new movement barrier in three planes and femoral head new posterior glide reached. Again, repeat the same 3 times in one session.

**Sustained stretch**: As shown in figure 8, the position of the patient for treatment is the same as the assessment position as explained above; after reaching the movement barrier in three planes, the therapist's left pisiform/olecranon is placed on the femoral head and posterior glide or hip flexion slack is taken with 12 kg force. Following this, the pillow is added under the right leg, as shown in figure 8, is kept to further increase the adduction and internal rotation of the hip. This position is kept for about 2-5 minutes, according to the patient's tolerance and condition of dysfunction.

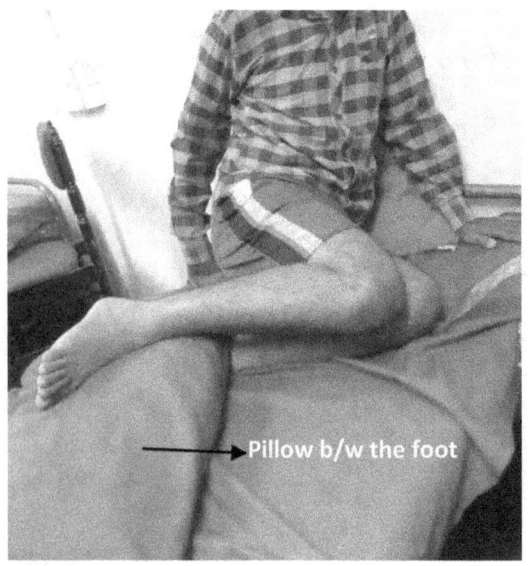

Figure 8: A sustained stretch of the right hip into internal rotation, adduction and flexion.

**Progressive strengthening:** is advised according to patient condition and tolerance

**c) Flexion lag: with abduction, external rotation, and adduction, internal rotation loss**

Assessment and treatment of this dysfunction of the hip include both **a)** and **b)** assessment and treatment of hip dysfunctions, which are already covered above.

## Spring test and treatment of hip joint extension lag dysfunctions:

2. Hip extension lag: a) with adducted, internally Rotated
   b) with abducted, externally Rotated
   c) with adduction, external rotation, and adduction, internal rotation loss

### a) Hip extension lag: with adducted and internally rotated.

**Spring test:**

**Position of the patient**: is prone with affected right hip abducted, externally rotated, and the knee is flexed as shown in figure 9.

**Position of the therapist and procedure:** The therapist approaches the patient from the right side, and the left-hand wraps around the medial side of the knee of the affected leg; the hip is externally rotated (transverse plane), abducted (coronal plane), and extended (sagittal plane) to reach an inter movement-barrier zone. After reaching the three planar movement barrier, the therapist's right olecranon/pisiform is placed over the posterior surface of the head of the femur. Then the femoral head anterior glide/extension slack is taken with 12 kg force, and additionally, 8kg force is applied to test the spring/end feel. If it does not, spring indicates the dysfunction.

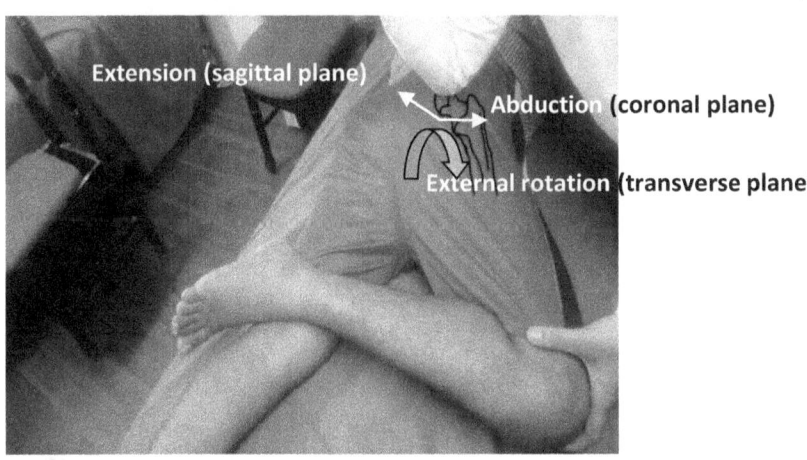

Figure 9: Spring test and treatment of hip extension lag with adducted and internally rotated.

### Treatment:

**Mobilization**[5, 6]: As shown in figure 9, the position of the patient for treatment is the same as the assessment position as explained above; after reaching the movement barrier in three planes, the therapist's right olecranon is placed on the posterior surface of the femoral head, and anterior glide/hip extension slack is taken with 12kg force. Further femoral head anterior glides are done according to the grades of mobilisation. 5 glides are given 3 times in one session. Each time 5 seconds of rest is given.

**Muscle energy technique**: As shown in figure 9, the position of the patient for treatment is the same as the assessment position as explained above; after reaching the movement barrier in three planes, the therapist's right-hand olecranon is placed on the posterior surface of the femoral head, and anterior glide or hip extension slack is taken with 12 kg force. Following this, the patient is asked to flex the hip, and simultaneously, the therapist resists producing an isometric contraction. After 5 sec of relaxation, a further new movement barrier in three planes is reached. Again, repeat the same 3 times in one session.

**Sustained stretch**: As shown in Figures 10 and 11, the patient should be supine lying, and the affected right hip is taken into abduction, external rotation, and extension, and the knee is flexed about 90 degrees so that the right leg is placed over the left leg. A log is placed under the posterior aspect of the femoral head to assist anterior and inferior glide. To further reinforce the glide and stretch, weight is kept over the medial aspect of the knee. This position is maintained for 2-5min according to patient condition and tolerance.

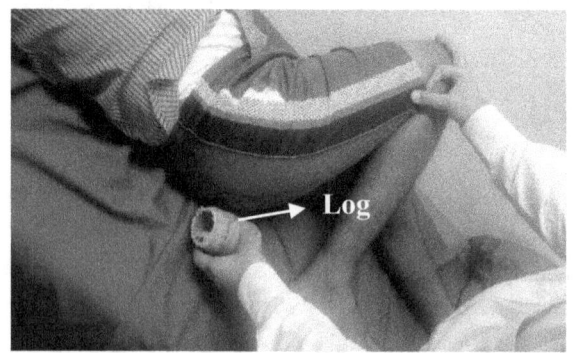

Figure 10: Sustained stretch and glide of the hip into the external rotation, abduction and extension with the log.

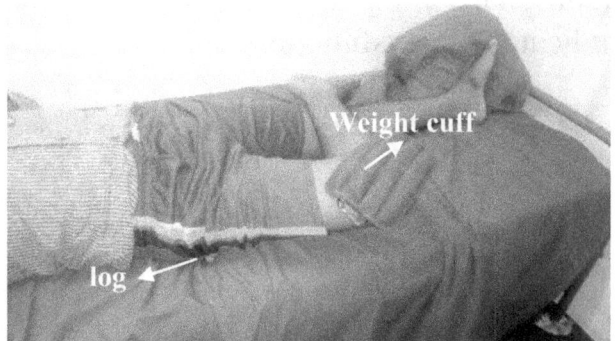

Figure 11: log is placed at the posterior surface of the femoral head for anterior and inferior glide. Weight can be added to reinforce the glide.

**Progressive strengthening of the hip:** is advised according to the patient's condition and tolerance

### b) Hip extension lag: with abducted and externally rotated.
**Spring test:**

**Position of the patient**: is a prone with affected right hip adducted, internally rotated, extended, and the knee is flexed as shown in figure 12.

**Position of the therapist and procedure:** The therapist approaches the patient from the right side and the left-hand wraps around the medial side of the affected leg knee. Then hip internal rotation (transverse plane), adduction (coronal plane), and extension (sagittal plane) inter movement-barrier zone is reached. Simultaneously, the therapist's right olecranon is placed over the posterior surface of the head of the femur to take anterior glide/extension slack with 12 kg force, and additionally, 8kg force is applied to test the spring/end feel. If it does not, spring indicates the dysfunction.

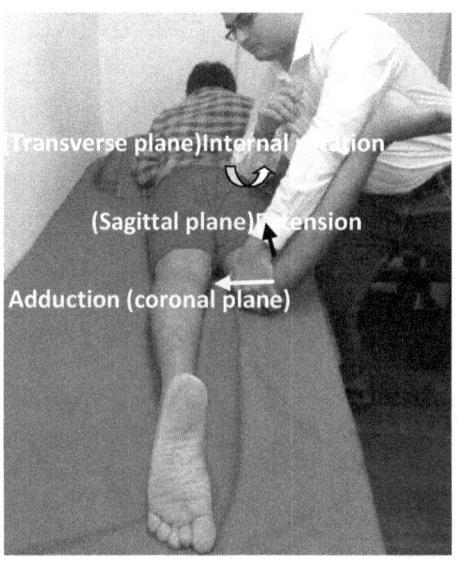

Figure 12: Spring test and treatment of hip extension lag with abducted and externally rotated.

## Treatment:

**Mobilization:** As shown in figure 12, the position of the patient for treatment is the same as the assessment position as explained above, and after reaching the movement barrier in three planes, the therapist's right olecranon is placed on the posterior surface of the femoral head, and anterior glide/hip extension slack is taken with 12kg force. Further femoral head anterior glides are done according to the grades of mobilisation. 5 glides are given 3 times in one session. Each time 5 seconds of rest is given[8, 9].

**Muscle energy technique**: As shown in figure 12, the position of the patient is the same as the assessment position as explained above, and after reaching the movement barrier in three planes, the therapist's right olecranon is placed on the posterior surface of the femoral head, and anterior glide/hip extension slack is taken with 12 kg force. Following this, the patient is asked to flex the hip, and simultaneously, the therapist resists producing an isometric contraction. After 5 sec of relaxation, a further new movement barrier in three planes is reached. Again, repeat the same 3 times in one session.

**Sustained[7] stretch**: As shown in Figures 13 and 14. The position the Patient is prone. The affected right hip slack is taken into internal rotation (transverse plane), adduction (coronal plane), and hip extension (sagittal plane). Then pillow is kept under the anterior distal femur of the patient to further assist in extension (sagittal plane), and after reaching the internal rotation barrier of the hip, a weight cuff of 1-3kg is kept over the medial surface of the foot of the patient to assist and maintain further internal rotation of the hip. This sustained stretch and glide can be kept for 2-5 minutes, according to the patient's condition and tolerance. As shown in figure 14, sustained glide can be maintained manually by the therapist by placing the therapist's left hand over the patient's medial surface of the foot to reinforce internal rotation, and right-hand olecranon/pisiform can be placed over the posterior surface of the femoral head to glide anteriorly.

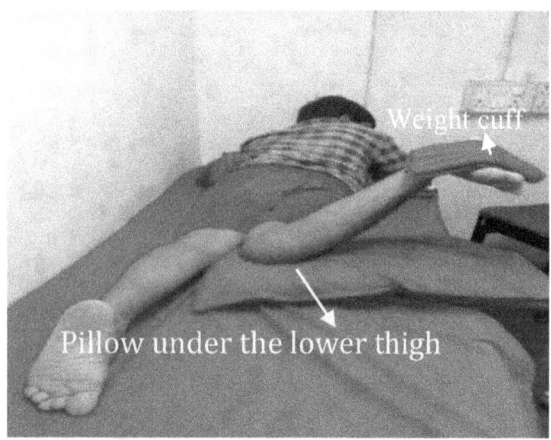

Figure 13: Sustained hip glide and stretch into adduction, internal rotation and extension. Hip extension is assisted by the pillow. Hip internal rotation assisted by weight cuff.

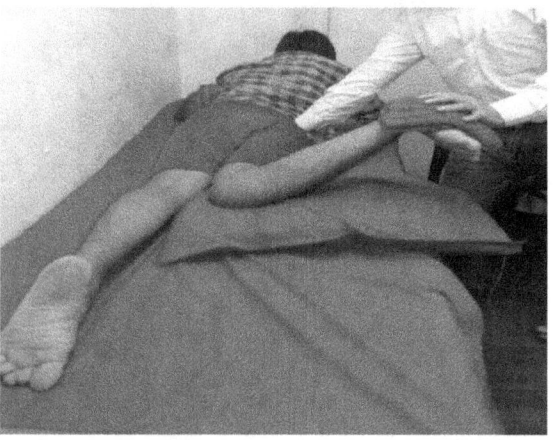

Figure 14: Sustained hip glide and stretch into adduction, internal rotation and extension, passively done by the therapist.

**Progressive strengthening:** is advised according to the patient's condition and tolerance

### c). Hip extension lag: with abduction, external rotation, and adduction, internal rotation loss

Assessment and treatment of this dysfunction of the hip include both **a)** and **b)** hip dysfunctions, which are already covered above.

### 3. Both extension and flexion lag of hip dysfunctions: include assessment and treatment of both 1 and 2 of hip dysfunctions that are already covered.

# Chapter 15: Hip joint- Biomechanics, Pathomechanics and Treatment

## Pathomechanics: hip extension dysfunction (2. b) → knee joint dysfunction → Medial Knee Arthritis/ "varus knee."

| Hip dysfunction (2.b): Extension lag with proximal femur externally rotated and abducted |
|---|

| Femoral head posterior leads to knee flexion, femoral head external rotation with inferior glide in acetabulum leads to external rotation, abduction of the femur. That will lead to varus pressure at the knee. |
|---|

| Knee dysfunction: extension lag with proximal tibia externally rotated and lateral glide/shifts. Medial compression and lateral gapping of the knee joint lead to the weight-bearing axis of the limb shifting to the medial to the knee. |
|---|

| That puts varus pressure over the knee during the weight-bearing stance phase of the gait cycle, leading to medial knee arthritis /" varus knee". |
|---|

⇩

| External rotation of the tibia leads to supinated foot |
|---|

The above flow chart shows step-by-step pathomechanics from hip extension (**2 b**) dysfunction to medial knee arthritis/varus knee; in hip extension lag, the femoral head is posterior, leading to knee flexion. And when the hip is externally rotated and abducted, the femoral head is externally rotated and glides inferiorly in the acetabulum. The acetabulum is cup-shaped, and the femur is abducted when the femoral head glides inferior. That will lead to varus pressure at the knee, shifting the weight-bearing axis of the limb medial to the knee joint. That intern gradually leads to the proximal tibia rotating externally and gliding laterally. Therefore, If hip dysfunction is not diagnosed early and treated, in the long run, it puts the knee under varus stress during the weight-bearing stance phase of the gait cycle, leading to medial knee arthritis/ "varus knee." The external rotation of the tibia leads to a "supinated foot".

**Pathomechanics: hip extension dysfunction (2a) → knee joint dysfunction → lateral knee arthritis/"valgus knee."**

> Hip dysfunction (2.a): Extension lag with femoral head internally rotated and adducted.

⇩

> Femoral head posterior leads to knee flexion, femoral head internal rotation with superior glide in acetabulum leads to internal rotation, abduction of the femur. That puts valgus pressure on the knee.

⇩

> Knee dysfunction (2a): extension lag with proximal tibia internally rotated and medially shifted.
> -Medial gapping and lateral compression of knee joint leads to weight-bearing axis shifting lateral to knee joint

⇩

> Valgus pressure over the knee during the weight-bearing stance phase of the gait cycle leads to lateral knee arthritis/ " valgus knee".

⇩

> Tibia internal rotation leads to pronated foot

The above flow chart shows step-by-step pathomechanics from hip extension (**2 a**) dysfunction to medial knee arthritis/valgus knee. That is, in hip extension lag, in which the femoral head is posterior, which leads to flexion at the knee. And when the hip is internally rotated and adducted, the femoral head is internally rotated and superior in the acetabulum. As the acetabulum is cup-shaped and when the femoral head glides superior, the femur is adducted, leading to valgus pressure at the knee, and the weight-bearing axis of the limb shifts laterally to the knee joint. That intern gradually leads to proximal tibia rotating internally and gliding medially. Therefore, if this hip dysfunction is not diagnosed early and treated, in the long run, it puts the knee under valgus stress during the weight-bearing stance phase of the gait cycle, therefore, leading to lateral knee arthritis/"valgus knee." The internal rotation of the tibia leads to a "pronated foot".

**Pathomechanics: hip extension dysfunction (2c) → knee joint dysfunction → Severe extension lag knee arthritis."**

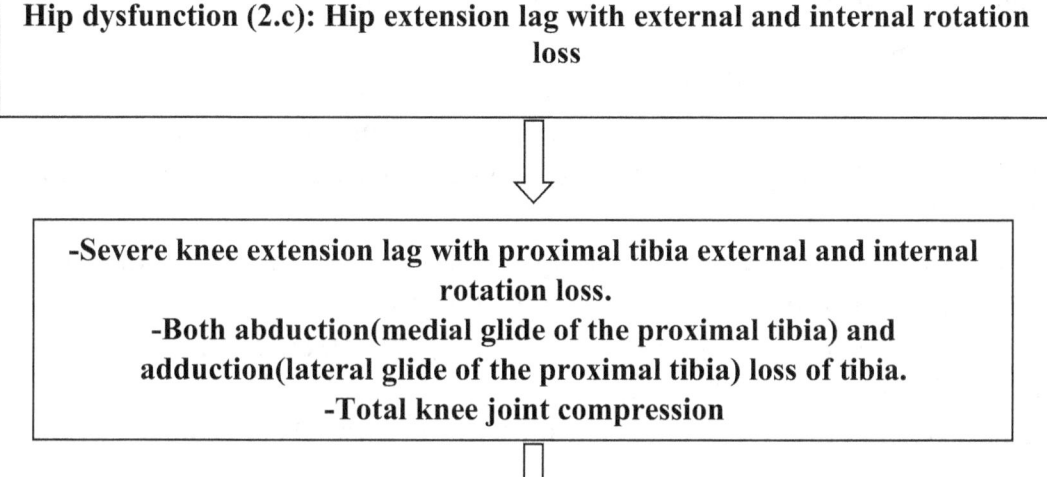

The above flow chart shows step-by-step pathomechanics from hip extension (**2 c**) dysfunction to severe knee extension lag arthritis. Hip extension lag with external and internal rotation loss leads to external and internal ration loss of tibia along with abduction and adduction loss. That intern gradually leads to severe knee extension lag with total joint compression at the knee. Distal tibia external and internal rotation loss gradually leads to supination and pronation loss of a foot.

**References:**

1. Sharon, Thomas, et al.,. Integrative manual therapy for upper and lower extremities, 2008, p 17.
2. David j magee, James e zachazewski, et al,. Pathology and intervention in musculoskeletal rehabilitation. 680; chapter 18 hip pathologies diagnosis and interventions.
3. Wright, Alexis, and Michael A. O'Hearn. "Differential Diagnosis and EarlyManagement of Rapidly Progressing Hip Pain in a 59-Year-Old Male." The Journal of Manual & Manipulative Therapy 20.2 (2012): 96–101. PMC. Web. 10 Dec. 2016.
4. Abbott, J.H., Robertson, M.C., Chapple, C., Pinto, D., Wright, A.A., Leon de la Barra, S. et al., Manual therapy, exercise therapy, or both, in addition to usual care, for osteoarthritis of the hip or knee: a randomized controlled trial. 1: clinical effectiveness. Osteoarthritis & Cartilage. 2013;21:525–534.
5. PT Classroom - A Review of Hip Joint Mobilization Techniques ׀ by Jennifer Hill, MPT, CSCS & Chai Rasavong, MPT, MBA; http://www.cyberpt.com/hipjointmobilization.asp
6. Hall & Brody: Hip Joint Mobilization, Therapeutic Exercise: Moving Toward Function, 2nd Edition © 2005, Lippincott Williams and Wilkins
7. Michael P. Remain, restricted hip mobility: clinical suggestions for self-mobilization and muscle re-education; Int J Sports Phys Ther, v. 8 (5); 2013 Oct, PMC3811738; https://www.ncbi.nlm.nih.gov/pmc/articles/PMC3811738/
8. Mark Buckingham; Functional Mobilization Techniques for the Lower Extremities; http://video.nata.org/gettingfunctional/handouts/handout5.pdf
9. https://www.youtube.com/watch?v=CTDmQzgtuYQ
10. https://www.youtube.com/watch?v=iTfDvFCPZ_w

# Index

## A

activities of daily life (ADL)., 30
**Acute stage**, 110
acute/chronic stage, 110
**Anatomy of patella**, 195
**Ankle- mechanics**, 249
**Arthrokinematics**, 133, 134, 139
**Assessment and treatment of PTF**
    1.Fibular head anterior-lateral 200, 214
    2. Posterior medial 2002, 214
    3. Both anterior & posterior glide loss 204, 214
    4. Superior 205, 214
    5. Inferior 208, 214
    6. Inferior & Superior glide loss 211, 214
**Assessment and treatment of tibio-femoral joint**
    1. Flexion lag 156, 174
    2. Extension lag 166, 174
    3. Extension & Flexion lag176, 174
**Assessment tools**
    1. Objective methods 138, 158
    2. Subjective Methods 140, 158
    3. Palpation 141, 158
    4. Spring test 143, 158
**Assessment-dynamic VS static**, 164
**Atrophy**, 33, 36, 37

## B

Below knee kinetic chain- knee, 247
**Benefits of Resistance Training**, 42
**Biomechanics of patella**, 198
BMD, 36, 38

## C

**Calisthenic Tests**, 47
**Characteristics of soft tissue injury**, 111
Cross fiber friction massage, 122

## D

**Design graded strengthening**, 49
**DTF- Deep Transverse friction massage**, 122
**Dynamic biomechanics of patella**, 199
dysfunctions, 24
Dysfunctions of Tibio-femoral joint
    1. Extension lag 123, 143
    2. Flexion lag 124, 143
    3. Both flexion and extension lag 124, 143

## E

**Effects of pressure variations**, 99
**Etiologies of pressure variations**, 96
examination of soft tissue injury, 118
**Examining Soft Tissue Injuries**, 117
**External topographic anatomy**, 92
Extrinsic factors
    Ergonomics & Environment 54, 73
    Foot wear.53, 73
    Gravity 55, 73
    Modalities 54, 73
    Orthotics 53, 73

## F

Femoral head-accessory movements
    Anterior +cepalide glide, 295
    anterior,posterior glide,, 295
    coudal & cephalide glide, 295
    Posterior glide + caudal glide, 295
fitness levels, 23
**FITT principle**
    Frequency 29, 51
    Intensity of training 29, 51
    Time- sets & repetitions 30, 51
    Type 31, 51
Foot
    spring test and treatment
        1. D/F Lag +inverted&adducted 241, 251
        2. D/F Lag +Everted&abducted 263, 251
**Foot dysfunctions**
    1. Dorsi/f loss +inverted&adducted 240, 249
    2. Dorsi/f loss + everted&abducted 240, 249
    3. Dorsi/f loss + both invertn,adductn+evertn,abd'n loss 240, 249
Foot -palpatory bony landmarks, 248
Foot-pronation, 246, 294
Foot-supination, 246
**Free weight squat**, 57
FTPTV, 89, 90, 96, 97, 98, 105

## G

gait cycle, 145, 146, 147, 151, 246, 291, 292, 308, 309
**Graded resistance strengthening**, 41

## H

**Hip dysfunctions-Spring test and treatment**
    1. Flexion lag 296, 299, 303
    2. extension lag 301, 299, 303

3. Both flexion & extension lag 305, 299, 303
**hip Dysfunctions-Type II**
1. Flexion lag 294, 296
2. Extension lag 294, 296
3. Both extension & flexion lag 294, 296
**Hip -palpatory landmarks**, 297

# I

**INJURY**, 31
a) Injury 10, 31
b) Death 12, 31
**injury zone**, 28
**Injury[12] /Dysfunction**, 28
**Internal gross anatomy**, 92
**Intertarsal- mechanics**, 249

# K

KNEE JOINT DYSFUNCTION
Patho-mechanics(gross), 140
knee motion causes, 89
Condylar cartilage nutrition 79, 89
Joint stability 80, 89
Pressure changes in the joint 69,70, 89
Synovial fluid influx & outflux 70, 89
Vascular flow 81, 89
**Knee soft tissue mobilization**
Anterior lateral side 217, 229
DTF-Deep transverse friction 216, 229
Medial 224, 229
Posterior 227, 229
knee tissue strength assessment
1. Warm up 35, 57
2. Choosing specific exercise 35, 57
3. Apply FITT principle 37, 57
4. Find 1RM 37, 57
Knee: Soft tissue palpation
I) Anterior,Medial,Lateral- knee 213, 227
II) Posterior knee 214, 227

# L

**Laws of Biomechanics**, 132
**level of stress on tissues**
Level of stress on tissues, 68
**Lunges**, 58

# M

**Machine squat**, 58
**maximum threshold level**, 28, 29, 30, 31, 37
**Mechanics of PTF joint**
Related to foot dysfunctions 199, 213
Related to knee dysfunctions 199, 213

**Mechanisms of Injury**, 110
**Movement and Alignment Factors**
Motor Control 49, 69
Muscle performance 49, 69
Physical activity 52, 69
Posture and alignment 50, 69

# O

osteokinematics, 133

# P

**PALPATION: KNEE**, 228
**palpatory landmarks of the Knee**, 172
**Patellar dysfunctions**
Medial, Lateral 190, 205
patellar tilt 190, 205
Superior,Inferior 190, 205
**Patellar mobilization**
1. Grade one 194, 208
2. Grade two 195, 208
pathomechanics
genu recurvatum, 153
Foot dysfunctions to genu valgum 290, 291
Foot dysfunctions to genu varum 289, 291
Hip dysfunction to genu varum, 308
Hip dysfunctions to genu valgum 316, 309
**Pathomechanics**
From gait analysis-genu valgum, 151
From gait analysis-genu varum, 151
**Pathomechanics of**
genu valgum, 151
genu varum, 151
**Patho-mechanics of patella**
Adhesions of soft tissue of patella 191, 200
Static factors 190, 200
pathomechanics of soft tissue dysfunction, 113
Physical stress, 23
**Physical Stress on a tissue VS Strength of the tissue**, 24, 25
VS Tissue adaptation 13, 24
VS Tissue strengthening 16, 24
**physical stress theory**, 24, 69
Physiological factors
Age 56, 76
Deficiency 56, 76
Obesity 57, 76
Systemic pathology 57, 76
**Prevention**, 28
a) Hypertrophy/substage1 7, 29
b) Maximum threshould zone 9, 29
**Proximal tibio-fibular joint**, 8, 129, 212
**PTF dysfunctions**, 213
Both anterior & posterior glide loss 200, 213

Fibular head anterior lateral 200, 213
Fibular head posterior medial 200, 213
Superior & inferior 200, 213
Superior & Inferior glide loss 200, 213

## S

**Safe /prevention zone**, 28
**Soft Tissue Adhesions and Manupiltion**, 121
**Strength VS Endurance**, 47
Sub acute/overuse stage, 110
**Sustained anterior glide of the tibia**, 190
Synovial mechanics, 89

## T

**Test for tissue strength 22**
    One RM 22, 44
**Test your muscular endurance**, 47
**The psychological factors**, 76
**tibio-femoral joint**
    Biomechanics, 8, 130
    Close chain mechanics, 138
    Open chain mechanics, 138
**Tibio-femoral joint**, 7, 129, 134, 141, 142, 143, 144, 145, 158
**Tibio-femoral joint dysfunctions**
    Patho-mechanics(specific), 145
**tissue adaptation in hypertrophy**, 37, 38
**Tissue adaptation in hypertrophy**, 37
**Tissue adaptation in maintenance**, 36
**tissue death**, 25, 26, 32, 33, 34, 36, 37, 113, 140
**Tissue endurance**, 40
**Tissue fitness**, 40, 41
**Tissue strength**, 25, 40, 54, 70
**TISSUE VS TISSUE ADAPTATION**
    Atrophy & Death 14, 33
    Hypertrophy 14, 33
    Maintenance 14, 33
**Treatment techniques used in MT**
    1. Joint mobilisation & Sustained glide 148, 166
    2. MET 150, 166
    3. Taping 150, 166
    4. DTF 150, 166
    5. Graded strengthening 150, 166
    6. orthotics 151, 166
Type II Movement of Hips, 295

## V

variable Factors, 68
    response of tissue to physical stress, 68
Variable Factors
    Extrinsic Factors 53, 69
    Movement and alignment factors 40, 69
    Physiogical Factors 55, 69
    Psychological Factors 55, 69

## Δ

$\Delta P = P$ atm $- P$ articular space, 92

**For Further Information on Courses and Educational Materials, Please Contact:**

NAVEEN INSTITUTE OF ORTHOPAEDIC MANUAL THERAPY
(Physio 4 Knee and Pain)
The main branch: Shop no 13 & 14, Agarwal Chambers, King Koti Road, Hyderabad, India.
Branch 2: Flat- 402, Block no- 5, Malaysian township, Hyderabad, India.
Cell: 9392403507
www.physio4kneenpain.com; e-mail: nimt@physio4kneenpain.com

**NAVEEN INSTITUTE OF ORTHOPAEDIC MANUAL THERAPY** is the learning, research, and resource centre for Orthopaedic Manual Therapy. Continuing education seminars and workshops are offered throughout India. The following courses are offered and available for all Physiotherapists.

**Orthopaedic Manual therapy for**

1. Lower limb
2. Upper limb
3. Pelvis and cervical, thoracic, lumbar spine
4. Rib cage and thoracic spine dysfunctions and their relation to Asthma
5. Headache and migraines: regarding mechanical dysfunctions of the upper cervical, temporomandibular joint, and occipital frontalis.

www.ingramcontent.com/pod-product-compliance
Lightning Source LLC
Chambersburg PA
CBHW080450220526
45465CB00006B/2227